Curriculum Development and Evaluation in Nursing Education

Sarah B. Keating, EdD, MPH, RN, C-PNP, FAAN, retired as endowed professor, Orvis School of Nursing, University of Nevada, Reno, where she taught Curriculum Development and Evaluation in Nursing, Instructional Design and Evaluation, and the Nurse Educator Practicum, and was the director of the DNP program. She has taught nursing since 1970 and received her EdD in curriculum and instruction in 1982. Dr. Keating was previously director of graduate programs at Russell Sage College (Troy, New York) and chair of nursing, San Francisco State University, dean of Samuel Merritt-Saint Mary's Intercollegiate Nursing Program (1995–2000), adjunct professor at Excelsior College, and chair of the California Board of Registered Nursing Education Advisory Committee (2003–2005). She has received many awards and recognitions, has published in numerous journals, and has been the recipient of 15 funded research grants, two from Health Resources and Services Administration (HRSA). Dr. Keating led the development of numerous educational programs including nurse practitioner, advanced practice community health nursing, clinical nurse leader, case management, entry-level MSN programs, nurse educator tracks, the DNP, and MSN/MPH programs. She served as a consultant in curriculum development and evaluation for undergraduate and graduate nursing programs and serves as a reviewer for substantive change proposals for the Western Association of Schools and Colleges (WASC) accrediting body. Dr. Keating published the first through third editions of *Curriculum Development and Evaluation in Nursing.*

Stephanie S. DeBoor, PhD, APRN, ACNS-BC, CCRN, is the associate dean of graduate programs, and assistant professor, Orvis School of Nursing, University of Nevada, Reno. She is a member of the University Curriculum Committee and teaches Nursing Education Role and Practicum, and Care of Clients With Complex Health Alterations. In addition, Dr. DeBoor is patient care coordinator and per diem RN at Northern Nevada Medical Center, Sparks, Nevada. She is the recipient of several honors, including the American Association of Colleges of Nursing (AACN) 2013–14 Fellowship Leader for Academic Nursing Program, and was honored as the Most Inspirational Teacher, UNR (2009, 2010, and 2012). Dr. DeBoor has published articles in *Journal of Nursing Education, Journal of Nursing Care Quality,* and *American Journal of Critical Care.*

Curriculum Development and Evaluation in Nursing Education

FOURTH EDITION

Sarah B. Keating, EdD, MPH, RN, C-PNP, FAAN

Stephanie S. DeBoor, PhD, APRN, ACNS-BC, CCRN

Editors

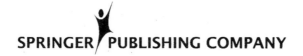

Springer Publishing Company, LLC
11 West 42nd Street
New York, NY 10036
www.springerpub.com

Acquisitions Editor: Margaret Zuccarini
Senior Production Editor: Kris Parrish
Compositor: Westchester Publishing Services

ISBN: 978-0-8261-7441-3
ebook ISBN: 978-0-8261-7442-0
Instructor's Manual ISBN: 978-0-8261-7438-3
Instructor's PowerPoints ISBN: 978-0-8261-7439-0

Instructor's Materials: Qualified instructors may request supplements by emailing textbook@springerpub.com

17 18 19 20 21 / 5 4 3 2 1

Library of Congress Cataloging-in-Publication Data
CIP data is available from the Library of Congress.

Contact us to receive discount rates on bulk purchases.
We can also customize our books to meet your needs.
For more information please contact: sales@springerpub.com

Printed in the United States of America by McNaughton & Gunn.

Contents

Contributors

Kimberly Baxter, DNP, APRN, FNP-BC   Assistant Professor and Associate Dean of Undergraduate Programs, Orvis School of Nursing, University of Nevada, Reno

Stephanie S. DeBoor, PhD, APRN, ACNS-BC, CCRN   Assistant Professor and Associate Dean of Graduate Programs, Orvis School of Nursing, University of Nevada, Reno

Susan M. Ervin, PhD, RN, CNE   Assistant Professor, Orvis School of Nursing, University of Nevada, Reno

Sarah B. Keating, EdD, MPH, RN, C-PNP, FAAN   Professor and Dean Emerita, San Francisco State University, San Francisco, California, and Samuel Merritt University, Oakland, California

Felicia Lowenstein-Moffett, DNP, APRN, FNP-BC, NP-C, CCRN   Assistant Professor, Orvis School of Nursing, University of Nevada, Reno

Heidi A. Mennenga, PhD, RN   Assistant Professor, South Dakota State University, College of Nursing, Brookings, South Dakota

Patsy L. Ruchala, DNSc, RN   Dean Orvis School of Nursing, University of Nevada, Reno

Michael T. Weaver, PhD, RN, FAAN   Professor and Associate Dean for Research and Scholarship, College of Nursing, University of Florida, Gainesville

Preface

It is gratifying to reflect upon nursing education and its tremendous growth over the past decade since the first edition of this text was published (2006). Even more astonishing is the fact that nursing is moving into higher levels of education by creating more accessible pathways for existing nurses to continue their education and, at the same time, increasing opportunities for students to enter into practice at the baccalaureate and master's levels. Nursing educators are recognizing the complexity of the health care system and the health care needs of the population and moving advanced practice and leadership roles into the doctoral level, offering programs that create nursing researchers, scholars, and faculty to keep the profession current and ready for the future.

As with previous editions of the text, Stephanie and I organized the chapters in what we consider logical order so that nursing educators and graduate students may use it to guide their activities as they review an existing program and assess it for its needs to determine if revision of the curriculum or perhaps a new program or track is indicated. A discussion of the finances related to curriculum development and budget management provides practical, but necessary, information for support of curriculum development activities. This edition places a fictitious case study of a needs assessment and subsequent program development in the Appendix. It provides an opportunity for readers to review the processes involved in curriculum development and there are additional data in the study for readers to develop curricula other than the one presented. The case study brings into play international possibilities for nursing programs to build collaborative nursing curricula through the use of web-based, online platforms.

The core of the text is Section III, which begins with a description of the classic components of the curriculum, discusses learning theories, educational taxonomies, and critical thinking as they apply to nursing, and then proceeds to describe the current undergraduate and graduate programs available in nursing in the United States. A unified nursing curriculum and its implications follow those chapters and the section ends with the impact of technology, informatics, and online learning. An overview of program evaluation, regulatory agencies, and accreditation follows the section to close the loop on the processes of curriculum development and evaluation. It is necessary for nursing educators to be familiar with the various systems that either regulate, accredit, or set standards to ensure the quality of educational programs. Nursing educators need to be aware of not only state board regulations and professional accreditation standards, but also those that reflect upon their home institutions, such as regional accrediting bodies. Participating in these activities as well as routinely assessing and evaluating the program as it is implemented ensures the quality of the end product and the integrity of the curriculum. A case study depicting the preparation for an accreditation report and visit illustrates the activities necessary for achieving accreditation.

The final section of the text reviews the literature for research on nursing education as it relates to curriculum development and evaluation. Research questions are raised from the review and suggestions offered for further study based on the National League for Nursing's identification of research priorities for nursing education. It is gratifying to see the increase in studies over the past decade but additional work needs to be done, especially replication of studies for generalizability and theory building. The final chapter of the text summarizes the chapters and raises issues and challenges for nursing educators.

It has been a pleasure to work with Stephanie who will be taking over the text in future editions. She is an expert nursing educator, administrator, and clinician, but most importantly, a dear friend and colleague of mine. For this edition, with an eye to the future, the contributors are young, experienced, expert nursing faculty and clinicians. They represent various nursing education levels, other disciplines' knowledge, clinical specialties, and the geographical regions of the United States. I am extremely grateful to them and to Stephanie. I know that the future of nursing and its education is promising and secure.

Sarah B. Keating

The face of nursing education is changing at a rapid pace. There is an increasing desire to advance education toward graduate programs. Technological expansions resulted in increased access to education via online and distance-learning programs. Face-to-face, on-site programs are challenged to remain relevant and solvent when online programs offer the same level of education at a faster and more economically enticing price. In addition, courses are offered in ways that meet the needs of the working student. Curriculum development and evaluation are an art and science that go beyond the methodologies of teaching. This text provides content essential for nursing education students, novice educators in academe, and experienced nursing faculty to meet the challenges they face in this changing environment. It describes the evolution of current nursing curricula and provides the theories, concepts, and tools necessary for curriculum development and evaluation in nursing.

I am honored to have had this opportunity to coauthor this text with Sarah. She has been my mentor and biggest supporter, and is now a cherished friend. I would like to believe that I may somehow coax her to contribute to the next edition, although she denies that is even a remote possibility. I am humbled, and excited to accept the torch that is being passed to me. I will treasure this gift. It gives me great pride to contribute to nursing knowledge and support those who pursue nursing education as their future path.

Stephanie S. DeBoor

Qualified instructors may obtain access to ancillary materials, including an instructor's manual and PowerPoints, by contacting textbook@springerpub.com.

SECTION I

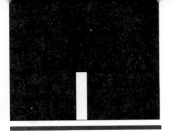

Overview of Nursing Education: History, Curriculum Development and Approval Processes, and the Role of Faculty

Sarah B. Keating
Stephanie S. DeBoor

OVERVIEW OF CURRICULUM DEVELOPMENT AND EVALUATION IN NURSING EDUCATION

The fourth edition of this text devotes itself to the underlying theories, concepts, and science of curriculum development and evaluation in nursing education as separate from the art and science of teaching and instructional processes. The textbook is targeted to both novice and experienced faculty and nursing education students. The curriculum provides the goals for an educational program and guidelines for how they will be delivered and ultimately, evaluated for effectiveness. Some major theories and concepts that relate to instructional strategies are discussed but only in light of their contributions to the implementation of the curriculum plan.

To initiate the discourse on curriculum development, a definition is in order. For the purposes of the textbook, the definition is: *a curriculum is the formal plan of study that provides the philosophical underpinnings, goals, and guidelines for delivery of a specific educational program*. The text uses this definition throughout for the *formal* curriculum, while recognizing the existence of the *informal* curriculum. The informal curriculum consists of activities that students, faculty, administrators, staff, and consumers experience outside of the formal planned curriculum. Examples of the informal curriculum include interpersonal relationships, athletic/recreational activities, study groups, organizational activities, special events, academic and personal counseling, and so forth. Although the text focuses on the formal curriculum, nursing educators should keep the informal curriculum in mind for its influence and use to reinforce learning activities that arise from the planned curriculum.

To place curriculum development and evaluation in perspective, it is wise to examine the history of nursing education in the United States and the lessons it provides for current and future curriculum developers. This section sets the stage through an examination of nursing's place in the history of higher education and the role of faculty and administrators in developing and evaluating curricula. Nursing curricula are currently undergoing transformation, especially with the tremendous growth in the delivery of courses and programs through the Internet and the application of technology to instructional strategies. Today's emphases on the learner and measurement of learning outcomes, integration into the curriculum of safety and quality concepts, evidence-based practice, translational science, and research provide exciting challenges and opportunities for nursing educators. Today and tomorrow's curricula call for an integration of processes that are learner and consumer focused and at the same time, ensure excellence by building in outcome measures to determine the quality of the program. In addition, there is a need for research on curriculum development and evaluation to provide the underpinnings for evidence-based practice in nursing education.

HISTORY OF NURSING EDUCATION IN THE UNITED STATES

Chapter 1 traces the history of American nursing education from the time of the first Nightingale schools of nursing to the present. The trends in professional education and society's needs impacted nursing programs that started from apprentice-type schools to a majority of the programs now in institutions of higher learning. Lest the profession forgets, liberal arts and the sciences in institutions of higher learning play a major role in nursing education and set the foundation for the development of critical thinking and clinical decision making so necessary to nursing care.

Chapter 1 reviews major historical events in society and the world that influenced nursing practice and education, as well as changes in the health care system. The major world wars of the 20th century increased the demand for nurses and a nursing education system that prepared a workforce ready to meet that demand. The emergence of nursing education that took place in community colleges in the mid-20th century initiated continuing debate about entry into practice. The explosive growth of doctor of nursing practice (DNP) programs in recent times and their place in defining advanced practice, nursing leadership, and education bring the past happenings into focus as the profession responds to the changes in health care and the needs of the population.

CURRICULUM DEVELOPMENT AND APPROVAL PROCESSES IN CHANGING EDUCATIONAL ENVIRONMENTS

Chapter 2 discusses the organizational structures and processes that programs undergo when changing or creating new curricula and the roles and responsibilities of faculty in realizing the changes. Administrators provide the leadership for organizing and carrying out evaluation activities. To bring the curriculum into reality and out of the "Ivory Tower," faculty and administrators must include students, alumni, employers, and the people whom their graduates serve into the curriculum building and evaluation processes.

The chapter describes the classic hierarchy of curriculum approval processes in institutions of higher learning and the importance of nursing faculty's participation within the governance of the institution. The governance of colleges and universities usually includes curriculum committees or their equivalent composed of elected faculty members. These committees are at the program, college-wide, and/or university-wide levels and through their review, provide the academic rigor for ensuring quality in educational programs.

It is a cardinal rule in academe that the curriculum "belongs to the faculty." In higher education, faculty members are deemed the experts in their specific disciplines, or in the case of nursing, clinical specialties or functional areas such as administration, health care policy, case management, and so forth. Nursing faculty must periodically review a program to maintain a vibrant curriculum that responds to changes in society, health care needs of the population, the health care delivery system, and the learners' needs. It is important to measure the program's success in preparing nurses for the current environment and for the future. Currency of practice as well as that of the future must be built into the curriculum, because it will be several years before entering cohorts graduate. In nursing, there is an inherent requirement to produce caring, competent, and confident practitioners or clinicians. At the same time, the curriculum must meet professional and accreditation standards. While it may be unpopular to think that curricula are built upon accreditation criteria and professional standards, in truth, integrating them into the curriculum helps administrators and faculty prepare for program approval or review and accreditation.

Both new and experienced faculty members have major roles in curriculum development, implementation, and program evaluation. While there is a tendency to see only the part of the curriculum in which the individual educator is involved, it is essential that instructors have a strong sense of the program as a whole. In that way, the curriculum remains true to its goals, learning objectives (student-learning outcomes), and the content necessary for reaching the goals. Following the curriculum plan results in an intact curriculum and at the same time provides the opportunity for faculty and students to identify gaps in the program or the need for updates and revisions. Such needs are brought to the attention of other instructors and the coordinators of the courses or levels for assessment and action through curricular review and change processes.

CHAPTER 1

History of Nursing Education in the United States

Susan M. Ervin

CHAPTER OBJECTIVE

Upon completion of Chapter 1, the reader will be able to:

- Compare important curricular events in the 19th century with those in the 20th and 21st centuries
- Cite the impact that two world wars had on the development of nursing education
- Differentiate among the different curricula that prepare entry-level nurses
- Cite important milestones in the development of graduate education in nursing
- Associate the decade most pivotal to the development of one type of nursing program, that is, diploma, associate, baccalaureate, master's, or doctoral degree
- Evaluate the impact of the history of nursing education on current and future curriculum development and evaluation activities

OVERVIEW

Formal nursing education began at the end of the 19th century when events such as the Civil War and the Industrial Revolution emphasized the need for well-trained nurses. Florence Nightingale's model of nursing education was used to establish hospital-based nursing programs that flourished throughout the 19th and well into the 20th century. With few exceptions, however, Nightingale's model was abandoned and hospital schools trained students with an emphasis on service to the hospital rather than education of a nurse. Early nurse reformers such as Isabel Hampton Robb, Lavinia Dock, and Annie W. Goodrich laid the foundation for nursing education built on natural and social sciences and, by the 1920s, nursing programs were visible in university settings. World War I and World War II underscored the importance of well-educated nurses and the Army School of Nursing and the Cadet Army Corps significantly contributed to the movement of nursing education into university settings.

Associate degree programs developed in the 1950s as a result of community college interest in nursing education, and Mildred Montag's dissertation outlined the preparation of the technical nurse to be prepared in these settings. The situation of nursing in community colleges, along with the American Nurses Association (ANA) proposal that nursing education be located within university settings, sparked a tumultuous period in nursing education. By the latter half of the 20th century, graduate education in nursing was established with master's and doctoral programs growing across the country. Graduate education continues to strengthen the discipline as it moves through the 21st century.

EARLY BEGINNINGS

Nursing education changed over the past 150 years in response to landmark events such as wars, economic fluctuations, and U.S. demographics. The initial milestone that catalyzed formal nursing education was the Civil War. Prior to the Civil War, most women provided nursing care to family at home. Older women who had extensive family experience and needed to earn a living might care for neighbors or contacts who were referred by word of mouth (Reverby, 1987). Although nursing practice was outside the norm for women, during the Civil War approximately 2,000 untrained but well-intentioned patriotic women moved from the home to the battlefield to provide care to soldiers. Sadly, lack of education, inadequate facilities, and poor hygiene contributed to more soldier deaths than bullets. The need for formal education for nurses became evident. Other catalysts for formal nursing education included the transition of hospitals from places for the destitute to arenas for the application of new medical knowledge and the industrial revolution that resulted in increased slums and disease (Rush, 1992).

Earliest Attempts at Formal Training

Florence Nightingale is considered to be the founder of modern nursing. She created a model of nursing education that has persisted for over 100 years. She believed that education was necessary to "teach not only what is to be done but how to do it [and] . . . why such a thing is done" (Nightingale, 1860). The New England Hospital for Women and Children was the first American school to offer a formal training program in 1872. Although it was not based on the Nightingale model, the school offered a 1-year curriculum. In addition to 12 hours of required lectures, students were taught to take vital signs and apply bandages. Interestingly, students were not allowed to know the names of medications they gave to patients and the medication bottles were labeled by numbers. In 1875, the curriculum was extended to 16 months (Davis, 1991). Linda Richards, considered to be America's first trained nurse, entered this school on the first day it opened. Subsequent to her graduation, Linda Richards spent her career organizing training schools for nurses. She supervised the development of the Boston Training School for Nurses at Massachusetts General Hospital as well as at least five other schools (Kalisch & Kalisch, 2004).

First Nightingale Schools

Nightingale's educational model proposed that nursing schools remain autonomous, not under the auspices of affiliated hospitals, and were to develop stringent educational standards (Anderson, 1981; Kelly & Joel, 1996). Education, rather than service to the hospital, should be the focus. In 1873, three schools opened in the United States that provided nursing education patterned on Nightingale's model: Bellevue Training School in New York City, the Connecticut Training School in Hartford, and the Boston Training School in Boston. The Bellevue Training School opened with a 2-year curriculum. The first year consisted of lectures and clinical practice, and the second year focused on clinical practice (Kalisch & Kalisch, 2004). Although practice was primarily service to the hospital (in opposition to Nightingale's model) and learning was hit and miss, there were some interesting firsts at Bellevue. These included interdisciplinary rounds, patient record keeping, and adoption of the first student uniform (Kelly & Joel, 1996).

The Connecticut Training School opened with four students and a superintendent of nurses. By the end of the first year there were nearly 100 applicants and by the end of the second year, graduates entered the field of private-duty nursing. By its sixth year of operation, the school developed a handbook titled *New Haven Manual of Nursing.* The Connecticut School is credited with the advent of the nursing cap; the wearing of large caps was instituted to contain the elaborate hairstyles of the time that did not belong in the "sickroom" (Kalisch & Kalisch, 2004). The initial goal of the Boston Training School, the third American school, was to offer a desirable occupation for self-supporting women and to provide private nurses for the community. Initially, there was minimal focus on didactic or clinical instruction. In 1874, Linda Richards became the third super-intendent of the school, reorganized the school, initiated didactic instruction, and, in general, "proved that trained nurses were better than untrained ones" (Kelly & Joel, 1996, p. 27).

The Early 20th Century

By the beginning of the 20th century, over 2,000 training schools had opened. With few exceptions, Nightingale's principles of education were abandoned and school priorities were "service first, education second" (Kelly & Joel, 1996). The 3-year program of most nursing schools consisted primarily of on-the-job training, courses taught by physicians, and long hours of clinical practice. Students provided nursing service for the hospital. In return, they received diplomas and pins at the completion of their training. Students entered the programs one by one as they were available and their services were needed. The patients were mostly poor, without families and/or homes to provide care. From the institution's standpoint, graduates were a by-product rather than a purpose for the train-ing school (Reverby, 1984).

Nightingale's text, *Notes on Nursing: What It Is and What It Is Not,* was published in 1859 and, for decades, was the sole text on nursing. If other textbooks were available to students, they were authored primarily by physicians. The first U.S. nurse–authored text, *A Text-Book for Nursing: For the Use of Training Schools, Families and Private Students,* was written by Clara Weeks (later Weeks-Shaw, 1902), an 1880 graduate of the New York Hos-pital and founding superintendent of the Paterson General Hospital School (Obituary, 1940). The possession of such a text led to decreased dependence of graduates on their course notes, supplied information that would otherwise have been missed because of cancelled lectures or student exhaustion, reinforced the idea that nursing required more than fine character, and exerted a standardizing effect on training school expectations.

It is interesting to note that hospital training schools did not represent the sole path of nursing education in the early 20th century (V. Bullough, 2004). Perhaps as a harbin-ger of the 21st century, distance learning provided an alternative educational path. Cor-respondence schools emerged and were regarded by many as a satisfactory alternative to hospital schools. The best known of these schools was Chautauqua School of Nurs-ing in the state of New York. Founded in 1900, it offered a three-course correspondence course that included general nursing, obstetrical, and surgical nursing. It attracted stu-dents for a variety of reasons. They may have been too old (older than 35 years of age) for hospital schools, were married (hence not eligible for hospital schools), or lived in com-munities where no hospital school of nursing was available. Fledging accrediting and registration bodies forced the closure of the school in the 1920s (V. Bullough, 2004).

REPORTS AND STANDARDS OF THE LATE 19TH AND EARLY 20TH CENTURIES

As the number of nursing schools and the number of trained nurses increased, the need for organization and standardization of education and practice was recognized.

The International Congress of Charities, Correction and Philanthropy met in Chicago as part of the Columbian Exposition of 1893. Isabel Hampton, the founding principal of the Training School and Superintendent of Nurses at Johns Hopkins Hospital, played a leading role in planning the nursing sessions for the Congress. She presented a paper, "Educational Standards for Nurses," which argued that hospitals had a responsibility to provide actual education for nursing students; the paper also urged superintendents to work together to establish educational standards (James, 2002). Hampton's paper included a proposal to extend the training period to 3 years in order to allow the shortening of the "practical training" to 8 hours per day. She also recommended admission of students with "stated times for entrance into the school, and the teaching year . . . divided according to the academic terms usually adopted in our public schools and colleges" (Robb, 1907). Hampton instigated an informal meeting of nursing superintendents that laid the groundwork for the formation of the American Society of Superintendents of Training Schools (ASSTS) in the United States and Canada, which later, in 1912, was renamed the National League of Nursing Education (NLNE). This was also the first association of a professional nature organized and controlled by women (V. Bullough & Bullough, 1978).

The year 1893 marked the publication of Hampton's *Nursing: Its Principles and Practice for Hospital and Private Use*. The first 25 pages were devoted to a description of a training school, including physical facilities, library resources, and a 2-year curricular plan for didactic content and clinical rotations (Dodd, 2001). In 1912, the ASSTS became the NLNE and their objectives were to continue to develop and work for a uniform curriculum. In 1915, Adelaide Nutting commented on the educational status of nursing and the NLNE presented a standard curriculum for schools of nursing. The curriculum was divided into seven areas, each of which contained two or more courses. There was a strong emphasis on student activity including observation, accurate recording, participation in actual dissection, experimentation, and provision of patient care (Bacon, 1987). In 1925, the Committee on the Grading of Nursing Schools was formed. The grading committee worked from 1926 to 1934 to produce "gradings" based on answers to survey forms. Each school received individualized feedback about its own characteristics in comparison to all other participating schools (Committee on the Grading of Nursing Schools, 1931).

In 1917, 1927, and 1937, the NLNE published a series of curriculum recommendations in book form. The *Standard Curriculum for Schools of Nursing* was the first, the second *A Curriculum,* and the third *A Curriculum Guide.* The first was developed by a relatively small group, but the second and third involved a long process with broad input. The published curricula were intended to reflect a generalization about what the better schools were doing or aimed to accomplish. As such, they give a picture of change over the 20-year period, but cannot be regarded as providing a snapshot of a typical school. Each volume represents substantial change from the previous, and while the same course topical area exists in all three, the level of detail and specificity increases with each decade. Indeed, the markedly increased length and wordy style of the 1937 volume appropriately carries the title "Guide."

Each *Curriculum* book increased the number of classroom hours and decreased the recommended hours of patient care, in effect making nursing service more expensive. Each *Curriculum* increased the prerequisite educational level: 4 years of high school (temporary tolerance of 2 years in 1917), 4 years of high school in 1927, and 1 to 2 years of college or normal school in addition to high school by 1937 (NLNE, 1917, 1927, 1937).

While the NLNE advocated for changes in nursing education, there remained a need for a national association of trained nurses. Bellevue Training School founded the first alumnae association in 1889 and by 1890 there were 21 alumni associations in the United

States. (Kalisch & Kalisch, 2004). In 1896, with the assistance of Isabel Hampton, a national association of trained nurses became a reality. The Nurses' Associated Alumnae of the United States and Canada was established. A constitution and bylaws were prepared and, 1 year later, adopted by the organization and Ms. Robb became the first elected president. Not one of the original attendees was a registered nurse as there were no licensing laws in place at the time (www.nursingworld.org). In 1911, the Nurses' Associated Alumnae became the American Nurses Association (Kalisch & Kalisch, 2004).

Diverse Schools of Nursing

Mary Mahoney, the first African American nurse, entered the New England Hospital for Women and Children School of Nursing on March 23, 1878. Her acceptance at this school was unique at a time in American society when the majority of educational institutions were not integrated (Davis, 1991). This lack of integration, however, did not deter African American women from entering the profession of nursing. In 1891, Provident Hospital in Chicago was founded, which was the first training school for African American nurses (Kelly & Joel, 1996).

Howard University Training School for Nurses was established in 1893 to train African American nurses to care for the many Blacks who settled in Washington, DC, after the Civil War. The school transferred to Freedman's Hospital in 1894 and by 1944 had 166 students (Washington, 2012). This rapid expansion was experienced by other African American nursing programs (Kalisch & Kalisch, 1978). Freedman's Hospital School transferred to Howard University in 1967 and graduated its last class in 1973. Howard University School of Nursing has offered a baccalaureate degree since 1974 and initiated a master's degree in nursing in 1980. After the *Brown vs Board of Education* decision in 1954, schools of nursing that served predominantly African American students began to decline and, by the late 1960s, nursing schools throughout the United States were fully integrated (Carnegie, 2005).

The first Native American School of Nursing was Sage Memorial Hospital School of Nursing, which was established in 1930. Located in northeastern Arizona, at Ganado, it was the first accredited 3-year nursing program on a reservation (Charbonneau-Dahlen & Crow, 2016). It was part of Sage Memorial Hospital, built by the National Missions of the Presbyterian Church, which provided care for Native Americans (Kalisch & Kalisch, 1978). By 1943, students enrolled in the school came from widely diverse backgrounds including Native American, Hispanic, Hawaiian, Cuban, and Japanese. In the 1930s and 1940s, such training and cultural exchange among minority women was not found anywhere else in the United States (Pollitt, Streeter, & Walsh, 2011). The school of nursing operated through 1951; decreased funding and an increased emphasis on baccalaureate education contributed to its closure. In 1993, the first reservation-based baccalaureate nursing program was opened by Northern Arizona University at the same location as Sage Memorial School (Charbonneau-Dahlen & Crow, 2016).

Men in Nursing Education

One little known legacy of the Civil War is the inclusion of men in nursing. Walt Whitman, known for his poetry, was a nurse in the Civil War. He cared for wounded soldiers in Washington, DC, for 5 years and was an early practitioner of holistic nursing, incorporating active listening, therapeutic touch, and the instillation of hope in patients (Ahrens, 2002). There were few nursing schools in the late 19th century that accommodated men; a few schools provided an abbreviated curriculum that trained men as "attendants." The McLean Asylum School of Nursing in Massachusetts was among the first to provide nursing education for men. Established in 1882, the 2-year curriculum prepared graduates to work in the mental health facilities of the time. Treatments in those facilities included application of restraints (e.g., strait jackets) and "tubbing" (placing the patient in a bathtub with a wooden cover locked onto the tub so only the patient's head was exposed) and it was believed the tubs required the physical power men possessed (Kenny, 2008).

The first true formal school of nursing for men was established at Bellevue Hospital in New York City in 1888 by Darius Mills. One of the best-known schools of nursing for men was the Alexian Brothers Hospital School of Nursing. It opened in 1898 and was the last of its kind to close in 1969 (LaRocco, 2011). Although the school admitted only religious brothers for most of its early history, in 1927 it began to accept lay students. In 1939, the school began an affiliation with DePaul University so students could take biology and other science courses to apply toward a bachelor's degree. By 1955, the school had obtained full National League for Nursing (NLN) accreditation and by 1962, 13 full-time faculty members and eight lecturers educated a graduating class of 42 students. This was the largest class in the school's history and one of the largest classes in any men's nursing school in the country (Wall, 2009). By the mid-1960s, men were being admitted to most hospital nursing programs and the school graduated its last class in 1969.

Diverse ethnic and racial groups account for more than one-third of the U.S. population (U.S. Census Bureau, n.d.) and nursing education strives to ensure the profession reflects the diversity of the nation. In 2016, 31.5% of baccalaureate nursing students were non-White (10.6% African American, 10.5% Hispanic, 0.5% American Indian, 7.4% Asian/Pacific Islander, 2.4% two or more races); in graduate programs 33.6% (master's) to 34.6% (doctoral) students were non-White. Twelve per cent of baccalaureate and nursing students are men (AACN, 2016).

MARCHING INTO SERVICE: NURSING EDUCATION IN WARTIME

Prior to World War I, nurses served in both the Civil War and the Spanish American War, which occurred between April and August 1898. In contrast to the Civil War, only nurses who graduated from an established training school were eligible to serve in the Spanish American War. Disease again caused significant fatalities with yellow fever claiming lives of both soldiers and nurses (Kalisch & Kalisch, 2004). Following the Spanish American War, the need for trained nurses was reinforced and both the Army Nurse Corps and the Navy Nurse Corps were established in the early 1900s.

World War I

When the United States entered World War I, admissions to nursing schools increased by about 25% (Bacon, 1987). The two phenomena that impacted nursing education during World War I were the development of the Vassar Training Camp and the founding of the Army School of Nursing. The Vassar Training Camp for Nurses was established in 1918. Its purpose was to enroll female college graduates in a 3-month intensive course that addressed natural and social sciences and fundamental nursing skills. Following this course, students completed the final 2 years of school in one of 35 selected schools of nursing (Bacon, 1987). Of the 439 college graduates who entered the Vassar Camp, 418 completed the course, went on to nursing school, replaced nurses who had entered the armed services, and helped fill key leadership roles in nursing for the next several decades (Kalisch & Kalisch, 1978). Although short-lived, the Vassar Training Camp provided the opportunity to build nursing competencies on a college education foundation and contributed to the eventual move of nursing education into the university setting (Bacon, 1987).

In 1918, Annie W. Goodrich, president of the ANA, proposed the development of an Army School of Nursing. This was in response to extremely vocal groups who believed that, because of the war, the educational preparation of nurses should be shortened. With the backing of the NLNE and the ANA in addition to nursing leaders such as Frances Payne Bolton, the secretary of war approved the school and Annie Goodrich became its first dean. She developed the curriculum according to the *Standard Curriculum for Schools of Nursing* published by the NLNE in 1917 (Kalisch & Kalisch, 1978).

World War II and the Cadet Nurse Corps

World War II, with its demands for all able-bodied young men for military service, mobilized available women for employment or volunteer service. From mid-1941 to mid-1943, with the help of federal aid, nursing schools increased their enrollments and postdiploma nurses completed post–basic course work to fill the places of nurses who enlisted. Some inactive nurses returned to practice (Roberts, 1954). Despite the effort necessary to bring about this increase, hospitals were floundering and more nurses were needed for the military services. Congress passed the Bolton Act, which authorized the complex of activities known as the Cadet Nurse Corps (CNC) in June 1943. It was conceived as a mechanism to avoid civilian hospital collapse, to provide nursing to the military, and to ensure an adequate education for student nurse cadets (Kalisch & Kalisch, 1978).

Hospitals sponsoring training schools recognized that CNC schools would out-recruit non-CNC schools, thereby almost certainly guaranteeing their closure or radical shrinkage. Thus, they signed on, despite the fact that hospitals had to establish a separate accounting for school costs, literally meet the requirements of their state boards of nurse examiners to the satisfaction of the CNC consultants, and allow their students to leave for federal service during the last 6 months of their programs, when they would otherwise be most valuable to their home schools. Visiting consultants looked at faculty numbers and qualifications, clinical facilities available for learning, curricula, hours of student clinical and class work, the school's ability to accelerate course work to fit into 30 months, and the optimal number of students the school could accommodate. Schools were pressed to increase the size of their classes and number of classes admitted per year, to use local colleges for basic sciences to conserve nurse instructor time, and to develop affiliations with psychiatric hospitals, for educational reasons, and secondarily to free up dormitory space for more students to be admitted (Robinson & Perry, 2001).

Students, who were estimated to be providing 80% of care in civilian hospitals, experienced a changed practice context. In addition to providing direct care, students now decided what could safely be delegated to Red Cross volunteers and any available paid aides. With grossly short staffing, nurses had to set priorities carefully. All of these circumstances altered student learning. The intense work of the consultants, who provided interpretation and linkage between the U.S. Public Health Service (USPHS) in Washington and each school, and their strategy of simultaneously naming deficiencies and identifying improvement goals, was a critical factor in the success of the programs as well as improvement in nursing education. Without the financial resources of the federal government to defray student costs, to assist with certain costs to schools, and to provide the consultation, auditing, and public relations/recruitment functions, the goals could not be met.

Other Wars

Nurses continued to serve in wars including Korea, Vietnam, Desert Storm, and the ongoing Middle East crisis. Educational incentives, notably the Army Student Nurse Program and the Reserve Officer Training Corps programs, assist student nurses with educational expenses in exchange for specific years of active duty service (Vuic, 2006).

THE EVOLUTION OF CURRENT EDUCATIONAL PATHS FOR ENTRY INTO PRACTICE

By the interwar period, the university became the dominant institution for postsecondary education (Graham, 1978). From 1920 to 1940, the percentage of women attending college in the 18- to 21-year-old age range rose from 7.6% to 12.2%. Men's attendance rose more quickly, hence the percentage of women in the student body dropped from 43% in 1920 to 40.2% in 1940 (Eisenmann, 2000; Solomon, 1985). In the first decade of the 1900s, technical institutes such as Drexel in Philadelphia, Pratt in Brooklyn, and Mechanics in Rochester, as well as Simmons College in Boston and Northwestern University in Chicago, offered course work to nursing students (Robb, 1907). The designers of the 1917 *Standard Curriculum for Schools of Nursing* gave some thought to the relationship of nursing education to the collegiate system. They suggested that the theoretical work in a nursing school was equivalent to 36 units, or about 1 year of college, and the clinical work another 51 units. Few voices actively campaigned for the alignment of nursing education with institutions of higher learning even as late as the 1930s, despite the recommendation of the Rockefeller-funded Goldmark (1923) report, *Nursing and Nursing Education in the United States,* in the early 1920s. Initially, education at the university level was envisioned solely for the leaders of training schools.

Educators wanted independent schools of nursing with a concentration on educational goals and emancipation from hospital student apprentice, work-study curricula. These educators looked hopefully at the Yale University School of Nursing, funded by the Rockefeller Foundation starting in 1924, and headed by the determined and respected Annie W. Goodrich. Similarly encouraging was the program at Case Western Reserve University, endowed by Francis Payne Bolton in 1923. Vanderbilt was endowed by a combination of Rockefeller, Carnegie, and Commonwealth funds in 1930. The University of Chicago established a school of nursing in 1925 with an endowment from the distinguished but discontinued Illinois Training School (Hanson, 1991). Dillard University established a school in 1942 with substantial foundation support and governmental war-related funds. Mary Tennant, nursing adviser in the Rockefeller Foundation, pronounced the Dillard Division of Nursing "one of the most interesting developments in nursing education in the country" (Hine, 1989). Although these were milestone events, endowments did little to dissipate the caution, if not hostility, toward women on American campuses. Neither did they cure all that was ailing in nursing education. They funded significant program changes, but even these would not meet the accreditation standards of later decades (Faddis, 1973; Kalisch & Kalisch, 1978; Sheahan, 1980).

Baccalaureate Education

The diverse baccalaureate curricula of the 1930s multiplied by the 1950s. As one educator wrote in 1954, "Baccalaureate programs still seem to be in the experimental stage. They vary in purpose, structure, subject matter content, admission requirements, matriculation requirements, and degrees granted upon their completion. Some schools offering baccalaureate programs still aim to prepare nurses for specialized positions. Others, advancing from this traditional concept, seek to prepare graduates for generalized nursing in beginning positions" (Harms, 1954).

Although a few programs threaded general education and basic science courses through 5 years of study, the majority structured their programs with 2 years of college courses before or after the 3 years of nursing preparation, or book-ended the nursing years with the split 2 years of college work (Bridgman, 1949). Margaret Bridgman, an educator from Skidmore College who consulted with a large number of nursing schools, made favorable reference to the "upper division nursing major" in her volume directed toward both college and nursing educators (Bridgman, 1953). Bridgman recommended that postdiploma students be evaluated individually and provisionally with a tentative grant of credit based on prior learning, including nursing schoolwork, and successful completion of a term of academic work. The student's program would be made up of "deficiencies" in general education and prerequisite courses and then courses in the major itself. Credit-granting practices varied considerably from place to place, so a nurse could easily spend 1½ to 3 years earning the baccalaureate.

Given the constant expansion of knowledge relevant to nursing, it was doubly difficult for programs with a history of a 5-year curriculum to shrink to 4 academic years in the 1960s and early 1970s. The expanded assessment skills expected of critical care nurses, together with the master's-level specialty emphases and certificate nurse practitioner (NP) programs, stimulated the inclusion of more sophisticated skills in baccalaureate programs in the early to mid-1970s (Lynaugh & Brush, 1996). In response to nursing service agitation to narrow the gap between new graduate skills and initial employment expectations, and much talk about "reality shock," baccalaureate programs structured curricula to allow a final experience in which students were immersed in clinical care to focus on skills of organization and integration.

In the 1980s and early 1990s nursing experienced another shortage. Because of the severity of this shortage, accelerated or fast-track baccalaureate nursing and entry-level master's programs were developed (Keating, 2015). The purpose of these programs was to attract students with nonnursing degrees, build on learning experiences provided by these degrees, and provide a path to licensure in 11 to 18 months for the baccalaureate with an additional 12 to 24 months for the master's level (AACN, 2015).

Accreditation

From the standpoint of the ordinary nursing school, the possibility of actual accreditation became a reality in the 1950s. The NLNE developed standards for accreditation and made pilot visits from 1934 to 1938. By 1939, schools could list themselves to be visited in order to qualify to be on the first list published by NLNE. Despite the greatly increased work, turnover, and general disruption created by the war, 100 schools mustered both the courage and energy required to prepare for accreditation evaluation and judged creditable by 1945. Many schools that qualified for provisional accreditation, however, were due for revisiting by the end of World War II. The National Organization for Public Health Nursing (NOPHN) had been accrediting post–basic programs in public health since 1920 but more recently had considered specialty programs at both baccalaureate and master's levels and the public health content in generalist baccalaureate programs (Harms, 1954). By 1948, these organizations, along with the Council of Nursing Education of Catholic Hospitals, ceded their accrediting role to the National Nursing Assessment Service (NNAS), which published its first combined list of accredited programs just 1 month before the survey-based interim classification of schools was published by the National Committee for the Improvement of Nursing Services (NCINS) in 1949 (Petry, 1949).

The NNAS, much like the cadet nurse program before it, elected a strategy designed to entice schools with at least minimal strengths to improve. It published the first list of temporarily accredited schools in 1952, giving these schools 5 years to make improvements and qualify for full accreditation. During the intervening time, it provided many special meetings, self-evaluation guides, and consultant visits to the schools. By 1957, the number of fully accredited schools increased by 72.4% (Kalisch & Kalisch, 1978). Changes in hospital school programs were catalyzed and channeled by accreditation norms (Committee of the Six National Nursing Organizations on Unification of Accrediting Services, 1949). But ultimately, the forces that drove change were primarily external, ranging from public expectations of postsecondary education mediated through hospital trustees and physicians, to competition among programs for potential students, who now had access to information about accreditation. By 1950, all states participated in the state board test pool examination, another measuring rod that induced improvement or closure of weaker schools.

Despite the influential Carnegie- and Sage-funded *Nursing for the Future* in 1948, which recommended a broad-based move of nursing education into general higher education, nursing's earliest centralized accreditation mechanism concentrated considerable energy on improving diploma schools, as had the Grading Committee before it (E. L. Brown, 1948; Roberts, 1954). Why this seeming mismatch between aspirations and effort? Partly, it sprang from realism: Students were in hospital schools, whether ideal or not, so they needed the best possible preparation because nursing services would reflect this quality. Further, the quality of many of the baccalaureate programs left a great deal to be desired and their capacity for more students was limited, so these could not be promoted as an immediate or ideal substitute for diploma programs. Although by 1957 there were 18 associate degree programs (Kalisch & Kalisch, 1978), no one foresaw the speed of their multiplication in the next decade. Finally, nursing's collective sense of social responsibility burdened it with finding ways to continue to provide essential services, both within the hospital and elsewhere, as its educational house moved from the base of the hospital to the foundation of higher education (Lynaugh, 2002).

Associate Degree Education

The NLNE held discussions during the middle and late 1940s with community colleges to discuss the possibility of associate degree nursing education (Fondiller, 2001). In 1945, the American Association of Junior Colleges (AAJC) showed an interest in nursing; at this point curriculum and recruitment were the two major challenges. In January 1946, a committee was established with representation from the Association of Collegiate Schools of Nursing (ACSN) to consider nursing education in community colleges. Between 1949 and 1950, the committee, along with NLNE and ACSN, discussed nursing education at this level. The focus was to be the "Brown" report, that is, *Nursing for the Future*, authored by Esther Lucille Brown, a social anthropologist with the Russell Sage Foundation (E. L. Brown, 1948). The immediate context for the committee, from the nursing side, was significant. In 1947, the board of NLNE adopted the policy goal that nursing education should be located in the higher education system. Also in 1947, the faculty at Teachers College, Columbia University (TCCU) launched a planning process that involved Eli Ginzberg, a young economist, who asserted that nursing could be thought of as a whole set of functions and roles rather than a single role or type of worker. He posited that nursing needed at least two types of practitioners, one professional, and one technical (Haase, 1990). Starting in fall 1947, Brown began her conferences with nursing leaders and visits to more than 50 schools, completing her report so that it could be disseminated in September 1948. She believed that perhaps a "graduate bedside nurse" needed more preparation than a practical nurse, but less than a full-fledged professional nurse. In early 1949, NLNE sought funding for the joint work with community colleges, and found the Russell Sage and W.K. Kellogg Foundations responsive with substantial support (Haase, 1990).

The committee reported that community colleges could develop one of two types of nursing programs: (a) a 2-year program that would be transfer oriented to a university program that offered a baccalaureate degree, or (b) a 3-year program leading to an associate of arts (AA) or an associate of science (AS). In 1951, Mildred Montag, whose dissertation proposed a new type of technical nursing program embedded in junior colleges, joined the committee. She was subsequently appointed to the Joint Committee in 1951 and became the project director for the anonymously funded Cooperative Research Project (CRP) in Junior and Community College Education for Nursing in early 1952 (Haase, 1990). The CRP pilot programs were 2 years long, or 2 years plus a summer. Initially, they were one-third general education and two-thirds nursing, but they moved toward equal proportions of each by the end of the project. The curricula, although controlled by faculty in each school, tended to focus on variations in health in their first year, and then deviations from normal (physical and mental illness), in the second year. These "broad fields" were accompanied by campus nursing laboratory learning and by clinical learning experiences in a wide variety of settings, but with a major hospital component. Students in the pilot programs were somewhat older than diploma or baccalaureate students, and some were married (a nonstarter in many diploma programs), and had children. Men were a small percentage of the students, but tripled the representation in diploma programs. State board examination pass rates for graduates of the pilot group were comparable to those of other programs. Montag intended, at that time, that this program would be self-contained, but stressed that graduates of this program could pursue baccalaureate education. She also recommended single licensure for nurses from all educational programs, although 25 years later, she rescinded that recommendation (Fondiller, 2001).

From the mid-1950s to the mid-1970s, when the associate degree program growth rate peaked, the number of programs doubled about every 4 years. By 1975, there were 618 associate degree programs in nursing, constituting 45% of basic nursing programs. Diploma programs constituted 31% of basic programs, although the vast majority of nurses in practice still originally came from diploma programs (Haase, 1990; Rines, 1977). By 1959, W.K. Kellogg Foundation assistance to the expansion of associate degree nursing education totaled more than $3 million. The Nurse Training Act of 1964 and subsequent federal legislation funding nursing also contributed to program growth (Scott, 1972). By the 1990s, associate degree programs produced nearly 60% of newly licensed registered nurses.

Over the years, associate degree education lengthened in time, due in part to the expanding knowledge base needed to be "a bedside nurse." There were pressures from elsewhere on campus to expand general education and pressures due to sequencing requirements of the nursing faculty. Much time was devoted to communicating with hospital nursing service representatives to identify students' competencies at graduation so that new graduate orientations and staff development plans articulated with them. Curricular offerings were fine-tuned to ensure that these baseline competencies were met. When "the bedside" noticeably moved out of the hospital in the early 1990s, questions about preparation for practice in the home care context became urgent, but the familiar condition of the hospital "nursing shortage" laid these to rest.

Programs of the 1950s in university settings had to cope with the entrenched traditions of both hospitals and universities as they struggled to make changes. By contrast, associate degree nursing programs began with a clean slate. They were initially welcomed by community colleges. The lure of having an additional supply of nurses promoted at least grudging cooperation from clinical agencies, although hospital nursing staff and administrators in many places had misgivings about the curricular arrangements and limited clinical experience of students.

Associate degree–prepared nurses of the early 1980s found expectations and mechanisms for matriculating into baccalaureate programs much more clearly defined than described by Bridgman 30 years earlier, and indeed, some baccalaureate programs were designed specifically for associate degree graduates. The ever-expanding body of nursing knowledge forced repeated decisions about which content was most essential and what clinical settings would bring about the best learning. By the 1990s, as hospital censuses plummeted and sick patients shuttled back and forth between home and ambulatory settings, programs were forced to consider increasing community-based clinical experience with its attendant challenges to find placements and provide geographically dispersed instruction.

Tumultuous Times in Nursing Education

The turbulence and cultural upheaval that characterized the mid-1960s through the 1970s was reflected in nursing education. Within nursing, a rift grew between those who believed an incremental approach would eventually get nursing education optimally situated and those who believed that the eventual goal should be clearly specified far in advance so that changes could take the goal into account. Nurses involved in day-to-day patient care and many diploma educators tended to cluster in the first group; the premise was that practice roles in nursing were rarely based on educational preparation. Graduates of all programs held the same license (Fredrickson, 1978). Those nurses, particularly educators, who were in national or regional leadership positions were in the second group. The latter group focused on the professional end of the nursing continuum, working to achieve the fullest possible academic and professional recognition for nursing so that its advocacy and action would have broad credibility and influence. They attempted to define differentiation of practice among the three levels of education (diploma, associate degree, and baccalaureate) and advocated for legislation that recognized differences among graduates (Orsolini-Hain & Waters, 2009).

The ANA 1965 position paper, "Educational Preparation for Nurse Practitioners and Assistants to Nurses," seemed like a logical step in this differentiation of practice (ANA, 1965). After all, for more than 15 years the NLNE, reconstituted and combined with the NOPHN, ACSN, and National Association of Industrial Nurses (NAIN) in 1952 to be the NLN, had been saying that education for nursing belonged in institutions of higher education. The idea that nursing was a continuum, composed of vocational, technical, and professional segments, had been talked about intermittently in those same circles during that entire period.

Unfortunately, the position paper dropped like a bomb on people who had never heard these conversations. It was said to ignore diploma schools and nurses altogether, classify associate degree–prepared nurses as technical nurses, and downgrade vocational/practical nurse preparation. Fundamental questions such as the "fit" of the three-part typology with the range of nursing work, the location and nature of the boundaries between the segments of the continuum, and the regulatory and licensure implications of such a plan could hardly be debated because of the emotionality that surrounded the specter of the loss of access to the RN title for associate and diploma nurses and what appeared to be the hijacking of the term "professional."

Regardless of nursing program background, the term professional had been applied to all that was good. General usage, likewise, cast "professional" in positive terms. Students who did a project or handled a situation "professionally" knew it was well done; students who "looked professional" knew they had met certain standards (however little clean shoelaces may have had to do with actual professionalism); and students who studied to be "professional nurses" would qualify to take the state board examination, and in the years just before the position paper, thought they would give comprehensive, individualized care to patients. "Technical" just did not have the same ring to it; technical sounded limited and mechanical; technical" sounded "less than." However knowledgeable, talented, and essential technical workers were in the discourse of educational macroplanners and economists, the word translated poorly to the world of nursing.

The crisis was gradually defused, partly by action on the recommendations of the next committee to study nursing, the National Commission for the Study of Nursing and Nursing Education (1970), which was commonly known as the Lysaught Commission, which reported in 1970. Among the recommendations in Abstract for Action were

1. Statewide planning for the number and distribution of nursing education programs
2. Career mobility for individual nurses
3. Cooperation of nursing service and education in working to improve patient care

As the world around community colleges changed so that more and more people, particularly women, resumed formal education after a hiatus, and senior colleges had good experience with community college graduates who sought baccalaureate degrees, the concepts of "career mobility" and "articulation" came into nursing discourse. By 1972, the NLN prepared a collection titled "The Associate Degree Program—A Step to the Baccalaureate Degree in Nursing." However, according to Patricia Haase, a historian of associate degree programs, it was also true that "[i]t was assumed by some in baccalaureate education that the curricula of the two nursing programs were not related, that they occupied two separate universes" (Haase, 1990).

In the early 2000s, partnerships between community colleges and universities set the stage for increased articulation between associate and baccalaureate programs. They developed shared curricula, admissions standards, and application processes that facilitate movement of graduates from associate degree programs into baccalaureate education. The Oregon Consortium for Nursing Education (OCNE) was the first in the country to develop such an approach (Tanner, Gubrud-Howe, & Shores, 2008) and acted as a model for articulation agreements between associate and baccalaureate nursing programs across the nation.

Master's Education

Master's programs were few and relatively small in the 1950s. The 1951 report of the NNAS Postgraduate Board of Review noted that in some instances, the same set of courses led to a master's degree for students who held a baccalaureate and to a baccalaureate for students who had no prior degree. Some of the clearly differentiated master's programs had so many prerequisites that few students qualified for admission without clearing multiple "deficiencies" by taking additional course work. The report opined that few programs focused on nursing "in its broadest sense," as contrasted to teaching and administration (National Nursing Accrediting Service Postgraduate Board of Review, 1951).

A Work Conference on Graduate Nurse Education, sponsored by the NLN Division of Nursing Education in fall of 1952, concluded that master's graduates needed competencies in interpersonal relations, communication skills, their selected functional area (e.g., teaching or administration), promotion of community welfare, and "sufficient familiarity with the principles and methods of research to conduct and/or participate in systematic investigation of nursing problems and evaluate and use research findings" (Harms, 1954). However, a 1954 study comparing six leading schools' master's curricula identified wide variability in actual practice. Program lengths were nominally 1 year for students without deficiencies; however, this actually ranged from 24 to 38 semester credits. Although research was an agreed-upon master's focus, only one of the six schools had one course that by title could be identified as addressing this area (Harms, 1954).

Given the relatively few students seeking admission, and the small size of programs, regional planning became important, particularly in the South and western United States. In regional activity that was the precursor to the formation of the Southern Council on Collegiate Education for Nursing (SCCEN), it was agreed in 1952 that six universities— Universities of Alabama, Maryland, North Carolina, Texas, Vanderbilt, and Emory

University—would come together to plan five new master's programs to serve the South. This regional project in graduate education in nursing garnered funding from both the W.K. Kellogg and Commonwealth Foundations. By 1955, all six programs were admitting students (Reitt, 1987).

In western states, the Western Conference of Nursing Education was convened in early 1956 by the Western Interstate Commission for Higher Education (WICHE). Nursing educators, nurse leaders in various other positions, and nonnurse representatives from higher education gathered to advise WICHE on the development of nursing education programs in the area. A 2-month study of nursing education in western states, conducted by Helen Nahm, laid the groundwork for the meeting. This report provided the group with the essence of hundreds of interviews conducted with educators in nursing and related fields in the eight states, as well as nurse manpower data by state for 1954. Respondents reportedly believed that graduate programs in nursing should contain more work in social science fields, advanced preparation in physical and biological science fields, strong foundations in education, courses basic to research, courses in philosophy, research in some area of nursing, and "graduate courses in a clinical nursing area which are truly of graduate caliber" (WICHE, 1956). Subsequently, the Western Interstate Council for Higher Education in Nursing (WICHEN) sponsored joint work that developed early master's-level clinical content and terminal competencies in the early and mid-1960s (J. M. Brown, 1978; WICHE, 1967).

Enrollment in master's programs almost doubled between 1951 and 1962, growing from 1,290 to 2,472 (Harms, 1954; Kalisch & Kalisch, 1978). During the 1960s, clinical area emphases replaced functional specializations as the organizing frames for curricula. This shift in focus to nursing itself not only clarified and enriched baccalaureate curricula in later decades (Lynaugh & Brush, 1996), but also freed doctoral-level training to focus directly on nursing knowledge development.

Political pressure for access to care, interacting with the shortage and maldistribution of physicians and recognition that nurses could competently do a subset of physician work, led to federal support for the spread of NP programs (B. Bullough, 1976; National Commission for the Study of Nursing and Nursing Education, 1971). Until the mid-1970s most NP preparation was offered as non-degree–related continuing education. The first national conference on family NP curricula convened in January 1976. At that point, programs ranged from 4-month certificate-level offerings to specialties set within master's programs, with divergent characteristics depending on rural or urban settings. Certificate programs accounted for 71% of NP program grants funded by the Division of Nursing of the USPHS that year. Just 9 years later, in 1985, 81% of NP program grants went to master's-level programs without any change in the authorizing law and presumably the award criteria. Multiple factors drove or accommodated this change. Practice settings had higher expectations, fears of educators about preserving the essence of nursing subsided, sufficient numbers of potential students saw value in a graduate degree, and faculty members who reconceptualized the curricula were persuasive. Not insignificantly, federal funds were available to assist with the costs of transition (Geolot, 1987).

Most large master's programs had multiple specialties by the mid-1980s, but these only weakly correlated with the major specialty organizations and with certification mechanisms (Styles, 1989). The clinical expertise and interest of nursing faculty, links to local resources, community needs for a particular specialty, and federal/state/local voluntary organization financial initiatives to address specific health problems all drove the pattern of specialty development (Burns et al., 1993). Nursing specialty organizations, reflecting current practice perspectives, exerted a substantial influence on specialty curricular content in their respective areas. The rapid expansion (27%) in the number of master's programs in the last half of the 1980s (Burns et al., 1993) may have spurred creative naming of specialties for purposes of student recruitment. Efforts to rationalize the relationships of the specialties to one another and where possible, to achieve common use of resources, were the natural response to this proliferation.

By the 1990s, clinical specialist content was combined with NP approaches. Advanced practice nurses of both types were beginning to question whether the two roles were, after all, so different from one another (Elder & Bullough, 1990). Changes in health care financing and delivery were prompting clinical nurse specialist programs to include content to prepare graduates to deal with cost and reimbursement dimensions of care for populations (Wolf, 1990), and pressuring practitioner programs to prepare graduates to care for patients with less stable conditions. By the end of the first decade of the 21st century, this trend coalesced into an advanced practice regulatory model that has standardized graduate-level educational requirements (ANA, 2017; Trossman, 2009).

In 2001, the Institute of Medicine (IOM) published a report calling for increased attention to the provision of safe patient care environments. In response to that report, in 2003 to 2004, the clinical nurse leader (CNL) was envisioned. The CNL is a role that provides leadership at the point of care. Advanced practice preparation and clinical leadership competencies, both acquired at the master's level, prepare this nurse leader to ensure the delivery of safe, evidence-based care that is targeted toward quality patient outcomes. The American Association of Colleges of Nursing (AACN) developed standards for the CNL and has a certification program for graduates of CNL programs (AACN, 2017; Reid, 2011).

The Essentials of College and University Education for Professional Nursing (AACN, 1986), with its ambitious goals for a substantial liberal arts and sciences background, reflected both nursing's self-understanding and changing external circumstances. Applicant interest and professional vision converged to support the development of programs at the master's level for nonnurse college graduates. Students completed prelicensure generalist preparation before focusing in a specialty or delimited area, leading to the master's as the first professional degree (Wu & Connelly, 1992). Very few such programs existed in the prior two decades (Diers, 1976; Plummer & Phelan, 1976). *The Essentials of Master's Education for Advanced Practice Nursing* codified the broad areas of agreement about master's preparation among educators (AACN, 1996) and this, together with accreditation mechanisms and a shared external environment, nudged programs toward common curricular characteristics.

The 1986 *Essentials* document foreshadowed another turning point in the long evolution of organized nursing thinking about the placement of basic generalist professional preparation within the standard degree structures of higher education. Given projections of health care system demand for nurses over the next three decades, the need for more comprehensively prepared nurses at the microsystem level due to increased care complexity, and concurrent flagging applicant interest in bachelor's programs with contrasting brisk interest in first professional degree master's programs, it seemed that the time had come to begin to move basic generalist professional preparation to the master's level (AACN, 2003, 2007). Early adopter programs began translating the curriculum template in the planning documents into the unique contexts of each school and cooperating nursing service provider(s). Variants were designed for both BSN and nonnurse college graduate applicants (AACN, 2013). Accreditation and individual graduate certification reinforced curriculum similarity across institutions, and many hope that practice settings will adopt differentiated practice roles that will eventually support regulatory recognition (AACN, 2008, 2010).

Doctoral Programs

The first doctoral programs tailored for the preparation of nursing faculty began in the 1920s and 1930s. Columbia University and New York University (NYU) offered an EdD and a PhD in their departments of education. There was, at this time, little coursework specific to nursing (Carter, 2009). By the 1950s, educators began to focus on the development of doctoral work in nursing. The need for doctorally prepared faculty to teach master's students, who it was hoped would graduate and teach in the multiplying baccalaureate programs, fueled part of the interest in this topic. But for leaders already involved in higher education, it was painfully clear that nursing needed some capacity for its own research that would focus on questions related to nursing interventions to create a coherent body of tested knowledge and improve care.

In 1954, with Martha Rogers as chair of the Department of Nursing Education at NYU in 1954, the doctoral program was redirected to become a PhD in nursing. University of Pittsburgh established a PhD with a focus in pediatric or maternal nursing in 1954. In contrast to Martha Rogers's view that theory was the starting point that would lead to knowledge development in the "applied" field of nursing, Florence Erickson and Reva Rubin at Pittsburgh believed that extensive exposure to clinical phenomena, along with skilled faculty guidance, would develop a true nursing science (Parietti, 1979). In the West, in the early WICHE/WICHEN conversations, the temporary need for help from other disciplines for research training was posited as a mechanism to build nursing knowledge and a critical mass of investigators (WICHE, 1956). The journal *Nursing Research* became available in 1952 as a mechanism for systematic communication (Bunge, 1962).

In 1955, the Nursing Research Grants and Fellowship Program of the USPHS allocated $500,000 for research grants and $125,000 for fellowships, the first such funding for nursing. From 1955 to 1970, 156 nurses were supported by special predoctoral research fellowships for doctoral study, and from 1959 to 1968, 18 schools of nursing received federally funded faculty research development grants to stimulate research capacity. The nurse scientist graduate training programs, which provided federal incentive funding to disciplines outside of nursing to accept nurses as students and provided fellowships to the students, were designed to create a critical mass of faculty and a climate conducive to establishing doctoral programs in nursing (Grace, 1978). The program continued from 1962 to 1976 and funded more than 350 nurse trainees (Berthold, Tschudin, Schlotfeldt, Rogers, & Peplau, 1966; Murphy, 1981).

Three additional doctoral programs were established in the 1960s (Boston University, 1960, doctor of nursing science [DNS], psychiatric/mental health focus; University of California, San Francisco [UCSF], 1964, DNS, multifocus; Catholic University, 1968, DNS, medical–surgical and psychiatric/mental health foci). The Boston program took a clinical immersion approach analogous to the University of Pittsburgh. UCSF's program was structured as a research degree, but identified clinical involvement as the base for knowledge development, influenced both by faculty with a strong clinical identity and by the grounded theory perspectives of the several social scientists who were a part of the faculty.

A federally funded series of nine annual ANA-sponsored research conferences was initiated in 1965 and WICHEN sponsored the first of its annual Communicating Nursing Research conferences in 1968, thus creating space for face-to-face research exchange. Medical Literature Analysis and Retrieval System (MEDLARS) made its debut in 1964, the first in a series of databases that would aid dissemination. Essential components for school of nursing research centers were identified (Gunter, 1966). A series of three federally funded conferences in Kansas City, Kansas, on nursing theory in 1969 to 1970 provided further opportunity to work through the divergent views of the relationships of theory, practice, and research to one another (Murphy, 1981).

In 1971, the Division of Nursing and the Nurse Scientist Graduate Training Committee (NSGTC) convened an invitational conference to address the type(s) of doctoral preparation. In this setting, Joseph Matarazzo, chair of the NSGTC, presented a paper arguing that nursing was ready as a discipline to launch PhD study, citing its body of knowledge and the qualifications of trainees (Matarazzo & Abdellah, 1971; Murphy, 1981). Comprehensive information about the state of nursing doctoral resources became available by the mid-1970s (Leininger, 1976) and by the late 1970s, national doctoral forums, open to schools with established programs, provided a mechanism for exchange of viewpoints about doctoral education. Three additional research journals began publication in 1978 (Gortner, 1991). "The Discipline of Nursing" (Donaldson & Crowley, 1978) was a milestone paper. It differentiated the discipline of nursing from the practice of nursing, but related the two as well, and proposed a productive interrelationship of research, theory, and practice. It shifted the terms of debate away from the dichotomous basic/applied categories.

The body of knowledge in nursing was still, relative to the old disciplines, rather modest in the late 1970s, but the progress in two decades was amazing, and the infrastructure to support further development was substantial (Gortner & Nahm, 1977). Students were focusing their dissertation research on nursing clinical issues (Loomis, 1984). However, the DNS and PhD degrees, the two dominant degree titles, though differently named, were indistinguishable in their objectives and end products (Grace, 1978). Finally, themes related to the challenge of mentoring students who are dealing with what is not known and fostering "humanship" between students and faculty to encourage student growth were beginning to come to print at the end of this decade (Downs, 1978).

Fifteen additional doctoral programs opened their doors during the 1970s (Cleland, 1976; Parietti, 1979). From 1980 to 1989 the number of programs grew from 22 to 50, prompting editorial comment, "as dandelions in spring, more and more doctoral programs are appearing" (Downs, 1984). Other observers surveying the situation recommended regional planning to sponsor joint programs, but conceded that the resources were in individual universities and states, and that the mechanisms for making such efforts were nonexistent. They predicted stormy waters for programs that launched without adequate internal and external supports in place (McElmurray, Krueger, & Parsons, 1982). At the end of the 1980s, doctoral educators were examining the balance between theory and research methods on the one hand and "knowledge" or "substance" in the curriculum on the other (Downs, 1988).

Programs expanded from 50 to 70 from 1990 to 1999. By the early 1990s, as the research programs were more numerous and robust in the older and larger schools, greater emphasis on research team participation (Keller & Ward, 1993) and mentoring into the range of activities doctoral graduates became visible themes (Katefian, 1991; Meleis, 1992). Postdoctoral study became more feasible and attractive (Hinshaw & Lucas, 1993).

The perennial question from the 1960s to the 1980s, that is, whether nursing should adopt the PhD or the DNS, was answered by the hundreds of individual choices of applicants and the program choices of numerous schools: By 2000, only 12% of nursing doctoral programs conferred the DNS, or variants thereof (McEwen & Bechtel, 2000). Much less clear, however, was the difference between the two. Concerns about attention to "substance," that is, organized analysis of the body of nursing knowledge, the adequacy of research programs to provide student experience, and preparation for the teaching component of graduates' expected academic roles, occupied curriculum planners in research-focused doctoral programs at the end of the century.

Questions about the desirability and feasibility of developing clinical or practice-focused doctoral programs in nursing were perennial but intermittent until the past decade (Mundinger et al., 2000), when the AACN in 2004 adopted a proposal that would move preparation for advanced practice nursing from the master's degree framework to the doctoral level by 2015 (AACN, 2004, 2009). Such programs are currently designed to articulate with both nursing baccalaureate and nursing master's (first professional degree and second). The four postbaccalaureate academic years include core areas for all students, as well as clinical specialty-focused study. The research-training component emphasizes the translation of research into practice, practice evaluation, and evidence-based practice improvement. Following from that, several possible forms of end-of-program practice-focused projects and project reporting formats demonstrate the student's synthesis and expertise, while laying the groundwork for future clinical scholarship (AACN, 2006). In 2017, there were 133 research-focused programs and 241 doctor of nursing practice (DNP) programs (AACN, 2017). What the long-term, steady-state allocation of nursing's academic resources should be for the two types of programs is yet to be determined. DNP–PhD programs were developed that enable nurses to combine skills gained in DNP education with research abilities offered through the PhD; some DNP–PhD programs also offer courses in pedagogy to assist in the transition from practitioner to faculty role.

DISCUSSION QUESTIONS

- The Nightingale model of nursing education was used to develop early nursing programs in the United States. What social and cultural phenomena were occurring in the United States during the 19th century that impacted the development of these, and subsequent, nursing education programs? Do similar phenomena impact nursing education today? If so, what are they and how do they impact education?
- Associate degree programs were developed in the 1950s as a result of Mildred Montag's dissertation. Their intent was to prepare a different type of nurse than the one who was prepared at the baccalaureate level. That was not the reality, however, and debate continues (into the 21st century) about educational programs for entry-level nurses. What might nursing education, at both the associate degree and baccalaureate levels, look like today if Montag's plan for a different type of nurse had been followed?
- AACN adopted a proposal in 2004 that would move preparation for advanced practice nursing from the master's to doctoral level by 2015. In order to facilitate a non-stop pathway from completion of the BSN to the DNP, programs have been implemented within schools of nursing. What effect might these programs have on other doctoral programs in nursing? DNP–PhD programs are being developed to assist advanced practice nurses transition from practice to research and academic settings. What are the risks and/or benefits of having these programs to nursing faculty and the students they teach?

LEARNING ACTIVITIES

Student-Learning Activity

Choose teams and debate the wisdom and feasibility of setting the doctoral degree as the minimum level of education for advanced practice nurses. Given hindsight gained from the efforts to transfer prelicensure education into university settings, how would you go about assisting state boards of nursing with this transition?

Faculty Development Activity

Trace your school of nursing's history and link major curricular changes to events external to the nursing programs.

References

Ahrens, W. D. (2002). Walt Whitman, nurse and poet. *Nursing, 32*, 43.

American Association of Colleges of Nursing. (n.d.). Clinical nurse leader (CNL). Retrieved from http://www.aacnnursing.org/CNL

American Association of Colleges of Nursing. (1986). *Essentials of college and university education for professional nursing.* Washington, DC: Author.

American Association of Colleges of Nursing. (1996). *The essentials of master's education for advanced practice nursing.* Washington, DC: Author.

American Association of Colleges of Nursing. (2003). Brief history of the CNL. Retrieved from http://www.aacnnursing.org/CNL-Certification/Commission-of-Nurse-Certification/History

American Association of Colleges of Nursing. (2004). AACN position statement on the practice doctorate in nursing October 2004. Retrieved from http://www.aacnnursing.org/Portals/42/News/Position-Statements/DNP.pdf

American Association of Colleges of Nursing. (2006). *The essentials of doctoral education for advanced nursing practice.* Retrieved from http://www.aacnnursing.org/Portals/42/Publications/DNP Essentials.pdf

American Association of Colleges of Nursing. (2007). *Clinical nurse leader education models being implemented by schools of nursing.* Retrieved from http://www.aacnnursing.org/Portals/42/AcademicNursing/CurriculumGuidelines/CNL-Competencies-October-2013.pdf

American Association of Colleges of Nursing. (2008). CNL frequently asked questions. Retrieved from http://www.aacnnursing.org/CNL/About/FAQs

American Association of Colleges of Nursing. (2009). DNP fact sheet. Retrieved from http://www.aacnnursing.org/News-Information/Fact-Sheets/DNP-Fact-Sheet

American Association of Colleges of Nursing. (2010). *New AACN data show growth in doctoral nursing program* [Press release]. Retrieved from http://www.professionalnursing.org/article/S8755-7223(11)00210-9/pdf

American Association of Colleges of Nursing. (2013). *Competencies and curricular expectations for clinical nurse leader education and practice.* Retrieved from http://www.aacnnursing.org/Portals/42/AcademicNursing/CurriculumGuidelines/CNL-Competencies-October-2013.pdf

American Association of Colleges of Nursing. (2016). *2016–2017 enrollment and graduation in baccalaureate and graduate programs in nursing.* Washington, DC: Author.

American Association of Colleges of Nursing. (2017). Fact sheet: The doctor of nursing practice (DNP). Retrieved from http://www.aacnnursing.org/Portals/42/News/Factsheets/DNP-Factsheet-2017.pdf

American Nurses Association. (1965). *Educational preparation for nurse practitioners and assistants to nurses: A position paper.* New York, NY: Author.

American Nurses Association. (2017). APRN Consensus Model. Retrieved from http://www.nursingworld.org/consensusmodel

Anderson, N. E. (1981). The historic development of American nursing education. *Journal of Nursing Education, 20,* 18–36.

Bacon, E. (1987). Curriculum development in nursing education, 1890–1952. *Nursing History Review, 2,* 50–66.

Berthold, J. S., Tschudin, M. S., Peplau, H. E., Schlotfeldt, R., & Rogers, M. E. (1966). A dialogue on approaches to doctoral preparation. *Nursing Forum, 5,* 48–104.

Bridgman, M. (1949). Consultant in collegiate nursing education. *American Journal of Nursing, 49,* 808.

Bridgman, M. (1953). *Collegiate education for nursing.* New York, NY: Russell Sage Foundation.

Brown, E. L. (1948). *Nursing for the future.* New York, NY: Russell Sage Foundation.

Brown, J. M. (1978). Master's education in nursing, 1945–1969. In J. Fitzpatrick (Ed.), *Historical studies in nursing* (pp. 104–130). New York, NY: Teachers College.

Bullough, B. (1976). Influences on role expansion. *American Journal of Nursing, 76,* 1476–1481.

Bullough, V. (2004). How one could once become a registered nurse in the United States without going to a hospital training school. *Nursing Inquiry, 11,* 161–165.

Bullough, V., & Bullough, B. (1978). *The care of the sick: The emergence of modern nursing.* New York, NY: Prodist.

Bunge, H. L. (1962). The first decade of nursing research. *Nursing Research, 11,* 132–137.

Burns, P. G., Nishikawa, H. A., Weatherby, F., Forni, P. R., Moran, M., Allen, M. E., & Booten, D. A. (1993). Master's degree nursing education: State of the art. *Journal of Professional Nursing, 9,* 267–277.

Carnegie, M. E. (2005). Educational preparation of Black nurses: A historical perspective. *The ABNF Journal, 16,* 6–7.

Carter, M. (2009). The history of doctoral education in nursing. In A. M. Barker (ed.), *Advanced Practice Nursing: Essential knowledge for the profession* (pp. 31–41). Boston, MA: Jones & Bartlett.

Charbonneau-Dahlen, B., & Crow, K. (2016). A brief overview of the history of American Indian nurses. *Journal of Cultural Diversity, 23,* 79–90.

Cleland, V. (1976). Developing a doctoral program. *Nursing Outlook, 24,* 631–635.

Committee of the Six National Nursing Organizations on Unification of Accrediting Services. (1949). *Manual of accrediting educational programs in nursing.* Atlanta, GA: National Nursing Accrediting Service.

Committee on the Grading of Nursing Schools. (1931). *Results of the first grading study of nursing schools.* New York, NY: Author.

Davis, A. T. (1991, April). America's first school of nursing: The New England Hospital for Women and Children. *Journal of Nursing Education, 30,* 158–161.

Diers, D. (1976). A combined basic-graduate program for college graduates. *Nursing Outlook, 24,* 92–98.

Dodd, D. (2001). Nurses' residences: Using the built environment as evidence. *Nursing History Review, 9,* 185–206.

Donaldson, S., & Crowley, D. (1978). The discipline of nursing. *Nursing Outlook, 26,* 113–120.

Downs, F. S. (1978). Doctoral education in nursing: Future directions. *Nursing Outlook, 26,* 56–61.

Downs, F. S. (1984). Caveat emptor. *Nursing Research, 33,* 59.

Downs, F. S. (1988). Doctoral education: Our claim to the future. *Nursing Outlook, 36,* 18–20.

Eisenmann, L. (2000). Reconsidering a classic: Assessing the history of women's higher education a dozen years after Barbara Solomon. In R. Lowe (Ed.), *History of education: Major themes* (Vol. 1, pp. 411–442). New York, NY: Routledge & Falmer.

Elder, R. G., & Bullough, B. (1990). Nurse practitioners and clinical nurse specialists: Are the roles merging? *Clinical Nurse Specialist, 4,* 78–84.

Faddis, M. (1973). *A school of nursing comes of age.* Cleveland, OH: Howard Allen.

Fondiller, S. H. (2001). The advancement of baccalaureate and graduate nursing education: 1952–1972. *Nursing and Health Care Perspectives, 22,* 8–10.

Fredrickson, K. (1978). *The AD graduate: Excellence in practice—fantasy or reality?* New York, NY: National League for Nursing.

Geolot, D. H. (1987). NP education: Observations from a national perspective. *Nursing Outlook, 35,* 132–135.

Goldmark, J. (1923). *Nursing and nursing education in the United States.* New York, NY: Macmillan.

Gortner, S. R. (1991). Historical development of doctoral programs: Shaping our expectations. *Journal of Professional Nursing, 7,* 45–53.

Gortner, S. R., & Nahm, H. (1977). An overview of nursing research in the United States. *Nursing Research, 26,* 10–33.

Grace, H. (1978). The development of doctoral education in nursing: An historical perspective. *Journal of Nursing Education, 17,* 17–27.

Graham, P. A. (1978). Expansion and exclusion: A history of women in higher education. *Signs, 3,* 759–773.

Gunter, L. M. (1966). Some problems in nursing care and services. In B. Bullough & V. Bullough (Eds.), *Issues in nursing* (pp. 152–156). New York, NY: Springer Publishing.

Haase, P. T. (1990). *The origins and rise of associate degree nursing education.* Durham, NC: Duke University.

Hanson, K. S. (1991). An analysis of the historical context of liberal education in nursing education from 1924 to 1939. *Journal of Professional Nursing, 7,* 341–350.

Harms, M. T. (1954). *Professional education in university schools of nursing* (Unpublished dissertation). Stanford University, Stanford, CA.

Hine, D. C. (1989). *Black women in white: Racial conflict and cooperation in the nursing profession, 1890–1950*. Indianapolis: Indiana University.

Hinshaw, A. S., & Lucas, M. D. (1993). Postdoctoral education—A new tradition for nursing research. *Journal of Professional Nursing, 9*, 309.

James, J. W. (2002). Isabel Hampton and the professionalization of nursing in the 1890s. In E. D. Baer, P. O. D'Antonio, S. Rinker, & J. E. Lynaugh (Eds.), *Enduring issues in American nursing* (pp. 42–84). New York, NY: Springer Publishing.

Kalisch, P. A., & Kalisch, B. J. (1978). *The advance of American nursing*. Boston, MA: Little, Brown.

Kalisch, P. A. & Kalisch, B. J. (2004). *American nursing: A history* (4th ed.). Philadelphia, PA: Lippincott Williams & Wilkins.

Katefian, S. (1991). Doctoral preparation for faculty roles: Expectations and realities. *Journal of Professional Nursing, 7*, 105–111.

Keating, S. B. (2015). Looking back to the future: Current issues facing nursing education from the reflections of a member of the silent generation. *Nursing Forum, 15*, 153–163.

Keller, M. L., & Ward, S. E. (1993). Funding and socialization in the doctoral program at the University of Wisconsin-Madison. *Journal of Professional Nursing, 9*, 262–266.

Kelly, L. Y., & Joel, L. A. (1996). *The nursing experience: Trends, challenges, and transitions* (3rd ed.). New York, NY: McGraw-Hill.

Kenny, P. E. (2008, June). Men in nursing: A history of caring and contribution to the profession. *Pennsylvania Nurse, 63* (Pt. 1), 3–5.

LaRocco, S. (2011, February). The last of its kind: The all-male Alexian Brothers Hospital school of nursing. *American Journal of Nursing, 111*, 62–63.

Leininger, M. (1976). Doctoral programs for nurses: Trends, questions, and projected plans. *Nursing Research, 25*, 201–210.

Loomis, M. (1984). Emerging content in nursing: An analysis of dissertation abstracts and titles: 1976–1982. *Nursing Research, 33*, 113–199.

Lynaugh, J. E. (2002). Nursing's history: Looking backward and seeing forward. In E. D. Baer, P. O. D'Antonio, S. Rinker, & J. E. Lynaugh (Eds.), *Enduring issues in American nursing* (pp. 10–24). New York, NY: Springer Publishing.

Lynaugh, J. E., & Brush, B. L. (1996). *American nursing: From hospitals to health systems*. Cambridge, MA: Blackwell.

Matarazzo, J., & Abdellah, F. (1971). Doctoral education for nurses in the United States. *Nursing Research, 20*, 404–414.

McElmurray, B. J., Kreuger, J. C., & Parsons, L. C. (1982). Resources for graduate education: A report of a survey of forty states in the Midwest, west and southern regions. *Nursing Research, 31*, 1–10.

McEwen, M., & Bechtel, G. A. (2000). Characteristics of nursing doctoral programs in the United States. *Journal of Professional Nursing, 16*, 282–292.

Meleis, A. I. (1992). On the way to scholarship: From master's to doctorate. *Journal of Professional Nursing, 8*, 328–334.

Mundinger, M. O., Cook, S. S., Lenz, E. R., Piacentini, K., Auerhahn, C., & Smith, J. (2000). Assuring quality and access in advanced practice nursing: A challenge to nurse educators. *Journal of Professional Nursing, 16*, 322–329.

Murphy, J. F. (1981). Doctoral education in, of, and for nursing: An historical analysis. *Nursing Outlook, 29*, 645–649.

National Commission for the Study of Nursing and Nursing Education. (1970). *An abstract for action*. New York, NY: McGraw-Hill.

National Commission for the Study of Nursing and Nursing Education. (1971). *Nurse clinician and physician's assistant: The relationship between two emerging practitioner concepts*. Rochester, NY: Author.

National League of Nursing Education. (1917). *Standard curriculum for schools of nursing*. Baltimore, MD: Waverly.

National League of Nursing Education. (1927). *A curriculum for schools of nursing*. New York, NY: Author.

National League of Nursing Education. (1937). *A curriculum guide for schools of nursing*. New York, NY: Author.

National Nursing Accrediting Service Postgraduate Board of Review. (1951). Some problems identified. *American Journal of Nursing, 51*, 337–338.

Nightingale, F. (1860). *Notes on nursing: What it is and what it is not*. New York, NY: D. Appleton & Co. Retrieved from http://www.digital.library.upenn.edu/women/nightingale/nursing/nursing.html

Obituary. (1940). Mrs. Clara S. Weeks Shaw. *American Journal of Nursing, 40*, 356.

Orsolini-Hain, L. & Waters, V. (2009). Education evolution: A historical perspective of associate degree nursing. *Journal of Nursing Education, 48*, 266–271.

Parietti, E. S. (1979). *Development of doctoral education for nurses: An historical survey*. Ann Arbor, MI: University Microfilms International.

Petry, L. (1949). We hail an important first. *American Journal of Nursing, 49*, 630–633.

Plummer, E. M., & Phelan, J. J. (1976). College graduates in nursing: A retrospective look. *Nursing Outlook, 24*, 99–102.

Pollitt, P., Streeter, C., & Walsh, C. (2011, Fall). A nurse's journey: Viola Garcia, RN: Lieutenant, nurse. *Minority Nurse*, 23–27. Retrieved from http://www.minoritynurse.com/article/nurses-journey#sthash.cTtXookM.dpuf

Reid, K. B. (2011). The clinical nurse leader: Point of care safety clinical. *Online Journal of Issues in Nursing, 16*(3), 1–12.

Reitt, B. B. (1987). *The first 25 years of the Southern Council on Collegiate Education for Nursing*. Atlanta, GA: Southern Council on Collegiate Education for Nursing.

Reverby, S. (1984). "Neither for the drawing room nor for the kitchen": Private duty nursing in Boston, 1873–1914. In J. W. Leavitt (Ed.), *Women and health in America* (pp. 454–466). Madison: University of Wisconsin.

Reverby, S. M. (1987). *Ordered to care: The dilemma of American nursing, 1850–1945*. New York, NY: Cambridge University.

Rines, A. (1977). Associate degree education: History, development, and rationale. *Nursing Outlook, 25*, 496–501.

Robb, I. H. (1907). *Educational standards for nurses*. Cleveland, OH: E. C. Koeckert.

Roberts, M. M. (1954). *American nursing: History and interpretation*. New York, NY: Macmillan.

Robinson, T. M., & Perry, P. M. (2001). *Cadet nurse stories: The call for and response of women during World War II*. Indianapolis, IN: Center Press.

Rush, S. L. (1992). Nursing education in the United States, 1898–1910: A time of auspicious beginnings. *Journal of Nursing Education, 31*, 409–414.

Scott, J. (1972). Federal support for nursing education, 1964–1972. *American Journal of Nursing, 72*, 1855–1860.

Sheahan, D. A. (1980). *The social origins of American nursing and its movement into the university: A microscopic approach*. Ann Arbor, MI: University Microfilms.

Solomon, B. (1985). *In the company of educated women*. New Haven, CT: Yale University.

Styles, M. M. (1989). *On specialization in nursing: Toward a new empowerment*. Kansas City, MO: American Nurses Foundation.

Tanner, C. A., Gubrud-Howe, P. & Shores, L. (2008). The Oregone Consortium for Nursing Education: A response to the nursing shortage. *Policy, Politics & Nursing Practice, 9*, 203–209.

Trossman, S. (2009). APRN regulatory model continues to advance. *The American Nurse, 41*(6), 12–13.

U.S. Census Bureau. (n.d.). American fact finder. Retrieved from https://factfinder.census.gov/faces/tableservices/jsf/pages/productview.xhtml?pid=ACS_15_5YR_CP05&prodType=table

Vuic, K. D. (2006). "Officer. Nurse. Woman." Army Nurse Corps recruitment for the Vietnam War. *Nursing History Review, 14*, 111–159.

Wall, B. M. (2009, May/June). Religion and gender in a men's hospital and school of nursing, 1866–1969. *Nursing Research, 58,* 158–165.

Washington, L. C. (2012). Preserving the history of Black nurses. *Minority Nurse,* 28–31.

Weeks-Shaw, C. (1902). *A text-book of nursing: For the use of training schools, families, and private students* (3rd ed.). New York, NY: D. Appleton.

Western Interstate Commission for Higher Education. (1956). *Toward shared planning in western nursing education.* Boulder, CO: Author.

Western Interstate Commission on Higher Education. (1967). *Defining clinical content: Graduate programs* (pp. 1–4). Boulder, CO: Author.

Wolf, G. A. (1990). Clinical nurse specialists: The second generation. *Journal of Nursing Administration, 20,* 7–8.

Wu, C.-Y., & Connelly, C. (1992). Profile of nonnurse college graduates in accelerated baccalaureate nursing programs. *Journal of Professional Nursing, 8,* 35–40.

CHAPTER 2

Curriculum Development and Approval Processes in Changing Educational Environments

Felicia Lowenstein-Moffett

Patsy L. Ruchala

CHAPTER OBJECTIVES

Upon completion of Chapter 2, the reader will be able to:

- Analyze facilitators for and barriers to effective curriculum development and redesign
- Apply knowledge of potential barriers to curricular innovations in obtaining approvals for innovative curricular redesign
- Participate in faculty development activities to increase knowledge and skills in curriculum development and evaluation
- Analyze the role and responsibilities of faculty in curriculum development and evaluation

OVERVIEW

Faculty plays a critical role in curriculum development, ongoing evaluation, and redesign, and must determine which best practices must be implemented in nursing education so that students master the knowledge and skills necessary for them to become proficient nurses. The innate complexity of nursing education, the need for collaboration with other disciplines within the college or university, the ever-changing and complex health care systems, and the requirements of regulatory and accreditation agencies can position curriculum development and redesign as a challenging process. Technology expanded in both academic and health care settings and changed the landscape of nursing education and faculty practices. In addition to navigating the internal approval processes for curriculum approval, meeting the requirements of regulatory and accrediting agencies also impacts the direction taken by faculty when developing or redesigning nursing curricula. This chapter provides an overview of the preparation and support necessary for curriculum development/change, innovations in curriculum development, and approvals and accreditations that inform the nursing curriculum. It discusses the essential role of faculty in nursing curriculum development and evaluation.

THE PROCESS OF CURRICULUM DEVELOPMENT

Determining the Need for Curriculum Development or Change

The idea of curriculum change can generally arise among a few faculty members or stakeholders who have a vested interest in the school of nursing and its outcomes. The group might hold beliefs that the curriculum is outdated and no longer adequate to prepare students to meet their professional roles in the current health care environment. This stimulus can be a catalyst for the evaluation and assessment of the goals, mission, philosophy, framework, and student-learning outcomes of the curriculum, as well as course content and learning activities that identify areas of needed curricular revision or new program development.

Preparation and Support for Curricular Change

Nursing education evolved from the use of a variety of theories from other disciplines as well as middle range theories developed specifically for their application to nursing practice. Roles in nursing continually develop to meet the needs of health care in order to better serve individuals, families, and the communities where they live (American Association of Colleges of Nursing [AACN], n.d.; Institute of Medicine [IOM], 2010; Quality and Safety Education for Nurses [QSEN], 2014). Nursing faculty must be active in the scholarship of teaching by evaluating the curriculum and programs in their institutions to ensure quality education (Oermann, 2014). The need for change in nursing education can be prodigious and dynamic with an emphasis on evidence-based practice, quality improvement, safety standards, leadership, competency frameworks, health care technology, and interprofessional education (Andre & Barnes, 2010; Callen & Lee, 2009; Phillips et al., 2013; Spencer, 2012; Stephens-Lee, Der-Fa, & Wilson, 2013).

Faculty, administration, and stakeholder support is imperative for curriculum change success. According to Billings and Halstead (2015), curriculum change is inevitable as new evidence, ideas, and health care policies emerge. Situations may arise as a result of changes in community needs, policy, or accreditation changes, programmatic funding and resources, personnel changes, or the simple acknowledgment that the existing curriculum is no longer effective for current and future students. For effective change to take place, faculty must realize its role and responsibility to create an organizational climate that supports curriculum development in a dynamic process of continual quality improvement.

In addition to recognizing and embracing the need for curriculum change, faculty members need the knowledge and skills to engage in this endeavor. The engagement of faculty in ongoing curriculum development and assessment should begin with an orientation to the university or college. Faculty must participate in regular program evaluation in order to evaluate if program objectives, outcomes, and the vision and mission are being accomplished. It is routinely expected that faculty will update courses with pertinent, timely information each time a course is taught. Updating individual courses over time, however, may impact the overall curriculum, resulting in content gaps.

Faculty members benefit from serving on their school's curriculum committee and engaging in ongoing, open dialogue about the continuous process of curriculum evaluation. Novice faculty or faculty who have not engaged in curriculum redesign benefit from mentoring by faculty with more experience in the curriculum processes (Bryant et al., 2015; Hagler, White, & Morris, 2011; Huybrecht, Loeckx, Quaeyhaegens, DeTobel, & Mistiaen, 2011). Support is necessary to implement proposed changes and include administrative assurance of needed resources: physical space, administrative assistant support, workload considerations, expert consultants; and internal administrative assurance and encouragement that the work toward curricular change is valued and needed by the

Figure 2.1 Example of curriculum approval process sequencing.

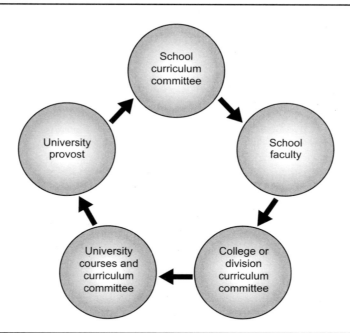

organization and, most importantly, for successful student outcomes. Successful curriculum change requires support from all levels of the organization, faculty, and students. Students bring a unique perspective to curriculum committee discussions, particularly when faculty members are charged to design a rigorous program while creating an environment conducive to a variety of student-learning preferences. Students at all levels of a program are constructive facilitators for successful implementation of a new curriculum.

A single faculty member or small group of faculty members can initiate curriculum assessment, development, and reform. Work begins at the level of the school curriculum committee. This may be a formal committee within the school or for smaller schools; it may consist of the entire nursing faculty. In most institutions of higher education, curriculum development and redesign must go through an extensive, multilevel approval process. Despite the number of levels in the approval process, a proposal for curriculum approval should be completed with the expectation that it will eventually be sent to the highest review body in the parent institution. Although this process varies at each institution, Figure 2.1 depicts an example for sequencing. Consideration should be given as to whether or not this is a proposal for undergraduate- or graduate-level curricular change as they may have different processes. When submitting a proposal for curricular change, completeness, accuracy, and acceptable institutional formatting are extremely important to successfully navigate all levels of the curriculum approval.

ISSUES RELATED TO CURRICULAR DEVELOPMENT OR REDESIGN

Faculty Development

It is the responsibility of the administrators and faculty in the school of nursing to build in faculty development activities to ensure the integrity of the curriculum and the quality of instruction in its implementation. These activities ultimately lead to the realization of the program goals and student-learning outcomes that ensure a quality nursing program. Curriculum development is in itself a faculty development activity (Elliott, 2015; Slimmer, 2012). With the current ongoing nursing faculty shortage (AACN, 2017a), schools of nursing are recruiting new faculty from health care institutions and recent graduates of master's or doctoral programs. Although many of these new faculty members have clinical expertise, they may lack experience in academe and have no experience in curriculum evaluation or design.

Orientation to the curriculum is one of the first steps for faculty development. It should not be assumed that all faculty members are familiar with the entire curriculum or underpinnings of the mission and vision, accreditation, and regulatory requirements. Other topics for faculty development related to curricular activities include the provision of knowledge on faculty governance; the processes of curriculum development and program evaluation; application of learning theories; instructional design and strategies including technology; and student assessment methods. To meet the role expectations of service and scholarship, workshops can be offered to review service opportunities within the institution and in the community for writing grants, supporting research, and preparing manuscripts for publications. Ideas that apply specifically to research related to curriculum development, program evaluation, and evidence-based practice in education can be shared in faculty meetings, workshops, and conferences that focus on the needs of the curriculum.

To be successful in developing and implementing curricular change, Billings and Halstead (2015) indicate that faculty members who understand the problems inherent in the current curriculum can effectively evaluate strategies for solving concerns within the curriculum. Scholarly literature and evidence can inform curriculum about the scholarship of teaching (Faison & Montague, 2013). The faculty members who have less experience in curriculum development may need to attain the knowledge and skills necessary to engage successfully in curriculum work. Faculty development opportunities for them include working with senior faculty, engaging in group discussion and debate, knowing that their contributions to the process will be heard and valued, and providing ongoing administrative support. These activities are all part of the mentoring of less experienced faculty to learn the process for curriculum change.

Experienced faculty members often observe trends in nursing and health care through their professional activities and literature reviews within their specialties, professional organizations, and academic responsibilities, and in clinical practice. Working with colleagues in the practice setting, supervising students or conducting research, and attending professional meetings and conferences are all stimuli for identifying changes and future implications for the nursing curriculum. New faculty members are usually immersed in assuming the new role of educator and, thus, may not have the time or experience to observe these implications for curriculum development and evaluation. At the same time, experienced faculty can take the opportunity to mentor new faculty and demonstrate the importance of assessing trends and changes in the health care system or education that influence the curriculum. As mentioned previously, the role of mentor to new faculty is a responsibility of practiced faculty and can be an expected formal assignment as part of an orientation plan or, informally, as part of the expectations for faculty.

Budgetary Constraints

Nursing has always been considered one of the more costly programs in institutions of higher education. In recent decades, the state of the national economy had a significant impact on all aspects of higher education, including nursing. Retirement of older faculty and the shortage of nurse educators stretch human, fiscal, and physical resources in nursing education. While the relentless echo of the growing need for more nurses at all levels of education continues, funding for many nursing programs has been significantly impacted. When developing or redesigning nursing curricula, an assessment of current and future resources is crucial. Budgetary constraints on hiring faculty and other resources, such as the availability and use of high-fidelity simulation, have a major impact on the curriculum design change and/or implementation of the curriculum. In 2016, over 64,067 qualified applicants were turned away from U.S. nursing schools due to insufficient numbers of faculty, clinical sites, classroom space, clinical preceptors, and budget constraints (AACN, 2017b). The creation of local and regional partnerships with nurse employers, foundations, and other stakeholders as a sustainability strategy needed by the nursing profession is highly encouraged in the current era of health care reform and budget constraints (AACN, 2012).

Amount of Curricular Content

Knowledge expansion relevant to nursing is another issue impacting curriculum development and change in the management of the curricular content. The nursing literature provides an overwhelming amount of evidence indicating that faculty and students are besieged with enormous amounts of content (AACN, 2017b; Lee, 2015; Mailloux, 2011). As the information explosion in health sciences education continues to flourish, an increasing amount of content is deemed essential to include in all nursing curricula (AACN, 2008, 2009; Accreditation Commission for Education in Nursing [ACEN], 2017; National Council of State Boards of Nursing [NCSBN], 2016; Skiba, 2012). One example of essential knowledge content in nursing curricula relates to the need to continuously improve the overall quality and safety of health care delivery in all areas of specialty areas. As nursing practice embraced the focus on improved quality and safety, it became clear that graduating nurses were missing critical competencies. The result was a major national initiative, QSEN, which centered on patient safety and quality topics, with a primary goal to address the challenge of preparing future nurses with the knowledge, skills, and attitudes necessary to continuously improve the quality and safety of the health care systems in areas where they practice (NCSBN, 2016; NLN, 2017). As the amount of essential knowledge and content increases, there tends to be an inherent faculty perception that they must teach everything to their students in great detail. Consequently, "content saturation" is a major problem in many nursing curricula. Giddens (2017) surmises that faculty should learn how to teach conceptually and, subsequently, minimize emphasis on the *amount* of content students learn. Erickson (2007) suggests a major paradigm shift in nursing curricula from an exclusively laborious, content focus to concepts and instructional designs that foster intellectual development. Curricula could focus on conceptual understanding of the complexities of human health rather than focus on lower level cognitive work such as memorization of vast amounts of content.

Technology

The advance of technology and its application to health care and the educational arena is quickly becoming standard practice in higher education (Lee, 2015). The lecture method as the gold standard for teaching has rapidly been supplemented and sometimes replaced by technology. The type of technology available for the classroom ranges from low- to very high-fidelity equipment. The methods of curriculum delivery and the use of technology must be addressed in any curriculum analysis, development, or redesign, including to what extent technology will be used, resources to obtain and sustain technology, and faculty development to use technology effectively to meet programmatic outcomes. For example, high-fidelity simulators are increasingly used as an adjunct or replacement to some of the clinical experiences in nursing programs. High-fidelity simulation requires a significant up-front investment as well as the cost for routine maintenance and upgrades of simulators, and for ancillary staff for simulation centers. In addition, effective use of high-fidelity simulation requires a significant investment for faculty development in the use of the equipment, as well as training on how to maximize learning outcomes and incorporate simulation experiences into the curriculum.

Faculty Issues

The shortage of nursing educators has been discussed as an issue related to curriculum development and change, yet several other faculty issues arise that could impact curriculum development or redesign. Challenges to curriculum revision often occur when working with faculty members who insist on keeping the old familiar curricular paradigm (Grant, 2014; Powell-Cope, Hughes, Sedlak, & Nelson, 2008). Inherent in curriculum development and redesign is the human dimension of the nursing faculty and, subsequently, the interpersonal dynamics associated with every aspect of curriculum analysis and redesign (Oermann, 2014).

Fear of and resistance to change are the most influential barriers to progress in curriculum development and redesign. While not an exhaustive list by any means, the following have been identified as barriers to successful curriculum development and redesign:

- Differing faculty values about nursing education
- Fear of losing control of certain aspects of the curriculum
- Differing views about priorities in the curriculum
- Lack of embracing the need for curricular change
- Uncertainty about how to begin the change process
- Lack of resources
- Incivility
- Lack of rewards
- Feeling that the curricular change process is too overwhelming given the current resources, workload, and time constraints
- Feelings of inadequacy in the area of curriculum analysis, development, and redesign (Billings & Halstead, 2015)

The work of faculty with the curriculum must take into account not only a tumultuous and complex health care environment, but also the pressures to maintain currency in both clinical expertise and teaching technologies (Gaza & Shellenbarger, 2010). Cash, Daines, Doyle, and von Tettenborn (2009) identified these pressures as "tensions (that) underpin curriculum and the ways in which knowledge is constructed through the framing of educational (including clinical) experiences" (pp. 318–319). Many nursing faculty members are no longer employed in health care facilities, and, in many instances, this creates an "education–practice gap." Although clinical supervision of students helps some faculty stay connected to current clinical practices, many nursing faculty find it challenging to balance their full-time roles as academicians with the need for ongoing clinical practice. Faculty may find it difficult to access clinical practice experiences, even on a part-time basis, to maintain current practice knowledge and skills. Complex health care systems and practices, cost implications, and risk management considerations further complicate faculty practice arrangements. Faculty members struggle with work–life balance as they struggle to maintain academic, personal, professional, and home life, which, consequently, inhibits their willingness to take on additional responsibilities in curriculum design (AACN, 2005).

RESEARCH IN CURRICULUM DEVELOPMENT AND EVALUATION

Issues and Trends

Some of the major issues and trends affecting nursing education today as they apply to the nursing faculty role in curriculum development and evaluation are as follows:

- A current and looming nursing faculty shortage
- Increasing ratios of part-time to full-time faculty
- Fewer faculty members with formal preparation in education
- Increasing numbers of doctorally prepared graduates, especially doctor of nursing practice (DNP) graduates, who may not have the pedagogy required for the faculty role
- Rapid changes in instructional designs including online platforms, distance education, high-technology simulations, and other technological advances that are changing instructional design and the implementation of the curriculum
- Constant health care system changes that influence the preparation of nurses and, therefore, the role of faculty in keeping the curriculum relevant

Roberts and Glod (2013) address some of these issues in their paper regarding the dilemmas in nursing faculty roles. Historically, nursing education focused on the development of clinical skills in the care of patients. It then moved into the academic setting with an emphasis on the sciences, social sciences, and liberal arts integrated into the science and clinical skills of the profession. As a result, nursing found itself with many challenges surrounding the nursing faculty role. More recently, institutions that are research focused expect tenured/tenure-track faculty to generate research, as well as to fund their teaching positions with research grants. This results in increasing numbers of clinical faculty members who are part time and who have a minimized role in faculty governance activities and scholarship of teaching. Yet, these instructors are the bedrock of the prelicensure programs in delivering clinical supervision, while tenure-track or tenured faculty members deliver the didactic courses and teach in graduate-level courses, resulting in lower teaching loads to provide time for research and scholarly activities. This trend in nursing education has implications for how education will be delivered and curricula designed.

Research Implications for Evidence-Based Curriculum Development and Evaluation

scarce research on nursing education

Nursing faculty members have boundless opportunities for educational research as it relates to curriculum development and evaluation. There is a scarcity of recent research related to nursing education due to nursing's move to provide its own doctoral education, through either research-focused (PhD/DNSc) or practice-focused (DNP), applied science—doctoral degrees. Much of nursing research focuses on practice issues and health care policy, which is beneficial for the profession, health care, and the public. However, there is a paucity of research focused on nursing education, its processes, and outcomes.

ROLES AND RESPONSIBILITIES OF FACULTY

Implementation of the Curriculum

Implementation is a critical component of curriculum development and/or redesign and is the responsibility of the faculty. To ensure that the curriculum is implemented as planned, intense oversight is necessary. Rapid changes in technology and economics, along with the ever-increasing information explosion and the need for multiculturalism, dictate that ongoing review and redesign of nursing curricula must occur at regular intervals. One of the greatest challenges is to resist the temptation to make changes to the new curriculum too quickly before it has been thoroughly evaluated for effectiveness.

All faculty members should be thoroughly acquainted with the total curriculum, specifically its mission, philosophy, organizational framework, student-learning outcomes, and plan of study. Full-time faculty should have a working knowledge of these components for all levels of the school of nursing programs. While teaching opportunities may focus on graduate studies or undergraduate levels, it is necessary for faculty members to know how each program informs one another and builds upon the other. It is not essential that part-time faculty members know the details of the entire curriculum, but they should understand the relationship of the course(s) they teach to the curriculum, its framework, and program goals.

Schools of nursing curricula generally have one organizational framework that acts as the roadmap for all levels of degree work and demonstrates the rationale for the preparation of professional nurses at each of the various levels. Critical to the integrity of the curriculum is that faculty members are able to identify the place that the courses in which they teach fit into the organizational and programmatic framework. Thus, the temptation to change course content is less likely to occur. A course coordinator can assume the responsibility for a new faculty member's orientation to the course and its relationship to the curriculum and also to periodic assessment of the delivery of the course content to ensure its germaneness to the curriculum. Periodic meetings of faculty members in the courses, levels, or programs to review teaching strategies, learning activities, and student-learning outcomes are vital to the implementation of the curriculum and to overall quality control.

Innovations in Nursing Education

A major aspect of the nursing curriculum development and redesign process is the consideration of current and future resources and needs for implementation, including the nature of the health care environment in which future nurses will work. It is widely noted in the literature that due to the complexities of today's health care system and health care delivery, transformation of nursing education with a health systems framework is necessary to adequately prepare nurses to practice safely (AACN, 2017b; IOM, 2010; National League for Nursing, 2017; NCSBN, 2009b; Phillips et al., 2013). Nursing education must have innovative approaches to prepare graduates at all levels of education for the nursing practice and health care leadership of the future. The NCSBN (2012) defined innovation as "a dynamic, systematic process that envisions new approaches to nursing education." Innovations reported in the nursing literature include the use of dedicated educational units for clinical education (Moscato, Miller, Logsdon, & Chorpenning, 2007), pedagogical approaches such as narrative pedagogy, conceptual thinking, and deliberate discussion (Brown, Kirkpatrick, & Mangum, 2008; Goodin & Stein, 2008, Mauro, Hickey, McCabe, & Ea, 2012; Nehring, 2008; Reese, Jeffries, & Engum, 2010). Innovations include the use of high-fidelity simulation as an adjunct to or replacement for clinical experiences and use of simulation and virtual reality to extend faculty (Cleary, McBride, McClure, & Reinhard, 2009). Other innovations in nursing education include partnering with clinical agencies or with other educational institutions to form a consortium for sharing resources for the delivery of nursing education.

Developing innovation in nursing education is an essential strategy to meet the needs of future nurses and the demands of today's health care environment. However, when planning an innovative curriculum, faculty should be aware of potential deterrents that may prolong the approval and implementation process. First and foremost are the barriers that educational institutions impose upon themselves such as multilevel institutional hierarchies and lengthy committee processes to obtain approval of curriculum changes (Bellack, 2008; Coonan, 2008). As a practice profession, nursing education's relationship with health care institutions is critical. Clinical practice settings, community partners, and educational institutions may have different outcome goals and thus barriers may stem from centralized power bases and linear thinking (Grant, 2014; Untershuetz, Hughes, Nienhauser, Weberg, & Jackson, 2008). In addition, there may be real or perceived regulatory barriers to innovative nursing education. In 2008, the NCSBN established the Innovations in Education Regulation Committee. The charge to this committee was to identify real and perceived regulatory barriers to educational innovations and to develop a regulatory model for innovative educational proposals (NCSBN, 2009a). Potential regulatory barriers to innovative nursing education may not be flexible enough to allow for nursing innovation including specified numbers of clinical or didactic hours in the nursing curriculum, faculty–student ratios, full- and part-time ratios of faculty, disallowance of dedicated educational units due to lack of faculty oversight or qualifications of nursing staff, and simulation limitations (NCSBN, 2009b, 2012). However, advanced knowledge of potential barriers may assist faculty in negotiating with internal or external stakeholders to overcome these obstacles and create a curriculum that is innovative, resource-friendly, and forward thinking in educating nurses for the future. Being mindful about compliance with the state nurse practice act and state nursing regulations before planning innovative curricular changes is very important (Hargreaves, 2008). It is always advisable to consult with the respective state board at the conceptual stages of planning for any innovative teaching strategy proposal to curriculum redesign.

Need for Revision or New Programs

As the curriculum is implemented, faculty members continually observe and assess the effectiveness of learning activities, methodologies, student-learning outcomes, and the relationship of courses to the curriculum. When gaps or concerns are detected, it is the faculty member's responsibility to report the observations to the course leader or level coordinator. Together, faculty should further investigate and analyze the concern and then with input from students and other stakeholders bring the matter to the curriculum committee (or academic committee that has responsibility for curricular change) for its consideration. A root cause analysis with suggestions for remediation should accompany the report to facilitate the needs identified for curricular evaluation and possible revision. Many times, faculty, students, and stakeholders identify the need for new programs based on their experiences and interactions in the health care system. The processes for bringing the information to the attention of the curriculum committee are the same, that is, a summary of the identified need accompanied with documentation and possible proposal for the development of a new track or program.

Faculty Activities Related to Curriculum Development, Evaluation, and Accreditation

Many of the roles and responsibilities of faculty in curriculum development have been reviewed. They include, on an individual level: familiarization with the components of the curriculum, developing and carrying out instructional designs and strategies that are congruent with the curriculum, observation, assessment, and reporting of needs for either curricular revision or development of new programs, participation on curriculum/academic/evaluation/accreditation committees, and developing or participating in scholarly activities that relate to curriculum development and evaluation. As academic faculty, the group should participate in orientation of new faculty members to ensure the integrity of the curriculum; review faculty governance structures to maintain faculty ownership of the curriculum; identify trends and issues in health care, curriculum development and evaluation; generate research ideas; identify program development grants; actively participate in the scholarship of teaching and learning; and build on ideas for evidence-based educational practice.

Accrediting agencies such as the ACEN (2013) and Commission on Collegiate Nursing Education (2017) standards/criteria include the educational preparation and qualifications for nursing faculty. As part of their role, faculty members should be familiar with these expectations and ensure that they meet the qualifications and expectations for the role of faculty. Participation in accreditation activities and program evaluation activities is expected for all faculty members. Program evaluation for the academic institution usually takes place every 5 years, while accreditation takes place from every 5 to 10 years, depending on the program's history, type of program, and level of accreditation granted. Knowing the curriculum components such as the mission, vision, philosophy, organizational framework, student-learning outcomes, and the program of study are crucial responsibilities of faculty in the evaluation and accreditation processes. They should be able to articulate where the courses in which they teach fall into the curriculum framework. The faculty should be familiar with processes of continual program analysis and identifying curriculum and individual course needs for possible revision when necessary to ensure quality and consistency of the program.

SUMMARY

Curriculum development and ongoing evaluation and redesign are core activities for nursing faculty. Faculty participation in planning for accreditation can expand their capacity to implement curriculum evaluation and design processes that have direct relevance on program outcomes. The significance of curriculum evaluation and design extends far beyond the curriculum itself. Determining how to best facilitate the curriculum process by working together as a group to identify and overcome potential barriers and being innovative to meet the challenges of educating future generations of practicing nurses in an ever-changing health system are key elements for successful curriculum development or redesign. Ongoing challenges of the collective volume of information in nursing and health sciences, the trend toward developing interdisciplinary curricula, closing the faculty–student gap in technology knowledge, and meeting the requirements of regulatory and accrediting agencies are all important issues to address as we develop nursing curricula for the future and embrace a continuous process improvement plan for curriculum design that will ensure quality education for nurses.

DISCUSSION QUESTIONS

- What are ways in which nursing faculty can be motivated to engage in curriculum redesign?
- Why do you think faculty members have the ultimate responsibility for curriculum development and evaluation? List at least five reasons for this responsibility.
- What real or perceived barriers do regulatory agencies impose on curricular development or redesign?
- Based on a current issue in nursing education, develop a research question for investigation into the issue and possible solutions. Explain why you chose the issue and what implications it has for the future of nursing education.

LEARNING ACTIVITIES

Student-Learning Activities

1. Imagine yourself in the role of a new faculty member in a school of nursing. List the topics that you believe you need to know in order to be an effective teacher. Prioritize the list and explain the rationale for the order of priority.
2. Determine how new or revised curricula of nursing programs are reviewed and acted upon by your local state board of nursing. Attend a State Board of Nursing meeting and describe how the process of nursing program approval relates to the board's mission of protection of the public's health and welfare in your state.

Faculty Development Activities

1. Assess your school's orientation and faculty development programs. Identify any gaps in the programs as they relate to curriculum development and evaluation. How would you develop or change the programs to meet the needs of new and experienced faculty?
2. Describe two innovations in curriculum and/or teaching strategies for implementation of your curriculum. What constraints or barriers can you identify that would delay or prohibit you from implementing these innovations?
3. Develop a list of five key facilitators and five key barriers to curriculum development and/or redesign in your school of nursing. How can you as a faculty member assist your school or other faculty members to overcome the barriers you identified?

References

Accreditation Commission for Education in Nursing. (2013). *ACEN accreditation manual*. Atlanta, GA: Author.

Accreditation Commission for Education in Nursing. (2017). ACEN history of ensuring educational quality in nursing. Retrieved from http://www.acenursing.org/acen-history

American Association of Colleges of Nursing. (n.d.). Clinical nurse leader tool kit. Retrieved from http://www.aacnnursing.org/Education-Resources/Tool-Kits/Clinical-Nurse-Leader-Tool-Kit

American Association of Colleges of Nursing. (2005). Faculty shortages in baccalaureate and graduate nursing programs: Scope of the problem and strategies for expanding the supply. Retrieved from http://www.aacnnursing.org/Portals/42/News/White-Papers/facultyshortage-2005.pdf

American Association of Colleges of Nursing. (2008). *The essentials of baccalaureate education for professional nursing practice*. Washington, DC: Author.

American Association of Colleges of Nursing. (2009). *The essentials of baccalaureate education for professional nursing practice: Faculty tool kit*. Washington, DC: Author.

American Association of Colleges of Nursing. (2017a). Nursing faculty shortage. Retrieved from http://www.aacnnursing.org/News-Information/Fact-Sheets/Nursing-Faculty-Shortage

American Association of Colleges of Nursing. (2017b). Fact sheet: The impact of education on nursing practice. Retrieved from http://www.aacnnursing.org/Portals/42/News/Factsheets/Education-Impact-Fact-Sheet.pdf

American Association of Colleges of Nursing—American Organization of Nurse Executives Task Force on Academic Practice Partnerships. (2012). AONE guiding principles. Retrieved from http://www.aone.org/resources/academic-practice-partnerships.pdf

Andre, K., & Barnes, L. (2010). Creating a 21st century nursing workforce: Designing a bachelor of nursing program in response to the health reform agenda. *Nurse Education Today*, *30*(3), 258–263.

Bellack, J. P. (2008). Letting go of the rock. *Journal of Nursing Education, 47*(10), 439–440.

Billings, D. M., & Halstead, J. A. (2015). *Teaching in nursing* (4th ed.). St. Louis, MO: Elsevier Saunders.

Brown, S. T., Kirkpatrick, M. K., & Mangum, D. (2008). A review of narrative pedagogy strategies to transform traditional nursing education. *Journal of Nursing Education, 47*(6), 283–286.

Bryant, A., Brody, A., Perez, A., Shillam, C., Edelman, L., Bond, S., . . . Siegel, E. (2015). Development and implementation of a peer mentoring program for early career gerontological faculty. *Journal of Nursing Scholarship, 47*(3), 258–266. doi:10.1111/jnu.12135

Callen, B. L., & Lee, J. L. (2009). Ready for the world: Preparing nursing students for tomorrow. *Journal of Professional Nursing, 25*(5), 292–298.

Cash, P. A., Daines, D., Doyle, R. M., & von Tettenborn, L. (2009). Quality workplace environments for nurse educators: Implications for recruitment and retention. *Nursing Economics, 27*(5), 315–321.

Cleary, B. L., McBride, A. B., McClure, M. L., & Reinhard, S. C. (2009). Expanding the capacity of nursing education. *Health Affairs, 26*(4), w634–w645.

Commission on Collegiate Nursing Education. (2017). *Achieving excellence in accreditation: The first 10 years of CCNE*. Washington, DC: Author.

Coonan, P. R. (2008). Educational innovation: Nursing's leadership challenge. *Nursing Economics, 26*(2), 117–121.

Elliott, R. (2015). Faculty development curriculum: What informs it? *Journal of Faculty Development, 28*(3), 35–45.

Erickson, L. (2007). *Concept-based curriculum and instruction for the thinking classroom*. Thousand Oaks, CA: Corwin Press, Sage.

Faison, K., & Montague, F. (2013). Paradigm shift: Curriculum change. *Association of Black Nursing Faculty Journal, 24*(1), 21–22.

Gaza, E. A., & Shellenbarger, T. (2010). The lived experience of part-time baccalaureate nursing faculty. *Journal of Professional Nursing, 26*(6), 353–359.

Giddens, J. (2017). *Concepts for nursing practice*. St. Louis, MO: Elsevier.

Goodin, H. J., & Stein, D. (2008). Deliberate discussion as an innovative teaching strategy. *Journal of Nursing Education, 47*(6), 272–274.

Grant, A. (2014). Neoliberal higher education and nursing scholarship: Power subjectification, threats and resistance. *Nursing Education Today, 34*(10), 1280–1282.

Hagler, D., White, B., & Morris, B. (2011). Cognitive tools as a scaffold for faculty during curriculum redesign. *Journal of Nursing Education, 50*(7), 417–422.

Hargreaves, J. (2008). Risk: The ethics of a creative curriculum. *Innovations in Education and Teaching International, 45*(3), 227–234.

Huybrecht, S., Loeckx, W., Quaeyhaegens, Y., De Tobel, D., & Mistiaen, W. (2011). Mentoring in nursing education: Perceived characteristics of mentors and the consequences of mentorship. *Nursing Education Today, 31*, 274–278.

Institute of Medicine. (2010). *The future of nursing: Leading change, advancing health*. Washington, DC: National Academies Press.

Lee, J. (2015). Effects of the use of high-fidelity human simulation in nursing education: A meta-analysis. *Journal of Nursing Education, 54*(9), 501–507.

Mailloux, C. F. (2011). Using the Essentials of Baccalaureate Education for Professional Nursing Practice (2008) as a framework for curriculum revision. *Journal of Professional Nursing, 27*(6), 385–389.

Mauro, A., Hickey, M., McCabe, D., & Ea, E. (2012). Attaining baccalaureate competencies for nursing care of older adults through curriculum innovation. *Nursing Education, 33*(3), 184–195.

Moscato, S. R., Miller, J., Logsdon, K., & Chorpenning, L. (2007). Dedicated education unit: An innovative clinical partner education model. *Nursing Outlook, 55*(1), 31–37.

National Council of State Boards of Nursing. (2009a). *Innovations in education regulation committee: Recommendations for boards of nursing for fostering innovations in education*. Retrieved from https://www.ncsbn.org/Recommendations_for_BONS.pdf

National Council of State Boards of Nursing. (2009b). *Tips for planning nursing education innovative approaches*. Retrieved from https://www.ncsbn.org/Tips_for_Faculty.pdf

National Council of State Boards of Nursing. (2012). *The initiative to advance innovations in nursing education: Three years later*. Retrieved from https://www.ncsbn.org/InitiavetoAdvanceInnovations.pdf

National Council of State Boards of Nursing. (2016). *FY 2015–16 Nursing Education Trends Committee*. Retrieved from https://www.ncsbn.org/2016_Nursing_Ed_Trends_Comm_Report.pdf

National League for Nursing. (2017). Advocacy teaching: Nursing is social justice advocacy. Retrieved from http://www.nln.org/professional-development-programs/teaching-resources/toolkits/advocacy-teaching

Nehring, W. (2008). U.S. boards of nursing and the use of high-fidelity patient simulators in nursing education. *Journal of Professional Nursing, 24*(2), 109–117.

Oermann, M. (2014). Defining and assessing the scholarship of teaching in nursing. *Journal of Professional Nursing, 30*(5), 370–375.

Phillips, J. M., Resnick, J., Boni, M. S., Bradely, P., Grady, J. L., Ruland, J. P., & Stuever, N. L. (2013). Voices of innovation: Building a model for curriculum transformation. *International Journal of Nursing Education Scholarship, 10*(1), 1–7.

Powell-Cope, G., Hughes, N. L., Sedlak, C., & Nelson, A. (2008). Faculty perceptions of implementing an evidence-based safe patient handling nursing curriculum module. *Online Journal of Issues in Nursing, 13*(3). doi:10.3912/OJIN.Vol13No03PPT03

Quality and Safety Education for Nurses. (2014). QSEN competencies. Retrieved from http://qsen.org/competencies/pre-licensure-ksas

Reese, C. E., Jeffries, P. R., & Engum, S. A. (2010). Using simulations to develop nursing and medical student collaboration. *Nursing Education Perspectives, 31*(1), 33–37.

Roberts, S. J., & Glod, C. (2013). Dilemmas in faculty roles. *Nursing Forum, 48*(2), 99–105.

Skiba, D. (2012). Technology and gerontology: Is this in your nursing curriculum? *Nursing Education Perspectives, 33*(3), 207–209.

Slimmer, L. (2012). A teaching mentorship program to facilitate excellence in teaching and learning. *Journal of Professional Nursing, 28*(3), 182–185.

Spencer, J. A. (2012). Integrating informatics in undergraduate nursing curricula: Using the QSEN framework as a guide. *Journal of Nursing Education, 51*(12), 697–701.

Stephens-Lee, C., Der-Fa, L., & Wilson, K. E. (2013). Preparing students for an electronic workplace. *Online Journal of Nursing Informatics, 17*(3), 1–10.

Unterschuetz, C., Hughes, P., Nienhauser, D., Weberg, D., & Jackson, L. (2008). Caring for innovation and caring for the innovator. *Nursing Administration Quarterly, 32*(2), 133–141.

S E C T I O N II

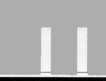

Needs Assessment and Financial Support for Curriculum Development

Sarah B. Keating

OVERVIEW

When contemplating a new educational program or revising an existing curriculum, a needs assessment is indicated. There are two purposes for conducting an assessment. The first is to validate the currency, academic and professional relevance, and continued need for an existing program. The second is to establish the feasibility for a new nursing program including the demand for it, available resources, academic soundness, and financial liability.

[handwritten margin notes: purpose N.A.; 1st validate; 2nd feasibility]

Even though justification for revising a current program usually exists, it is wise to survey constituents and collect information relative to the same factors that are examined in a needs assessment for a new program. This information either reaffirms assumptions about the curriculum on the part of program planners or identifies gaps or problems that indicate a need for change. The assessment is also useful for accreditation and program review purposes and can serve as the organizing framework for a master plan of evaluation (see Section IV). Chapter 3 discusses the essential components of a needs assessment and offers a model for collecting and analyzing information that is preliminary to new program development, expansion, or revision of an existing curriculum. Chapter 4 reviews the need for financial support, and the budgetary planning and management necessary for curriculum development and evaluation.

THE FRAME FACTORS MODEL   *[handwritten: P – I – E]*

Johnson (1977) presented a conceptual model for curriculum development, instructional planning, and evaluation that is similar to the nursing process. Although it is a simple and linear model, (P [planning]—I [implementation]—E [evaluation]), Johnson expands it into a complex step-by-step logical process. The process includes examining the frame factors or context within which the program exists, setting goals, identifying curriculum content, structuring the curriculum, planning for instruction, and finally, evaluation. Johnson speaks of frame factors as the context in which the curriculum exists. Furthermore, he classifies the context into natural, cultural, organizational, and personal elements (p. 36). This author chose the term of frame factors, external and internal, from Johnson's discussion and adapted it to curriculum development in nursing education. It includes the elements that Johnson identified and adds other components that specifically apply to nursing education, health care systems, and the profession.

Frame factors for this text are defined as the external and internal factors that influence, impinge upon, and/or enhance educational programs and curricula. As a conceptual model, it collects, organizes, and analyzes information that is useful for the development and

[handwritten: internal & external factors influencing curricula]

Figure II.1 Frame factors conceptual model.

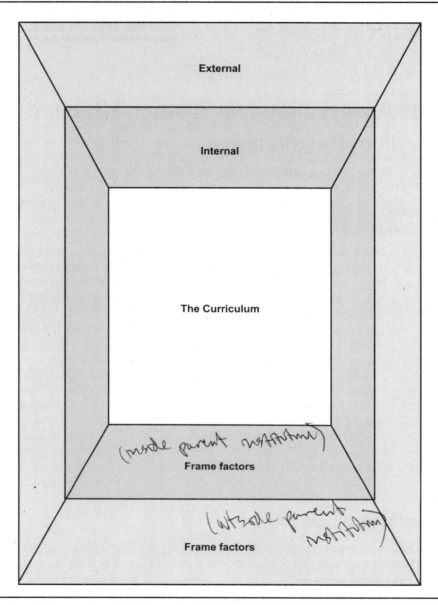

Source: Adapted from Johnson (1977).

evaluation of curricula. There are two major categories of frame factors: external and internal factors. *External frame factors are those that influence curriculum development from the larger environment and outside the parent institution. Internal frame factors are those factors that influence curriculum development and are within the environment of the parent institution and the program itself.* Figure II.1 illustrates the frame factors conceptual model.

Faculty should be involved in the needs assessment even though its principal role focuses on the need for curriculum improvement based on assessment of its implementation and program outcomes. Faculty members cognizant of the factors that impact and influence the program have an advantage in promoting the program by an awareness of the program's financial security, position within the health care system and the profession, and its role in meeting health care needs. In addition, data from the needs assessment are useful to individual faculty seeking grants and other funding to support research and program development activities.

It is recommended that nursing educators use the frame factors model when evaluating programs, considering revisions of existing programs, or initiating new ones. While administrators take the leadership role in conducting needs assessments, faculty should participate in the decisions for what type of and how much data to collect and for proposed changes that could affect the curriculum.

EXTERNAL AND INTERNAL FRAME FACTORS

Chapter 3 describes the factors that influence the curriculum from the environment external to the parent institution and the nursing education program. The factors include the community, population demographics, the political climate, the health care system, the characteristics of the academic setting, the need for the (nursing) program, the nursing profession, regulation and accreditation requirements, and external financial support. All of these factors influence the curriculum in positive and negative ways and while they may not be in the control of the faculty, they are important to recognize and analyze for their impact on the program. They can "make or break" a program. For example, lack of accreditation for a nursing program can prohibit its graduates from career opportunities and continuing education.

The environmental factors within the parent institution and the nursing program that influence the curriculum are termed the "internal frame" factors. They include: a description of the organizational structure of the parent academic institution; mission, philosophy, and goals; economic situation and its influence on the curriculum; resources within the institution (laboratories, classrooms, library, student services, etc.); and existing and potential faculty and student characteristics. Similar to the external frame factors, the internal factors influence the curriculum and play a major role in the development, revision, and expansion of programs. Faculty uses the information gleaned from the assessment to arrive at decisions regarding the curriculum. The same data collected for a needs assessment are in fact related to total quality management of the curriculum and contribute to the evaluation of the program. A case study that utilizes the external and internal frame factors needs assessment model and results in the development of a new program that is provided in the Appendix.

RELATIONSHIP OF NEEDS ASSESSMENT TO CONTINUOUS QUALITY IMPROVEMENT OF THE CURRICULUM

Establishing a new program is not an exercise that occurs in a vacuum. Information from outside and within the institution can indicate a possible need for a new program or revision or expansion of its existing offerings There are usually trigger mechanisms that initiate the need for change such as a drop in NCLEX® scores, budget cuts, or a nursing shortage. Rather than responding to these external stimuli in a reactive way, faculty and nursing educators should have a master plan of evaluation in place that continuously monitors the program and provides the data needed for planning for changes that are both timely and at the same time look to the future. Such activities are part of a process that provides the data for analysis and decisions leading to continuous improvement and the quality of the educational program. The factors discussed in the Frame Factors Model in this section of the text apply to evaluation strategies as well. While Section IV discusses program and curriculum evaluation, accreditation, and strategic planning; it is useful to incorporate the notion of evaluation as a process when conducting a needs assessment, not only in terms of the present plans for program start-up and changes, but also for planning for the future.

FINANCIAL SUPPORT AND BUDGET MANAGEMENT FOR CURRICULUM DEVELOPMENT AND EVALUATION

An awareness of the financial support and budgeting issues for curriculum development and evaluation is essential for nursing education administrators, managers, and faculty to ensure the success and continuation of the program. Chapter 4 provides practical guidelines for budget support, seeking funds to develop new programs through grants, endowments, and scholarships as well as managing the budget. It discusses the various roles of faculty, administrators, and staff in securing funds and planning and managing budgets for curriculum development and evaluation activities.

Reference

Johnson, M. (1977). *Intentionality in education*. Albany, NY: Center for Curriculum Research and Services.

CHAPTER 3

Needs Assessment: The External and Internal Frame Factors

Sarah B. Keating

CHAPTER OBJECTIVE

Upon completion of Chapter 3, the reader will be able to:

- Appreciate the value of a needs assessment for analysis of factors that influence a nursing education program and its implications for curriculum revision or development
- Identify major external and internal frame factors for a needs assessment
- Apply the guidelines for assessing frame factors to a simulated or actual curriculum development situation

OVERVIEW

Curriculum development activities in the academic setting usually relate to the revision of the educational program based on feedback from staff, clients, students, faculty, administrators, alumni, and consumers of the program's participants and graduates. Whether curriculum development involves a new program or revisions of an existing curriculum, program planners and faculty must evaluate the external and internal environmental influences that affect the curriculum, their impact on the current program, and what role they play in forecasting the future.

A needs assessment for curriculum development is defined as the process for collecting and analyzing information that contributes to the decision to initiate a new program or revise an existing one. Using the Frame Factors Conceptual model as described in the Overview of Section II, collected information is organized into two major categories: external and internal frame factors (Johnson, 1977). External frame factors are defined as those factors that influence curriculum in the environment outside of the nursing program and the parent institution. Internal frame factors influence curriculum from within the parent institution and the program itself. Figure 3.1 depicts the external frame factors that surround the curriculum when conducting a needs assessment, while Figure 3.2 illustrates internal frame factors.

EXTERNAL FRAME FACTORS

Description of the Community

The first step in developing or revising a curriculum is to provide a description of the community or context in which the program exists (or will exist). A needs assessment

Figure 3.1 External frame factors for a needs assessment for curriculum development in nursing.

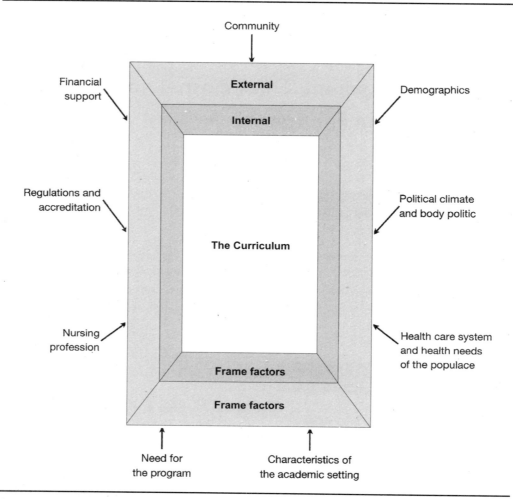

Source: Adapted from Johnson (1977).

ensures the relevance of the program to the community and predicts its eventual financial viability. Owing to the vast differences in communities served by academic institutions and for the purposes of this discussion, "community" is defined as an entity within a larger network or system. It can be identified by its cluster and distinctive functional structure within the system (Young, Allard, Hébert-Dufresne, & Dubé, 2015). Depending on the nature of the educational program, the community can be global or as narrow as a small town within a state. Most institutions of higher education in the United States identify themselves according to classifications found in the Carnegie Foundation for Advancement of Teaching Classification. The Carnegie classification was first published in 1970 with the most recent classification occurring in 2015 (Indiana University Center for Postsecondary Research, 2016). The 2015 designations are according to Basic, Undergraduate, and Graduate Instructional Program, Enrollment Profile and Undergraduate Profile, and Size and Setting. A listing with a detailed description of each type of classification is available at www.carnegieclassifications.iu.edu/downloads/CCIHE2015-FactsFigures.pdf.

Figure 3.2 Internal frame factors for a needs assessment for curriculum development.

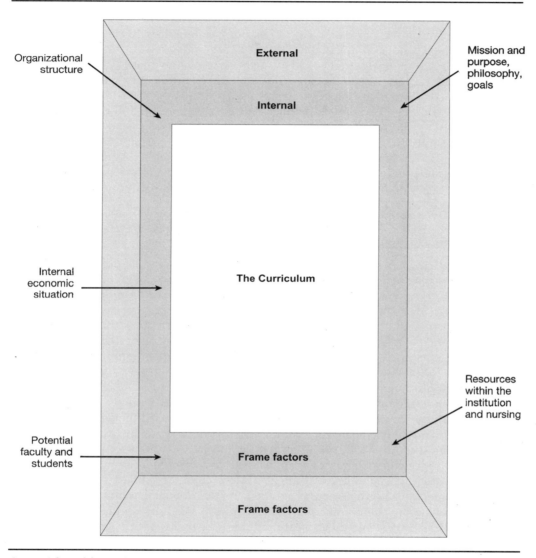

Source: Adapted from Johnson (1977).

Large universities or colleges with research notoriety often attract international scholars to campus or to an online program, while some state-supported and private programs attract students who live nearby and intend to spend their professional lives in their home community. With the growth of web-based programs including MOOCs (massive open online courses), campuses have become worldwide and attract students from many different countries and cultures who may never set foot on the physical campus. For some web-based programs that offer degree programs, there may be no physical campus, only a location in which the administration functions with student services, library resources, classroom participation, and so forth, available online. In those instances, a definition of the community to be served is according to its functional structure as a community, for example, a cadre of international nurses wishing to advance their education and practice in their home countries who enroll in an online degree program.

Both web-based and on-site campuses should survey major industries and educational systems in their communities (or networks, in the case of international and Internet programs) as possible sources for students into the program and for potential partnerships such as online resources, scholarships, and learning experiences. Industry has resources for scholarships, financial aid programs, hardware and software resources for web-based learning, and experts in the field who can serve as consultants, faculty, or adjunct faculty. Health care industries, in particular, should be participants in the needs assessment and curriculum planning to bring the reality of the practice setting and the community's health care needs into planning. For on-site campuses, the major religious affiliations linked to the institution, political parties, and systems such as transportation, communications, government, community services, and utilities in the community are additional external frame factors. These factors have an effect on the curriculum as to its relevance to the community and the support it needs to meet its goal. For example, state-supported schools are very dependent on government funding, while private schools must rely on tuition and endowments.

Demographics of the Population   *who will students serve?*

When considering a new program, or revising an existing curriculum, it is useful to have knowledge of the people with whom the faculty and students will work for clinical experiences and whom the graduates will eventually serve. "Demographics" are the data that describe the characteristics of a population (e.g., age, gender, socioeconomic status, ethnicity, education levels). The demographic information that is vital to program planners includes the age ranges and preponderance of age groups in the population, predicted population changes including immigrant and emigrant statistics, ethnic and cultural groups including major languages, educational levels, and socioeconomic groups. This information identifies potential students and their characteristics and the needs of the population that the students and graduates will serve.

Educational programs and curricula must be geared toward the needs of the learners. If the student body comes from the region surrounding the institution, the characteristics of the students should be analyzed for special learning needs. For example, if there are nurses seeking to advance their careers, the curriculum needs to focus on adult learning theories and modalities. Younger students about to embark on their first professional degree will need curricula that focus on their developmental needs as young adults as well as the content necessary for gaining basic nursing knowledge, clinical skills, and socialization into the professional role. Meeting the learning needs of different generations of learners is a major challenge for curriculum planning. Chapter 6 addresses this issue with several ideas on learning approaches and strategies for reaching various types of learners while implementing the curriculum.

Program planners should survey students coming to the institution from great distances or internationally as to what drew them to the program and if those factors are useful for program planning and recruitment. Faculty should identify potential students with needs for learning resources beyond the usual, for example a need for tutoring for students whose primary language is not English, or translators, if the program is broadcast internationally. It is useful to learn about the financial resources of the potential student body and if there is a need for major financial aid programs. Ethnicity and cultural values in the community and its beliefs about higher education have an impact on recruitment strategies and are especially important in light of the need for increasing the diversity of the nursing workforce and also the educational level of nurses worldwide. Another consideration related to demographics is the existence of potential faculty and identification of people who have the credentials to teach. Identifying potential faculty through partnerships with industry and the community is helpful if the program needs to recruit new faculty or seek adjunct faculty and preceptors for clinical experiences.

Political Climate and Body Politic

When assessing the community, part of the data describes the public governing structure. For example, if it is urban, it is useful to know if there is a mayor, a chief executive, and a city governing board. Likewise, if it is rural or suburban, vital information includes the type of county or subdivision government, who the chief executive is, if the officials are elected or appointed, and what is the major political party. If the program is geared toward an international clientele, the types and structures of the governmental involved and the place of nursing and education in government regulations are vital sources of information.

Equally, if not more important, is information about the *body politic*. A simple definition for the "body politic" is: the people power(s) behind the official government within a community. It is composed of the major political forces and the people who exert influence within the community. The assessors should identify the major players, their visibility, that is, high profiles or low profiles as the powers behind the scenes. Additional information is how those in power influence decisions in the community and how they exert their power by using financial, personal, political, appointed, or elected positions. Specific information that is useful to educators is how the key politicians view the college or university and during elections and other crucial times, if they recognize the power of its people (i.e., students, faculty, and staff).

Relative to nursing, the politicians' and the body politics' specific interests in the profession are helpful. For example, if they have family members who are nurses or they have been recipients of nursing care, they are more apt to support nursing education programs. All educational programs need the support of the community and its power structure. Therefore, the information from the assessment of the political climate is vital to planning for the future and seeking assistance when the call comes for additional resources or for political pressure and support to maintain, revise, or increase the program.

The Health Care System and Health Needs of the Populace

Providing nurses to care for the health care needs of the populace is of critical interest to the health care system and the consumers of care. It is obvious that information about these two factors is essential to program planning and curriculum development. To assess the international, national, or regional health care systems, it is necessary to identify the major health care providers, types of organizations, and financial bases for the delivery of health care. In the United States with the implementation of the Affordable Health Care Act (ACA) and its possible repeal or revision, it is unwise to discuss at length the U.S. health care delivery system. Assessors should check governmental and health care systems' websites for the current and projected future of the system. An overview of the ACA is available at www.hhs.gov/healthcare/rights/index.html through the U.S. Department of Health and Human Services.

A list of major U.S. health care organizations and their websites is provided for the readers' convenience in searching for the latest information regarding health care services. The following provides a list of major resources that can provide information on the health care system(s) for the locality, region, or nation that the educational program serves.

- Major governmental health care systems such as Medicare, Medicaid, Civilian Health and Medical Program of the Uniformed Services (CHAMPUS), Veterans Affairs (VA), and so forth

- Non-profit or for-profit health care systems and agencies and eligibility for services
- Sectarian and nonsectarian health-related agencies and eligibility for services
- City, county, regional, state, and national public health services
- Services for the underserved or unserved population groups
- Major primary health care systems and agencies and providers
- Voluntary health care agencies and their services
- Other community-based health-related services staffed by nurses, for example, schools, industry, state institutions, forensic facilities

The assembled list provides an overview of the health care system within which the program is located. It describes the health care resources that are available or not available to the population including the nursing school and institution's populations. It points out the gaps of services in the community and the possibilities for community partnerships including school-based services for the underserved and unserved populations. It identifies trends in health care services and anticipated changes for the future that can influence curriculum development.

It is useful to know if resources within the system such as health care libraries are available to students and faculty during clinical experiences or as resources for students enrolled in distance education programs. A review of the list pinpoints existing clinical experience sites and the potential for new ones. Personnel in the agencies with qualifications as preceptors, mentors, and adjunct faculty are additional resources for possible collaboration opportunities. Scholarship and research opportunities for students and faculty may emerge from the review and can influence curriculum development as well as foster faculty and student development.

An overview of the major health problems in the region contributes to curriculum development as exemplars for health care interventions. The National Center for Health Statistics website (www.cdc.gov/nchs) provides general information on leading causes of death and morbidity. Vital statistics, health statistics, and objectives for 2020 and information on the development of *Healthy People 2030* are located at the *Healthy People 2020* website (www.healthypeople.gov). For international facts on health in specific countries, the World Health Organization website (www.who.int/en) is a good place to start. It provides information about the various member countries' health systems and major health problems.

Characteristics of the Academic Setting

Other institutions of higher learning in the nearby community, region, or online competitors have an influence on the program and its curriculum. Identifying other institutions, their levels of higher education (technical schools, associate degree, baccalaureate, and higher degree), financial base (private or public), and affiliations (sectarian or nonsectarian) gives the assessors an idea of the existing competition and the need for programs to continue their graduates' education. Information about other institutions' intentions for the future enables developers to understand the gaps in the types of programs and the nature of the competition from other programs. For example, if the institution's curriculum offers a nurse practitioner program and two other programs in the region offer similar programs, perhaps the curriculum should be revised (e.g., as a specialty primary or acute care program such as an Adult Gerontology Acute Care Nurse Practitioner), discontinued, or possibly entered into a joint venture with the other schools. A private institution that is dependent on tuition and endowments may question whether it should continue to offer a curriculum that is redundant with a state-supported school. Other data to consider are the need for nurses in the area and its surroundings that the institution *nurse need more* (handwritten)

serves, and even though there are multiple programs, the success rates of graduates finding employment in the region.

A suggested resource for collecting data on other academic institutions internationally and in the United States is the Council for Higher Education Accreditation website (www.chea.org). National databases may be found at the National Center for Education Statistics website (www.nces.ed.gov). Another source for identifying other nursing programs in the region is the list of approved programs provided by the state board of nursing. A listing of the state boards and their websites and contact information may be found at the National Council of State Boards of Nursing website (www.ncsbn.org/index.htm).

The Need for the Program

An examination of the external environment informs the faculty about the increased or continued need for nurses. The following data points act as guides to document the need for the program.

- Characteristics of the nursing workforce and the extent of a nursing shortage, if it exists
- Predictions for future nursing workforce needs
- Adequate numbers of eligible applicants to the program, currently and in the future
- Specific areas of nursing practice experiencing a shortage
- Employers' projections for the numbers of nurses needed in the future
- Employers' views on the types of graduates needed

A brief survey of health care administrators can provide this information, although it is sometimes difficult to expect a good response rate owing to the current pressures on administrators. Another strategy is to conduct focus groups that take no more than 15 minutes in the health agencies. Instructors who use the facilities for students or clinical coordinators are excellent people for collecting the information. There are several resources to identify the national and regional need for nurses. They are the state nurses' associations that can be located through the American Nurses Association (www.nursingworld.org/FunctionalMenuCategories/AboutANA/WhoWeAre/CMA.aspx) and the U.S. Department of Health and Human Services (http://bhpr.hrsa.gov). For international information, the WHO website provides information on workforce issues worldwide as well as qualifications for nurses and nursing educators.

As described previously in the characteristics of the academic setting, knowledge of other nursing programs in the region and online is useful to avoid curriculum redundancies. The data on the need for the program demonstrate how many of its graduates are currently needed and in the future, the level of education necessary to provide the level of care required, and short- and long-term health care system needs. A current nursing workforce demand indicates the possibility for accelerated programs. Shortages in specialties indicate advanced practice curricula and increased opportunities for registered nurses to continue their education

The Nursing Profession

In addition to the need for nurses, it is important to learn about the nursing profession in the region or nation. Professional organizations are rich resources for identifying leaders, mentors, and financial support such as scholarship aid. Curriculum developers should survey faculty and colleagues for a list of the nursing professions in the region. Such organizations include local or regional affiliates of the ANA; the National League for Nursing (NLN); Sigma Theta Tau International; educator organizations such as the

American Association of Colleges of Nursing (AACN) and the National Organization of Associate Degree Nursing (NOADN); and the plethora of specialty organizations. Questions to gather information about the profession follow: Who are the nurses in the area? Are there professional organizations with which the program can link? What is the level of education for the majority of the nurses in practice? Are there nurses prepared with advanced degrees who could serve as educators or preceptors? Are scholarship and research activities in nursing and health care underway that present opportunities for students and faculty?

Regulations and Accreditation Requirements

Whether the program is new or under revision, state and national regulations regarding schools of nursing should be reviewed for their requirements and any recent or anticipated changes in them that affect the curriculum. Information on regulations is available through the state boards of nursing. For a listing of specific state boards of nursing, consult the NCSBN website (www.ncsbn.org).

National accreditation is not required of schools of nursing; however, it provides the standards for nursing curricula and demonstrates program quality. Sophisticated applicants to the school will look for accreditation. Alumni find it advantageous to graduate from an accredited institution when applying for positions in the job market, for future advanced education, and positions in the military. Many scholarships and financial aid programs require that students enroll in accredited institutions. Nursing has two major accrediting agencies and a few specialty-accrediting bodies. The Accrediting Commission for Education in Nursing accredits clinical doctorate, master's/postmaster's certificate, baccalaureate, associate, diploma, and practical nursing programs. Detailed information on its accrediting process and standards may be found at its website (www.acenursing .org). The Accrediting Commission for Education in Nursing also lists the standards for international programs at www.acenursing.org/resources. The Commission on Collegiate Nursing Education accredits baccalaureate and higher degree programs. Information on it may be found at www.aacn.nche.edu/ccne-accreditation. A fairly recent national nursing accrediting agency is the National League for Nursing Commission for Nursing Education Accreditation that accredits nursing programs from the licensed practical nurse/licensed vocational nurse (LPN/LVN) to the clinical doctorate. Its website may be found at www.nln.org/accreditation-services/overview.

In addition to accreditation, there are standards and competencies set by professional organizations that serve as guidelines or organizational frameworks for curricula. Several examples for prelicensure and graduate-level programs are those developed by the AACN in their *Essentials Series* for baccalaureate and higher degree programs. Access to these documents may be found at www.aacn.nche.edu/education-resources/essential-series.

Another external frame factor that influences the nursing curriculum in the United States is regional accreditation. The parent institution of a nursing program undergoes periodic review by its regional accrediting body. Members of the nursing faculty are involved in the regional accreditation process and should be mindful of the standards set by that organization as well as those set by the professional accrediting body. Information about the regional accrediting agencies may be found at the CHEA website (https:// www.chea.org/4DCGI/cms/review.html?Action=CMS_Document&DocID=38&Menu Key=main). Detailed descriptions of accreditation processes and standards for educational programs are described in Section IV of this text.

Financial Support Systems

An analysis of the finances of the program provides curriculum developers with vital information on the economic health of the program. Indicators of financial health influence how the curriculum will be delivered. Faculty should recognize signs that demonstrate the program's financial viability. If new sources of income for the program are indicated, possible resources need to be identified. The proposed revisions in the curriculum must be realistic in terms of cost. If it is a new program, adequate resources including start-up funds for its implementation must be available. If it is an existing program, faculty and administration should consider whether to continue it at its present level of financial support or increase or decrease support.

Analyzing external frame factors in light of proposed new programs or curriculum revisions helps faculty and administrators determine the type of new program needed or, in the case of an existing program, the extent to which changes in the curriculum are indicated. A review of the external frame factors provides a check with reality including the community in which the program is located, the industry for which the program prepares graduates, and the economic viability of the program. Other items of study include how the program is financed and the major sources of revenues such as fees, tuition, state support, private contributions, grants, scholarships, or endowments. Knowing if there are adequate resources to support the program to be self-sufficient is a critical element in the analysis of the financial viability. Although this type of information is within the responsibility of administration, curriculum developers must have a basic understanding of the financial support systems that impact curriculum development. Chapter 4 discusses the role of faculty and curriculum planners in procuring funds for support of curriculum development and evaluation and an overview of budgetary planning and management.

INTERNAL FRAME FACTORS

Internal frame factors include a description of the organizational structure of the parent academic institution; its mission and purpose, philosophy, and goals; internal economic situation and its influence on the curriculum; resources within the institution (e.g., laboratories, classrooms, library, academic services, instructional technology support, student services); and existing and potential faculty and student characteristics. The information related to these factors is analyzed for its relevance to the program and the findings are weighed as to their importance to the quality of the program, its existence, and possible changes.

Description and Organizational Structure of the Parent Academic Institution

When looking at the environment that surrounds a nursing education program, the parent institution in which it resides is examined in light of the scenario it sets for the program. The physical campus and its buildings create the milieu in which the program exists with the nursing program a reflection of its place within the institution or in the case of a web-based program, its Internet features. The nature of the institution influences the structure of the campus and for nursing education programs, can be located in health care agencies, academic medical centers, liberal arts colleges, large research universities, land grant universities, multipurpose state-supported or private universities, community colleges, or an independent Internet entity. In small private institutions, the school of nursing can be one of the largest and most influential constituents, while in statewide university systems, nursing can be a small department within a health-related college that is within the greater university. The history of the institution is important to know such as its growth or change over the years and the role the nursing program had in its political fortunes or misfortunes.

Educational institutions and health care agencies usually have organizational structures of a hierarchal nature. Faculty should analyze the structure of the parent institution as well as that of the nursing program to describe the hierarchal and formal lines of communication that guide the faculty in developing and revising programs. For example, as described in Chapter 2, curriculum proposals and changes must be approved first on the local level (the nursing curriculum committee and faculty), moved to the next level of organization such as a college curriculum committee and dean, and finally, to an all-college- or university-wide curriculum committee with its recommendations going to the faculty senate (or its like) for final approval. There can be administrative approval along the way from department heads, deans, and perhaps academic vice presidents or provosts, especially in regard to economic and administrative feasibility. Nevertheless, the major approval bodies are those that are composed of faculty and within faculty governance prerogatives.

At the same time, it is useful to include the major players within the faculty and administrative structures in order to discuss with them the plans and rationale for proposed new programs or curriculum revisions. Prior consultation with these key people can help smooth the way when the proposals are ready to enter the formal arena and they can give advice related to changes that might enhance approval or advice on the best presentation formats that facilitate an understanding of the proposal. These contacts can be of a formal or informal nature; however, a word of caution, to avoid disastrous results, never blindside an administrator or decision maker. It is wise to keep them informed of new proposals or possible changes to place them in the advocate role as the approval process wends its way through the system.

Mission, Philosophy, and Goals of the Parent Institution

The mission/vision and purpose, philosophy, and goals of the parent institution determine the character of the nursing program. Most institutions of higher education focus their missions and philosophies on three endeavors: education, service, and scholarship/ research. Nursing must examine the mission and philosophy of its parent institution to determine its place within these three basic activities. For example, a state-supported university may have as part of its mission and philosophy the education of the people of the state for professional, leadership, and service roles. Thus, the nursing program could focus its mission and philosophy on the preparation of nurses for leadership roles and provision of health care services to the people of the state. If the statewide system is the predominant preparer of nurses within the state as compared to independent colleges, then the additional mission or purpose might be to provide an adequate nursing workforce for the state.

In contrast, independent or private colleges and universities may have missions and philosophies that have a sectarian flavor such as preparing individuals with strong liberal arts foundations for public service or roles in the helping professions. Again, a nursing program's mission is usually compatible with this mission. Academic medical centers are yet another example of nursing's match to health disciplines that are housed in one institution and whose mission is to prepare individuals for the health professions. Community college or junior college missions usually focus on technical education or on prerequisite preparation for entering into upper-division-level colleges and universities.

Internal Economic Situation and Influence on the Curriculum

As stated previously, the economic health of the institution has a significant impact on the nursing program and curriculum. How much of the share of resources, income, and expenditures that the nursing program has can affect program stability and room for expansion. For example, nurse-managed clinics must be self-supporting or economic recessions can cause their demise. For state-sponsored programs, the parent institution is subject to the state economy during periods of recession and prosperity. Independent colleges, unless heavily endowed, depend on tuition, student fees, or other income-generating operations. Some parent institutions allow programs to charge a higher tuition rate for both in- and out-of-state students to cover the additional costs of developing and maintaining web-based programs.

All institutions depend upon endowments and financial aid programs for students including scholarships, loans, and grants. Nursing programs are eligible for many federal grants and have a history of securing other types of grants from private foundations, state-supported programs, and private contributions including those from alumni associations. These income-generating programs illustrate to the parent institution that the nursing program is viable and at the same time, the institution's reputation and ability to garner external financial resources help the nursing program secure funding.

Institutions usually have support systems for assisting faculty to write grants and to seek outside financial support. Nursing programs should have close relationships with these support systems and have a plan in place for securing additional funds. Faculty plays a major role in writing grants with the perks related to them if funded, of released time for program development and scholarship and research activities. Two sources for U.S. funding to support program development on the national level are the Health Resources and Services Administration (bhpr.hrsa.gov/nursing) and the National Institute of Nursing Research (www.ninr.nih.gov). The latter focuses on clinical research; however, it is possible that faculty may wish to conduct curriculum and educational program research. A listing of other resources can be found at proposalCENTRAL: https://proposalcentral.altum.com.

Assessment of the economic status of the parent institution and the nursing program provides a realistic picture of the potential for program expansion and curriculum revision. When developing curriculum, the first demand for financial support comes with the need for resources to conduct a needs assessment such as the costs of released time for those who are conducting the assessment, review of the literature, and surveys of key stakeholders. A cost analysis for revising a curriculum or mounting a new one requires a business case to justify the costs and to forecast its financial viability. Unless there is a nursing program financial officer, the nursing program administrator and faculty should work closely with the parent institution's business office or chief financial officer in developing the business case.

Resources Within the Institution and Nursing Program

An analysis of the existing resources within the institution and the nursing program supplies information related to possible program expansion and curriculum revisions. First, there should be adequate classrooms, learning laboratories, library staff and resources, computer facilities, clinical practice simulations, instructional technology support, and distance education resources for the current program. When planning for revisions of the curriculum or for new programs, the need for expansion of these facilities and additional staffing should be identified. If expansion is not possible, then creative approaches to scheduling for the maximum use of these facilities can be examined, for example, evening classes, weekend learning experiences, and online delivery of courses.

Academic support services such as the library, academic advisement, teaching-learning resources, and instructional technology contribute to the maintenance of a quality education program and are internal frame factors that should be assessed when developing new programs or revising existing ones. If there are to be new programs or expansion of current curricula, the library resources must be adequate. Library resources include not only those resources on campus but also services for off-campus programs and students. There should be Internet and web-based library access for students and faculty and this is especially true when the campus has a large commuter student population, distance education programs, or proposes new programs. Library and instructional technology support staffing must be large enough and knowledgeable about nursing education needs. Thus, faculty should have strong relationships with librarians and the instructional technology staff in order to build the resources needed to revise the curriculum or develop new programs.

Academic advisement services play an important role in program planning as new programs can require additional staffing. If the curriculum is revised, updates for academic advising are necessary so that the faculty and its support staff that provide the services have current information to impart to the students. Teaching-learning resources need to be available to keep faculty current in instructional strategies, particularly if the revisions to the curriculum have an effect on instructional design. For example, a baccalaureate program may decide to convert its RN program to a web-based delivery system. In this case, faculty needs training in preparing and implementing web-based courses.

Instructional support systems are part of planning as well since the nature of the proposed program or the revised curriculum may call for additional resources. These resources include programmed instructional units, audio-visual aids, hardware and software, computer technologies, high-fidelity and low-fidelity mannequins for simulated clinical situations, and so forth. They can generate large costs to the program and should be calculated into the business case and the costs associated with their maintenance and replacement expenses over time. Some instructional support systems include monthly or annual student fees as well. For new programs or revisions, these costs are often included in requests for additional student lab fees or external funding. If the updating or creation of new laboratory/simulation practice labs involves one-time-only costs, external funding through donations, grants, or endowments are possibilities.

Student support services are equally important to nursing education programs and are an integral part of the curriculum development process. Major student services include enrollment (recruitment, admissions, registrar activities, and graduation records), maintenance of student records, advising and counseling, disciplinary matters, remediation and study skills, work-study programs, career counseling, job placement, and financial aid. Depending on the size of the university or college, these services can be congregated into one department or subdivided into several. Their role in curriculum development is important, as expanding or changing educational programs require student services support. For example, if a new program is proposed, then the recruitment and admissions staff will need to be apprised of the program to best serve the needs of the new program in recruitment and admission activities.

Financial aid programs are crucial to the recruitment, admission, and retention of students and if the proposal brings in new revenues through grants or other financial support structures, the financial aid staff must be cognizant of the proposal. They can provide useful information to program planners and thus, a partnership between the student services staff and the nursing program staff is beneficial.

Work-study programs and job placement information can supplement the curriculum, if these programs are in concert with the educational plan and not in conflict with the program of study. An example of a conflict is a revised curriculum that calls for accelerated study and clinical experiences that disallow student employment and therefore prohibits enrollment in the work-study program. Another aspect is the potential influence of students' part-time employment on the curriculum and its role in intended and unintended outcomes on the educational experience. With the preponderance of adult learners in nursing programs, the reality of their outside employment while enrolled in studies must be taken into account.

The informal curriculum often takes place through the planned activities of the student services department. Again, partnerships between student services and nursing faculty increase the effectiveness of the formal curriculum. Students who could benefit from remediation or learning skills workshops should be referred to student services. Faculty members work with student services staff to identify the learning needs of nursing students and this is especially relevant when curriculum changes are taking place. Additionally, student services staff work with faculty concerning the special needs of students with learning disabilities and the accommodations they require without imperiling the student's individual needs nor the safety of the clients for whom the students provide care.

Existing and Potential Faculty and Student Characteristics

When proposing new educational programs or revising existing curricula, thoughts need to go into the characteristics of the existing faculty and the student body who will participate in the educational program. If a new program is proposed, the faculty composition is reviewed. There should be adequate numbers of faculty members to represent diversity in gender and ethnic backgrounds and to reach the desired faculty to student ratio. Depending on the nature of the program, clinical supervision of students requires a low student to faculty ratio but can differ according to program. For example, master's and doctoral students are usually RNs and therefore, may not need the close supervision required for entry-level students. Although, for some advanced practice roles, there is a need for close faculty supervision. However, in these latter cases, preceptorships or internships are the usual format and a faculty member can supervise more students in collaboration with the clinical preceptors. In entry-level programs, the student to faculty ratio is usually 8–10 to 1; however, in the senior year, it is possible to have preceptorships with approximately 12 to 15 students, depending on the nature of the clinical experiences. While lectures can accommodate many students, seminars and learning laboratories demand fewer numbers of students and therefore additional faculty. Enrollment in online courses can vary with as few as 10 to 12 at the graduate-level and seminar-type courses to didactic online courses that accommodate as many as 30 or more students. In the case of the latter, the format for the course is modified to adjust to the larger number of students and the resultant teaching load for the instructor.

Yet another consideration related to faculty is the match of knowledge to the subject matter, clinical expertise, and pedagogical skills. Information on the numbers and types of faculty members needed, their required educational levels, and scholarship and research history feed into decisions about curriculum development. For international, web-based programs, potential faculty from the participating countries must be surveyed and identified, as well as the conundrum for translation from English (if U.S.-based) into the predominant language spoken. As with faculty considerations, the characteristics of the student body and the types of students the faculty hopes to attract to the new program or the revised curriculum are important. If it is a new program, the potential applicant pool should be identified according to interest, numbers, availability, and competition with other nursing programs. If a new program is contemplated, its type dictates the kind of applicant pool that the program and the admissions department need to target.

The characteristics of the students in the program help tailor the curriculum according to their learning needs. For example, if it is an entry-level associate degree or baccalaureate program, the applicants may be a mix of new high school graduates, transfer students with some college preparation, and adult learners with some work experience. The curriculum is then planned to meet a diversity of learning needs from traditional pedagogical learning theories to adult learning theories. Diversity of racial, ethnic, and cultural characteristics is the other factor to consider and the educational program must plan to be culturally responsive to students as well as prepare professionals with cultural competence.

SUMMARY

While the external frame factors examine the macroenvironment surrounding the program, the internal frame factors look at factors that are closer to the program and include the parent institution as well as the nursing program itself. Factors to examine include the characteristics of the parent institution and its organizational structure. How the nursing program fits into this structure can determine the economic, political, and resource support for program changes. It sets the stage for the processes that the nursing faculty must undergo to gain approval for the proposed changes. The mission and purpose, philosophy, and goals of the parent institution influence the nature of the nursing program and, to ensure success, the nursing program must be congruent with those of the parent institution. The internal economic status and the available resources of both the parent institution and the nursing program are assessed for the financial viability as well as the necessary additional resources and support services for proposed revisions or new programs. Finally, the characteristics of the faculty and the potential student body are reviewed to determine their match to the proposed change.

This chapter introduced the steps for conducting a needs assessment in curriculum development and revision. Prior to revising or developing new curricula, an assessment of the factors that influence the educational program is necessary. Tables 3.1 and 3.2 serve as guidelines for identifying the frame factors, collecting the data for an assessment, and analyzing the findings to determine if there is a need for a new program or if changes are necessary for an existing program. Appendix A offers a case study illustrating a needs assessment and, based on the needs assessment, a proposed curriculum revision.

THOUGHT QUESTIONS

1. Conducting a needs assessment is time-consuming; discuss the pros and cons of using all faculty members, a representative task force, paid consultants, or a combination of all three to conduct the assessment.
2. How does the process of a needs assessment apply to both curriculum development and curriculum evaluation?

SUGGESTED LEARNING ACTIVITIES

Student-Learning Project

As a student group, examine the community around you for its potential for a nursing program. Use Tables 3.1 and 3.2 to collect data on the factors that you need to consider. After you collect the data, summarize your findings and compare them to the "Desired Outcomes" listed in the tables. Based on the findings, justify why or why not a new or revised nursing program is needed.

Faculty Project

Using Tables 3.1 and 3.2, assess your nursing curriculum. Collect data for each frame factor as it applies to the curriculum. Summarize your findings and compare them to the "Desired Outcomes" listed in the table. In light of your summary, is a curriculum revision or a new program indicated? Explain your reasons for the decision.

TABLE 3.1   Guidelines for Assessing External Frame Factors

Frame Factor	Questions for Data Collection	Desired outcomes
Description of the Community	Is the community setting conducive to academic programs? Describe its major characteristics, i.e., distance education and/or on-site, totally or partially web-based, international, national, urban, suburban, or rural.	The institution's campus is a safe and supportive environment for its students, faculty, and staff.
		Industries are stable and have a history of financial support for the institution and employ its graduates.
	What are the major industries related to the institution and do they offer financial support as well as employment opportunities for graduates?	The public, private, and professional school systems provide graduates for the institution and are of high quality. School counselors have strong relationships with the institution's admissions department.
	What are the major educational systems and what is the quality of the programs? How do they feed into the parent institution?	Community colleges and higher degree institutions collaborate and have articulation agreements for ease of transfer.
	What community services provide an infrastructure for the institution, i.e., transportation and communications services?	Students have access at reasonable cost to public transportation to and from home (for commuter students) and to stores and other community services.
		The community has multiple media communication networks of high quality for marketing, public relations, and educational purposes. Internet, postal service, and other delivery systems are reliable.
	What services provide an infrastructure for the institution, i.e., recreation, housing, utilities, and human and health services?	There are varied and multiple recreational sites for students' leisure activities.
		If there are no student health services, the community has quality health and human services for which students are eligible.
	What type of government is in place in the community and what are its politics? Is the government supportive of the institution in its midst and does it recognize its contributions to the community?	The governmental structure is supportive of the parent institution in its community.
		Key members of the parent institution serve on advisory boards for the local government.

(continued)

TABLE 3.1 Guidelines for Assessing External Frame Factors (*continued*)

Frame Factor	Questions for Data Collection	Desired outcomes
Demographics of the Population	What are the characteristics of the general population? What indications are there that the population supports higher education? Within the population, what is the potential for acquiring student, faculty, and staff for the program?	The population reflects multicultural and ethnic characteristics with a wide range of age groups. A majority of the population and the powers structures completed high school or higher levels of education and/or there is growing interest in and need for these levels of education. There is an adequate applicant pool for the program(s). There are potential qualified faculty and staff available.
Political Climate and Body Politic	Identify the type of government and its structure. Who are the political power brokers in the community? What are the relationships of the parent institution to the political power brokers?	Key politicians and community leaders support the institution and have working relationships with the people within the educational institution.
The Health Care System and Health Needs of the Populace	Identify the major types of health care systems and the predominant health care delivery patterns. Describe the major health care problems and needs of the populace in the educational program's region. Describe the role of nursing in the health care system.	Currently and for the future, there are ample clinical spaces for nursing student placements in the various health care systems and settings. Major health care problems and needs match the foci of the curriculum. Nursing, as part of the health care workforce, has a strong representation within the health care system.
Characteristics of the Academic Setting	Identify other institutions of higher learning in the region or on the Internet. Within those institutions, what types of nursing programs are offered, if any? Are there potential or existing competitors?	Other institutions of higher learning in the region or on the Internet have programs not in direct competition with the curriculum and can serve as feeder schools to the program. There are no known future plans that could conflict with the program.

The Need for the Program	Describe the nursing workforce in the region as well as the state and nation.	There is a demonstrated need for nurses in the region, state, and nation(s) currently and in the future.
	Describe the numbers and types of nurses needed in the region, state, and nation(s) for the future.	The numbers and types of nurses meet the goals and type(s) of preparation available in the educational program for the future.
The Nursing Profession	List the major professional nursing organizations in the region or nation.	There are at least two major nursing organizations in the region or nation to be served that support the program and provide collegial relationships for students and faculty.
	Describe the characteristics of nurses in the region.	The types of nurses in the region match the potential applicant pool for continued education and/or faculty and mentor positions.
Financial Support	Analyze the present financial health of the parent institution and the nursing program.	The institution and the nursing program are in solid financial condition and there are either guaranteed state or national support or substantial endowment funds from the local and greater communities for the future.
	Develop a list of existing and potential economic resources.	There are adequate economic resources for the present and the future of the program.
Regulations and Accreditation Requirements	Identify the state board of registered nursing or national regulations for educational programs.	The nursing education program meets the state board or national regulations and has or is eligible for approval.
	List accreditation agencies that impact the parent institution and the nursing education program.	The parent institution is accredited by its regional or national agency and the nursing program meets the standards of a national professional accrediting body.

TABLE 3.2   Guidelines for Assessing Internal Frame Factors

Frame Factor	Questions for Data Collection	Desired outcomes
Description and Organizational Structure of the Parent Academic Institution	In what type of educational institution is the nursing program located? What is the milieu of the parent institution in regard to the nursing program? What is the organizational structure of the parent institution? What place in the institution does the nursing program hold? What influence does it have? In what order must a program go through the approval process? Who are the major players in the various levels of approval processes? What are the layers of approval processes for program approval and curriculum revisions?	The nursing program matches the type of educational institution in its purpose, mission, and vision. There is a supportive organizational system for program planning and curriculum revision. The nursing program is recognized in the institution for its place in education, scholarship, and service to the community. A fair, participative, and comprehensive review process begins at the program level and moves through a logical sequence of the governing body for final approval that results in an economically sound and high-quality educational program.
Mission and Purpose, Philosophy, and Goals of the Parent Institution	What are the mission, philosophy, and goals of the parent institution? Are they congruent and supportive of the nursing program?	The mission and purpose, philosophy, and goals of the parent institution are congruent with and supportive of the nursing program.
Internal Economic Situation and Its Influence on the Curriculum	What is the operating budget of the nursing program? Is it adequate for the support of the existing program? Are there resources for program or curriculum development activities?	The nursing program has adequate resources for supporting its educational program from the parent institution. The nursing program has the resources for program or curriculum development activities.
	Does the program have a financial officer or administrative assistant who can develop a business plan for the proposed program or curriculum revision? If not, are there resources available from the parent institution?	The nursing program has a business plan, the resources, and administrative support for mounting a new program or revising the existing curriculum.
Resources within the Institution and Nursing Program	If the program is on-campus or a combination of on- and off-site, how many classrooms, clinical practice, simulation, and computer laboratories does the nursing program have and are they under its control? Can they accommodate additional students or newer technologies in the proposed program or curriculum revisions? Are there plans for these facilities in the proposal and are the costs calculated in the business plan?	The current physical facilities such as classrooms, offices, clinical practice and simulation laboratories, computer facilities, are adequate and can accommodate curriculum revisions or new programs OR there are plans for expansion in place that are part of the business plan and have the support of the financial bodies of the institution.

	For both off- and on-site, are the web and technology systems and staff in place for the institution and nursing program? Are they adequate and up-to-date? Are there plans for increasing and updating the systems and staff according to the revised or new program needs? What are the available resources for program planning and curriculum revision? Is there released time available for those involved? Is there staff support available? What teaching-learning continuing education programs are available to faculty? How many texts and journal holdings as well as electronic databases does the library have and will they meet the needs of students and faculty in the future? Is there adequate librarian and technical support? What are the available hours/days and staff support for students and faculty to access the library and other electronic communications?	There are technology systems and faculty and staff support systems that facilitate program planning and curriculum revisions. There are adequate instructional and technology support systems and staff available for the current program and for proposed future programs. The current and proposed library and electronic holdings are adequate to meet the needs of the nursing program and proposed curricular revisions. There are reasonable hours/days and staff support for students and faculty to access the library and other electronic communications.
Potential Faculty and Student Characteristics	Describe the characteristics of the current student body and the history of the applicant pool to the nursing program. Has the program been able to meet its enrollment targets in the past 5 years? If not, what strategies have taken place to meet the target? What are the characteristics of the student body for the proposed program or revised curriculum? Is there an adequate applicant pool to fulfill enrollment targets? Has the nursing program a partnership and plans with the admissions department for recruiting and retaining students? Describe the characteristics of the current faculty. Are the numbers of faculty sufficient? Do they meet program requirements, educational level, clinical expertise, scholarship/research, and teaching experience qualifications? Do they represent diversity? Are there plans to recruit additional faculty if indicated?	The parent institution and the nursing program have the resources to recruit, educate, and graduate the type of student body that the new program or curriculum revision requires. There is a sufficient number of qualified faculty members who represent diversity and meet faculty to student ratio standards as well as academic, accreditation, and professional requirements.
Analysis of the Data and Decision Making	Summarize the conclusions by generating a list of positive, negative, and neutral findings that can influence the curriculum and program planning.	Develop a final decision statement as to the feasibility for developing a new program or revising the curriculum based on the needs assessment and its findings of the external and internal frame factors.

References

Indiana University Center for Postsecondary Research. (2016). *The Carnegie Classification of institutions of higher education* (2015 ed.). Bloomington, IN: Author.

Johnson, M. (1977). *Intentionality in education* (distributed by the Center for Curriculum Research and Services, Albany, NY). Troy, NY: Walter Snyder Printer.

Young, J., Allard, A., Hébert-Dufresne, L., & Dubé, L. J. (2015). A shadowing problem in the detection of overlapping communities: Lifting the resolution limit through a cascading procedure. *Public Library of Science One, 10*(10), 1–19.

CHAPTER 4

Financial Support and Budget Management for Curriculum Development or Revision

Sarah B. Keating

CHAPTER OBJECTIVE

Upon completion of Chapter 4, the reader will be able to:

- Analyze the influence that financial costs and budgetary management have on curriculum development or revision
- Itemize the costs associated with curriculum development or revision
- Identify resources for the financial support of curriculum development and revision activities
- Analyze the roles of faculty, administrators, and staff in budgetary planning, management, and the procurement of funds for curriculum development and revision

OVERVIEW

Activities associated with curriculum development for new programs or revision of existing ones require financial support for the time spent by personnel on the project and its associated costs. The costs may be major or minor depending on the extent of the changes or new program development. For example, if it is a revision, it may not call for additional faculty but perhaps, renovation of the physical facilities and other instructional support needs. New programs usually require start-up costs associated with their initiation such as the time spent on developing the program prior to student admission, approvals from accreditation agencies and regulating bodies, and increased recruitment activities for students and new faculty. This chapter discusses the types of costs that occur, their impact on the proposed program or revision, budget planning and management, and possible resources for funding. The roles of administrators, faculty, and staff are described.

FINANCIAL COSTS AND BUDGETARY PLANNING

Financial Costs

The process for evaluating an existing program for possible revision and conducting a needs assessment for possible changes or creating a new program involves administrative, faculty, and staff time. Depending on the extent of the change or development of a new program, the time spent may be part of the usual role of these personnel. For example, faculty curriculum committee members review recommendations for change in the curriculum as part of committee activities, which in turn are part of the service role expectations for faculty. Another example is when planning and managing the budget, the administrator may find that one of the tracks in the overall program is losing money owing to low student enrollments, while another track is turning away applicants. Analyzing the problem and bringing it to the attention of the faculty is the next step to address the problem and is considered a usual administrative responsibility.

While activities associated with program changes normally take place in faculty curriculum committees and the time spent on these activities is considered a part of the faculty service role, faculty time spent over and above the usual service activities may be necessary. The costs associated with the additional time occur in the form of released time or a stipend for individual faculty members, or a consultant may be hired to coordinate the project. Staff support for the activities such as taking and recording minutes for meetings, coordination of participants' schedules for meeting times, collecting data for assessment, and so forth are included in the costs.

When calculating the costs associated with curriculum development, both direct and indirect costs must be considered. Direct costs are those that can be attributed to new costs and include: additional personnel; physical facilities such as offices, labs, classrooms, and furnishings; staff and instructional support equipment; web-based informatics and technology systems; computers and their hardware and software; office supplies; and so on. Indirect costs are those associated with the use of existing staff, physical facilities such as offices and meeting rooms, utilities, furnishings, and supplies that the institution provides from its resources. These indirect costs are usually estimated on a percentage basis of the total and can range from approximately 3% to 40% of the total costs. Personnel costs represent the largest expenditure for supporting curriculum change or development. However, there are a few other direct costs such as fees associated with data collection when conducting a needs assessment, office supplies, new computer hardware and software, and travel for data collection or consultation purposes.

Costs of Nursing Programs in Academe

Often nursing programs must defend themselves from other disciplines that assume that nursing education is an expensive proposition. Certainly, the nursing faculty to student ratio required for clinical supervision in health care agencies is costly. However, large theory classes where lecture prevails as the modality for entry-level programs and the use of online education, and clinical simulation help counterbalance the expense. Also, clinical instructors are often part time or serve as adjunct faculty who cost less than tenured or tenure-track faculty who are full time. Although the literature on the costs of program development is sparse, several articles were identified that discuss how to estimate the costs and benefits for a new program. The reader may find them useful when involved in curriculum development and planning.

Greene and Turner (2014) describe clinical academic partnerships in which schools of nursing and hospitals collaborated on the expenses associated with clinical education that benefitted students and cut costs associated with the clinical supervision of students by faculty. Another successful partnership between practice and academe is described by Stout, Short, Cintron, and Provencio-Vasquez (2015). The partnership consisted of an internship for senior baccalaureate in nursing students in the last semester of their senior year. Benefits listed for the hospital included an increase in baccalaureate-prepared graduates in the hospital and lower costs for orientation programs, while the university experienced highly satisfied graduates.

Advice for making a business case for a proposed program comes from Moore, Banks, and Neely (2014) in their description of how they proposed the development of the clinical nurse leader position in hospitals in the United States. They point out that the first step is to know who the audience is so that the proposal is targeted to that special interest group. The proposed program should be aligned with the institution's strategic goals and plans. To develop a business case for the program, the authors recommend a succinct description of who the program is for and its product, for example, who will the graduates be and what is their role in the delivery of health care services? The second step is to list the action items necessary such as recruitment of students, hiring of faculty, and so forth, followed by the plans for implementation of the program. Finally, a spreadsheet is created that lists the costs for mounting the program, maintaining it, and the estimated return on the investment including how it will be sustained over the long term. Examples of return on investment include increased student enrollments and therefore, increased income from tuition, fees, scholarships, and possible long-term grants and endowments for the program

Budgetary Planning and Management

The chief nursing officer (CNO; dean, director, or chair) of the educational program is responsible for managing the budget. Administrative support staff assists in the management of the budget allocation although, in some smaller nursing programs, these responsibilities may be included in the expectations for the CNO. Planning for the future, both annually and long term, is part of the CNO role. Schools of nursing and their parent institutions have strategic goals and plans for the future, usually within a 5-year framework. In addition, most schools have a master plan of evaluation. These plans, with their goals and objectives, provide guidelines for projected curriculum revisions, new program proposals, and program and accreditation activities. Thus, a section in the budget for curriculum development and evaluation should be part of the planning process. When planning annual budgets in association with the development of short- and long-term goals, administrators should involve faculty and staff to assist in the identification of current and potential needs for curriculum revision and the development of new programs and their related costs.

Specific items in budgets that relate to curriculum planning include faculty released time to identify possible revisions or new programs; released time for conducting a needs assessment; consultant fees if indicated for major revisions or new program development; expenses related to attendance at relevant conferences/workshops; and additional staff support, office supplies, and communications and technology support. According to the program's long-range goals or strategic plan, these costs may be for 1 year or several depending on the extent of the changes. As the planning process develops, indications for change or new programs require further planning for the future based on the costs for developing new programs and, perhaps, discontinuing programs that no longer meet the goals of the program. Table 4.1 lists the elements to consider in planning annual budgets as they apply to curriculum revision or development of new programs.

If a program decides to offer a new program based on the findings from a needs assessment, planning for a budget to start and maintain the program is a crucial step. Costs to develop the curriculum, including recruitment of students, and additional faculty, staff, physical facilities, and supplies must be part of the cost side of the budget, along with the revenue side of the budget to indicate sources of financial support. See Table 4.2 for a listing of the items to include in a budget when planning for a new program.

Several articles describe ways to finance new programs including associated physical facilities that require approval for new construction. Bavier and Bavier (2016) describe their roles as a dean of nursing and architect in the construction of new facilities for a

TABLE 4.1   Budget Elements for Curriculum Assessment and Planning

Item	Associated Costs	Potential Benefits	Risks	Total Cost
Faculty Released Time	% of released time necessary (salary)	Faculty development in curriculum planning and assessment Faculty ownership of the curriculum	Time away from teaching activities Development of barriers and resistance to curriculum change	$
Conference/ Workshop Attendance	Fees, travel expenses	Faculty development for curriculum planning	Time away from teaching activities	$
Consultant	Fees, travel, lodging	Expert assistance for identifying needs, redundancies, and nonproductive programs	Insufficient or inadequate product compared to expense	$
Staff	% of released time necessary (salary) *or* New temporary position	Experienced program management perspectives *or* 100% of time devoted to the activity	Time away from usual activities Temporary positions are difficult to fill	$ (salary and benefits)
Office Supplies	Computer accessories, paper, desk supplies, etc.	Support for the process	None	$
Needs Assessment	Access to data bases, travel to agencies, mailing costs, telephone charges, etc.	Documents needs Develops potential partnerships with outside agencies	Time-consuming Can be slanted Missing data	$
Reports	Time of personnel Office supplies	Record for documentation and planning purposes	Time-consuming	$
Total				$

nursing program. Included in the description are the processes associated with cost estimates, design, schematics, drawings of the proposed facilities, and dates for occupancy, as well as processes for moving in. Millett (2016) discusses an accelerated nursing degree program for students who are nonnursing college graduates and the support those students received from the Robert Wood Johnson Foundation in the form of scholarships. This helped maintain enrollments as these students seeking another undergraduate degree were not eligible for federal grant programs.

Yucha, Smyer, and Strano-Perry (2014) report on several strategies for maintaining and creating new programs in the case of budget cuts and faculty shortages. One method is to use affiliated hospital nursing staff for clinical supervision of students, the second is to create differential enrollment fees for nursing students to help allay program costs, and the third is the creation of a collaborative program with another nursing school to split the number of courses taught by faculty and thus, reduce costs. An interesting

TABLE 4.2   Elements for Budget Planning for New Programs

Item	Year 1	Year 2	Year 3	Year 4	Year[a] 5
COSTS					
Salaries and Benefits of Existing Faculty, Administrators, and Staff for Curriculum Development					
Salary and Benefits for Coordinator of Program					
Salary and Benefits for Program Faculty					
Consultant Fees and Costs					
Salary and Benefits for Support Staff					
Recruitment of Personnel					
Recruitment of Students					
Capital Improvements/Additions					
Supplies, Services, Technology, and Information Services and Staff					
Library Additions and Staff					
INCOME					
Student Enrollments/Tuition (Include Admissions, Anticipated Attrition Rate, and Graduations; Part Time, Full Time if Applicable)					
Student Fees					
Income from Grants, Endowments, Donations, Scholarships, Other					
TOTALS					

[a]Five-year budget planning recommended with annual review for adjustments.

perspective is offered by Roark (2015) who points out that sometimes, it is not necessary to offer financial compensation for program planners when operating within a tight budget situation. The author shows that a recent study found that around 60% of Americans preferred noncash awards to compensation in the form of motivation, appreciation, and recognition. Incentive programs improve relationships and the overall milieu within organizations.

SOURCES FOR FINANCIAL SUPPORT

There are three major sources of funding for curriculum development and planning other than the home institution's support in its regular budget. Depending on the nature of the home institution, the majority of funds for the budget come from the general funds (if state supported), tuition and fees, endowments, grants, and donations. When considering funds for curriculum development, the three major resources for funds are grants (private and public), partnerships with the community, and philanthropy (donations and endowments). Each of these sources is discussed with ideas from the literature for procurement of funds.

Grants

A major resource for program development and student and faculty support at the federal level comes from the Health Resources and Services Administration (HRSA), Division of Nursing (2017). Included in the program of grants are traineeships for advanced practice students, faculty loans, support for nurse-managed health care services, and program development. The program development funds, for the most part, focus on starting up new programs and a large part of the funds support curriculum development. It is not permanent funding and is intended as an incentive to increase the advanced practice nursing workforce and to support other types of advanced nursing education programs, for example, education and public health. For detailed information on this major resource go to the HRSA, Health Workforce, Nursing website (www.bhw .hrsa.gov/grants/nursing). Included in its programs are: advanced nursing education workforce; advanced education nursing traineeships: advanced nursing education; nurse anesthetist traineeships; nurse education, practice, quality, and retention; nurse education, practice, quality, and retention: veterans' bachelor of science degree in nursing program; nurse faculty loan program; and nursing workforce diversity. The costs for preparing a grant proposal must be factored into the planning process including faculty and staff time and additional related costs for preparation of the grant. Kulage et al. (2015) list the costs associated with the preparation of a grant submitted to the National Institute of Nursing Research (NINR). NINR (2017) supports research activities related to clinical practice and the advancement of nursing science, not program planning which can be more time-consuming than writing a program grant. However, Kulage, et al. present items that are included in grant writing.

In addition to federal grants, there are major private foundations and organizations interested in supporting nursing education programs. They include the Bill and Melinda Gates Foundation (www.gatesfoundation.org), Robert Wood Johnson Foundation (www .rwjf.org), the W.K. Kellogg Foundation (www.wkkf.org), the Josiah Macy Jr. Foundation (www.macyfoundation.org), the Gordon and Betty Moore Foundation (www.moore.org), and many others. A listing of other resources may be found at the proposalCENTRAL, website at https://proposalcentral.altum.com. Many universities and colleges offer courses in grant writing and there are a few that are online. One online site from the General Services Administration offers ideas for developing and writing grant proposals and may be found at www.nmfs.noaa.gov/trade/howtodogrants.htm.

Partnerships

There is a long history of partnerships between nursing education programs and health care agencies. The purpose for these partnerships is not only to provide clinical experiences for students, but also to support schools of nursing in preparing professionals for the workforce. These partnerships take many forms including work-study, internship, or residency experiences for students who may earn a modest salary and at the same time earn academic credits; contributions of nursing clinicians to the school as instructors; use of facilities for laboratory and simulation experiences; continuing education and research opportunities for both faculty and staff; and scholarship or loan programs for students in exchange for contracts to work for the agency upon graduation. The numbers and amount of financial support available from agencies seem to flow and ebb according to nursing workforce demands and the financial climate at the time.

A model for partnerships between health care systems and educational institutions is the Veterans Affairs (VA) Nursing Academy project that supplied $60 million to establish partnerships with the VA and baccalaureate schools of nursing. It funds faculty positions using expert clinicians from the VA system (or the community if there is a lack), provides clinical practice experiences for students, and recruits new graduates into the VA system. There are four established regions including the western, mid-west, south, and northeast regions of the United Stated. Benefits for the schools and the VA include current updates on clinical practice and an increase in the faculty workforce as well as the nursing workforce. This model serves as an example for other health care systems wishing to increase the nursing workforce and at the same time, participate in updating nursing curricula and addressing the nursing faculty shortage (Bowman et al., 2011).

An update on the VA program is described by Pearson, Wyte-Lake, Bowman, Needleman, and Dobalian (2015) who surveyed staff nurses on the VA units where students received their clinical training. The authors found a spillover effect on the nurses in that 80% of the staff ($n = 314$) did not think that the students' presence led to additional work, the majority were positive about the experience, and they either were enrolled or planned to enroll in higher education for themselves. The more exposure the staff had to the program, the greater their satisfaction and participation in the program. A recommendation from the study was that staff nurses need to have the learning objectives of the students, should have frequent interactions with the students, and should be encouraged to act as preceptors for the students.

Moch, Jansen, Jadack, Page, and Topp (2015) present ways in which nursing educators can obtain research funding and program development funds from health care agencies in the interest of client care. The steps and related processes to a plan for obtaining funds from the health care agencies include working with a business collaborator to establish a relationship with the potential funder, developing and presenting a concise business plan, communicating frequently with the funder, and planning for future collaboration. Details about this plan and associated processes are helpful for educators considering obtaining funding from affiliating agencies.

Partnerships between other schools of nursing and the institution's own programs in nursing can result in common campus activities such as orientation sessions, sharing of core courses that are common to program curricula, for example, statistical methods; blended clinical experiences that provide different, yet collaborative levels of care; and end-of-program projects that reflect varying levels of practice or role functions. These collaborative activities can lead to a savings in resources such as faculty and staff costs and facilities. Edward, Rayman, Diffenderfer, and Stidham (2016) describe a collaborative program between DNP and PhD programs that not only proved to be cost saving but improved collegial relationships between the two groups of students and led to research-practice collaborative models.

Philanthropy

Philanthropic funds come from donations to nursing programs. A large majority of these donations are earmarked for scholarships for students. However, there are times when programs receive donations for program development. Starck (2015) describes a fund-raising project that a school of nursing undertook to support an accelerated PhD program in nursing. A successful campaign consists of knowing the potential donors and having a personal connection. Contacts made with unknown people seldom succeed. The motivation of the donor for contributing to the program should be known, whether in response to a personal connection with the school, a desire to contribute to a good cause anonymously or not, and an opportunity to establish a memorial or tribute to someone close to the donor. When proposing a contribution to a project, it is important to point out the direct and indirect benefits for the donor from the gift and what impact it will have on the program and health care system currently, and in the future.

Alumni organizations are good resources for nursing programs and schools should encourage the support of alumni organizations through special functions such as reunions at the time of graduation, research events, and guest lectures. Fostering alumni participation can begin early in the professional socialization process through the nursing student association with faculty mentoring and support. A website for the Council for Advancement and Support of Education (www.case.org/About_CASE.html) provides information on fund raising and working with donors and alumni for the financial support of programs.

ROLE OF ADMINISTRATORS, STAFF, AND FACULTY IN FINANCIAL SUPPORT FOR CURRICULUM DEVELOPMENT ACTIVITIES

Administrators and Staff

When a curriculum revision is indicated or a new program is in the offing, additional administrator and faculty time is expected and usually it is over and above the normal job expectations. Therefore, released time and related costs are expected and must be planned for in the budget. Administrators, with faculty input, should include a line item for program planning in the budget to cover these anticipated costs. While indirect funds from a grant can provide for the released time spent on program planning, they usually are not available until after the fact, that is., the grant is approved and funded after initial activities take place. Depending on the institution's policies regarding indirect funds, administrators may have the discretion to use funds for program development generated from other grants. Otherwise, funds for program planning should be part of the regular budgeting process.

The administrator and the administrative staff have responsibility for the management of the school budget and records of expenditures for curriculum revision or new program development. The records are especially useful for illustrating how the expenditures tie to the purpose of the funding and the grant/project goals, and they provide documentation for accounting purposes. Each year, during the annual budget review and projections for the future, administrators, staff, and faculty should identify continuing and future funding needs for program development.

Faculty

Curriculum development and evaluation is an ongoing process built into the educational program activities. Nursing educators in the process of delivering the curriculum through instructional activities such as classroom lectures, seminars, conferences, laboratory practice, simulation activities, online teaching, and clinical supervision gather information on how well the curriculum is delivered. This ongoing assessment of teaching effectiveness and student-learning outcomes is part of the role of teaching and is a job expectation and therefore, as part of the usual responsibilities, is supported through faculty salaries. Yet another aspect of faculty work is participation in work groups such as course, level, and curriculum committee meetings. These activities are considered part of the service role for faculty and from a budgetary point of view, are a part of the salary paid to faculty and the expected responsibilities of the role. If major curriculum revisions or a new program are indicated, conducting a needs assessment and developing the curriculum can require faculty time over and above the usual expectations. In that case, the administrator and faculty in the program need to identify sources of funds to support the released time for these activities and to plan for them in the budget.

SUMMARY

This chapter discusses the importance of financial support for curriculum revision and program development. It reviews the costs, benefits, and budget planning and management activities associated with curriculum development and revision. Resources for funding these activities are offered and the roles of administrators, staff, and faculty in seeking funding, planning, and managing the budget are described.

DISCUSSION QUESTIONS

- What influences do finances and resources have on developing and maintaining a vibrant curriculum?
- What individual or group do you believe has the responsibility for procuring funds for program development and curricular revision? Provide a rationale.

LEARNING ACTIVITIES

Student-Learning Activities

Interview a member or chair of the curriculum committee for her or his perspectives on financial support for program development and curriculum revision. Interview questions you might consider asking are as follows:

1. How much time do you spend on curriculum activities?
2. Are you compensated in any way for this time or is it an expectation of your role? Do you believe faculty should have released time for curriculum development activities? Why or why not? How would you pay for overtime?
3. When was the last curriculum revision? Do you expect a revision in the near future? Are there plans for review and revision of the curriculum in the school strategic plan?
4. Do you participate in planning for future curriculum committee activities and development and are budgetary issues involved in the planning?
5. Are you aware of any resources to support curriculum change or new program development? If yes, what are these sources?

Faculty Development Activities

1. Survey your community/region for existing partnerships between nursing education programs and clinical agencies. Other than providing clinical experiences for students, are there any other financial support programs related to curriculum revision or new program development in the partnership?
2. Identify needs for and possible partnerships to support nursing education in your region. Indicate your strategies for developing the partnership and its maintenance over time.

References

Bavier, A., & Bavier, R. (2016). Creating nursing's new academic spaces: Making dreams come true. *Journal of Professional Nursing, 32*(3), 213–223.

Bowman, C. C., Johnson, L., Cox, M., Rick, C., Dougherty, M., Alt-White, A. C., . . . Dobalian, A. (2011). The Department of Veterans Affairs Nursing Academy: Forging strategic alliances with schools of nursing to address nursing's workforce needs. *Nursing Outlook, 59,* 299–307.

Edward, J., Rayman, K., Diffenderfer, S., & Stidham, A. (2016). Strategic innovation between PhD and DNP programs: Collaboration, collegiality, and shared resources. *Nursing Outlook, 64*(4), 312–320.

Greene, M., & Turner, J. (2014). The financial impact of a clinical academic practice partnership. *Nursing economics, 32*(1), 45–48.

Kulage, K., Schnall, R., Hickey, K. Travers, J., Zezulinski, K., Torres, F., . . . Larson E. L. (2015). Time and costs of preparing and submitting an NIH grant application at a school of nursing. *Nursing Outlook, 63*(6), 639–649.

Millett, C. (2016). Dollars and sense: The policy implications of financing an accelerated nursing degree. *Journal of Professional Nursing, 32*(5), S14–S23.

Moch, S., Jansen, D., Jadack, R., Page, P., & Topp, R. (2015). Collaborating with businesses to support and sustain research. *Western Journal of Nursing Research, 37*(1), 1308–1322.

Moore, P., Banks, D., & Neely, B. (2014). Making the business case for innovation. *Nursing management, 21*(8), 22–27.

National Institute of Nursing Research. (2017). Mission & strategic plan. Retrieved from https://www.ninr.nih.gov/aboutninr/ninr-mission-and-strategic-plan

Pearson, M., Wyte-Lake, T., Bowman, C., Needleman, J., & Dobalian, A. (2015). Assessing the impact of academic-practice partnerships on nursing staff. *BioMed Central Nursing, 14*, 28. doi:10.1186/s12912-015-0085-7

Roark, S. (2015). Why incentives are key to surviving tight safety budget challenges. *Occupational Health & Safety, 84*(9), 72.

Starck, P. (2015). Fundraising for accelerated study for the PhD in nursing: A community partnership. *Journal of Professional Nursing, 31*(3), 179–186.

Stout, C., Short, N., Aldrich, K., Cintron, R., Provencio-Vasquez, E. (2015). Meeting the future of nursing report™ recommendations: A successful practice-academic partnership. *Nursing Economics, 33*(3), 161.

Yucha, C., Smyer, T., & Strano-Perry, S. (2014). Sustaining nursing programs in the face of budget cuts and faculty shortages. *Journal of Professional Nursing, 30*(1), 5–9.

SECTION III

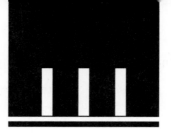

Curriculum Development Processes

Stephanie S. DeBoor

Sarah B. Keating

OVERVIEW OF CURRICULUM DEVELOPMENT PROCESSES

Prior to discussing curriculum development, it is useful to review the definition of curriculum. According to this text, *a curriculum is the formal plan of study that provides the philosophical underpinnings, goals, and guidelines for the delivery of a specific educational program.* Chapter 5 introduces the classic components of the curriculum and the process for its development followed by a chapter that describes the implementation of the curriculum through application of learning theories, educational taxonomies, critical thinking concepts, and learner-focused, instructional strategies. Specific chapters follow that describe undergraduate and graduate programs with the various pathways into the profession that are linked to them including a chapter on advanced practice and research-focused doctoral degrees. A chapter with a proposed unified curriculum summarizes the various educational pathways in nursing and the final chapter discusses the application of technology to the implementation of the curriculum through learning strategies, distance education, and the burgeoning growth of Internet programs.

Experienced educators will testify to the fact that as a curriculum ages, changes occur that were unintended in the original curriculum plan. These changes occur in response to feedback from students, faculty, and consumers; faculty's individual interpretations of the objectives and course content; changes in faculty personnel who are not familiar with the curriculum; changes in the practice setting; and the expansion of nursing knowledge. Unless there is continuous evaluation of the curriculum, the curriculum will eventually become so corrupted that it is barely recognizable.

Section IV that follows these chapters describes in detail the value of evaluation activities as they apply to approval, review, and accreditation of nursing programs. Still, it is wise in this section on curriculum development processes to recognize the need for continually monitoring the program, at least annually, to ensure that it is meeting the original mission, framework, goals, and objectives of the curriculum. The data collected from evaluation reviews and the recommendations issuing from them indicate to faculty the need for revising the curriculum, discontinuing certain programs within it, or initiating new tracks. If this exercise is conducted every year, maintaining the integrity of the curriculum becomes easy and there are fewer hoops to go through in seeking approval for major or minor changes. Annual review and minor revisions contribute to a curriculum that is current and is a living, vibrant organism that prepares nursing professionals for current and future markets.

PURPOSE OF CURRICULUM DEVELOPMENT

The overall purpose of curriculum development in nursing education is to meet the learners' needs by ensuring that it meets educational and professional standards and that it is responsive to the current and future demands of the health care system. To accomplish this long-term goal, the curriculum serves as the template for faculty to express its vision, mission, philosophy, framework, goals, and objectives of the nursing program. While curriculum development is the prerogative of the faculty, consumers of the program need to be involved in the process. Consumers include the students, their families, the health care system that utilizes its graduates, nursing educators and staff in the practice setting, and last, but not least, the patients who receive nursing care from students and graduates.

COMPONENTS OF THE CURRICULUM

The classic components of a school of nursing curriculum include (a) the mission and vision (for the future) of the program; (b) the philosophy of the faculty that usually contains beliefs about teaching and learning processes; critical thinking, scholarship, research, and evidence-based practice; and other selected concepts, theories, essentials, and standards that define the specific nursing education program; (c) the purpose or overall goal of the program; (d) a framework by which to organize the curriculum plan; (e) the end-of-program objectives or student-learning outcomes; and (f) an overall implementation plan (program of study). The components should be congruent with the parent institution's mission and philosophy. Chapter 5 discusses the components in detail and the pros and cons of frameworks to organize the curriculum plan including the use of nursing and other disciplines' theories and concepts and professionally defined standards or essentials of education. Chapter 6 reviews learning theories, educational taxonomies, and critical thinking concepts, and their application to implementation of the curriculum. These major theories, concepts, and models serve to guide educators as they develop mission and philosophy statements for the program and build the curriculum plan. They are considered again in detail as faculty applies them to the implementation of the curriculum through the processes of learner-focused instructional design and student evaluation. Chapter 6 discusses course development approaches to provide state–of-the-art active learning strategies to realize the mission and goals of the curriculum.

LEVELS OF NURSING EDUCATION

Chapters 7, 8, and 9 apply the components of the curriculum to the various levels of nursing education including the associate degree, the baccalaureate, master's, doctor of nursing practice (DNP), and research-based doctorates (e.g., the PhD and DNS). Each chapter provides a summary of the role that each level of education plays in the mission, philosophy, organizational framework, goals, and end-of-program objectives for its parent institution. The various pathways to completion and entry into practice, as well as advanced practice, are included. Issues that apply to each such as entry into practice, opportunities for further education, advanced practice, contributions to nursing education and the profession, evidence-based practice, and research are discussed. To summarize the various pathways into nursing at the entry and advanced practice levels, Chapter 10 proposes a unified curriculum for nonstop entry into practice ending with a doctorate. Parallel to it is the same curriculum that allows nurses to step out when they wish to enter practice and later, continue their education into advanced roles. The latter facilitates this movement by removing some of the barriers to continuing education that presently exist.

DISTANCE EDUCATION AND TECHNOLOGY

Chapter 11 examines informatics and technology and their influence on nursing education. It traces the history of distance education from the early home study programs to today's high technology–based programs delivered from home campuses to distant satellite campuses, as well as virtual campuses in cyberspace. The tremendous growth of online programs that offer not only individual courses, but also degree programs and their impact on campus-based programs are discussed. The chapter goes on to examine realistic clinical simulation programs that allow students to acquire basic, advanced, and critical-thinking nursing skills in a safe environment prior to actual clinical practice. Other high-tech devices and systems such as electronic record systems, smart phones, electronic tablets, and advanced communication systems add to the rapid changes in the delivery of education and the need for students and faculty to keep abreast of the newer innovations.

CHAPTER 5

The Classic Components of the Curriculum: Developing a Curriculum Plan

Sarah B. Keating

CHAPTER OBJECTIVES

Upon completion of Chapter 5, the reader will be able to:

- Recognize the various types of educational institutions and levels of nursing education
- Distinguish the formal curriculum from the informal curriculum
- Analyze the components of the curriculum according to their role in producing a curriculum plan
- Assess an existing curriculum or educational program by using the Table 5.1

OVERVIEW

This chapter provides an overview of types of educational institutions in higher education and how the various levels of nursing education fit into them. It continues with a discussion about the classic components of the curriculum from the mission to its implementation plan. Table 5.1 provides guidelines for assessing the key components of a curriculum or educational program.

TYPES OF INSTITUTIONS

Most institutions of higher education identify themselves according to classifications found in the Carnegie Classification of Institutions of Higher Education (2017). Carnegie classifies institutions into the following categories: doctoral, master's, baccalaureate, baccalaureate/associate's, associate's, special focus institutions, and tribal colleges. Within some of these categories are subcategories such as R1, R2, and R3 for doctoral programs according to the level of research; and M1 and M2 to differentiate between larger and medium programs at the master's level. Types of higher educational institutions are classified as "private" or "public," and "undergraduate" or "graduate." For the purposes of this text, the discussion about types of higher educational institutions includes private (nonprofit and for-profit) and public institutions (federal, state, or regionally supported), as well as community colleges, small liberal arts colleges, large multipurpose or comprehensive colleges and universities, research-focused universities, and academic health science/medical centers.

"Sectarian" and "nonsectarian" institutions are yet another classification with sectarian institutions reflecting a religious affiliation, for example, Catholic University, Southwest Baptist University, Brigham Young, and so on. While curriculum development activities are quite the same across types of institutions, the differences arise when examining the overall purpose and mission of the institution and the financial and human resources that are available for revising or initiating new programs.

LEVELS OF NURSING EDUCATION

The types of nursing education programs addressed in this text range from the associate degree to the doctorate level and many nursing curricula include step-in and step-out educational programs that provide career ladder opportunities for nurses. Associate degree programs are usually housed in community colleges. These colleges are regional, public-supported institutions; however, there are some privately funded 2-year colleges that include nursing programs. Baccalaureate, master's, and doctorate nursing programs are found in both state-supported and privately funded institutions. There are a few "single-purpose," nursing-only schools. Many of these schools are or were former diploma, hospital-based programs with the latter converting to associate degree or baccalaureates in nursing. Most hospital-based diploma programs are affiliated with higher degree programs, for example, community colleges and baccalaureate or higher degree programs. According to the National League for Nursing (NLN, 2014) Annual Survey of Schools of Nursing 2014, diploma programs account for 4% of all nursing programs in the United States with most located in the Midwest and the East.

For all types of programs, administrators and faculty should plan in advance for the financial support of curriculum development and evaluation activities and investigate possible external resources such as grants for curriculum changes and program development activities. Federally sponsored programs that are available for nursing program development and traineeships may be found at the Health Resources and Services Administration's (HRSA) website (www.bhw.hrsa.gov/fundingopportunities).

THE FORMAL AND INFORMAL CURRICULA

The *formal curriculum* is the planned program of studies for an academic degree or discipline. It includes the components of the curriculum that are discussed in this chapter and the curriculum plan is visible to the public through its publication in catalogs and recruitment materials, and on websites. The *informal curriculum* is sometimes termed the hidden curriculum, or cocurriculum, and is composed of extracurricular activities. These planned and unplanned influences on students' learning should be kept in mind as faculty assesses and develops the curriculum. Examples include special convocations with invited speakers, student organization activities that parallel course work, and outside-of-class meetings with students and faculty to enrich learning experiences. The cocurriculum incorporates planned activities such as collaboration with other academic units, student affairs meetings (information meetings, orientation, counseling sessions, etc.), field trips, work–study programs, service learning, and planned volunteer services in the community. Examples of extracurricular activities are athletics, social gatherings, and student organization events.

Some examples of the informal curriculum's influence in nursing are student services activities and counseling, special convocations, graduations, honor society meetings, study groups, student nursing association meetings, student-invited attendance at faculty meetings, participation in academic committees, and so on. Many schools of nursing schedule informal student–faculty meetings, holiday parties, and special events such as pinning ceremonies, honors convocations, and so on. These activities provide opportunities for student–faculty interchanges to enrich and supplement the formal classroom setting, as well as facilitate leadership opportunities for the students.

Effects of Student–Faculty Interactions on the Curriculum

Several studies have demonstrated the positive effects that student–faculty interactions have on the learning environment and ultimately, on the success of the curriculum's purpose. Cress (2008) found that positive learning environments in institutions of higher learning are established by strong student–faculty relationships to mitigate a negative climate created by other students, particularly toward students of color, females, and gay/lesbian groups. The positive relationships between faculty and students help create a positive learning environment. The article, Influencing Academic Motivation: The Effects of Student–Faculty Interaction (Teniell, Trolian, Jach, Hanson, & Pascarella, 2016), examined the leading factors from the Wabash National Study of Liberal Arts Education that most influenced student motivation in 4-year colleges. The student–faculty interactions that were positive included quality of interaction, frequency, research with the faculty, personal discussion, and out-of-class interactions. Smith (2015) discussed the influence of interactions between faculty and students in virtual classrooms on pedagogical, curricular, and instructional outcomes. The author offers specific strategies for orienting adjunct faculty to the challenges of teaching online and at the same time, maintaining contact with the institution, community, and colleagues.

THE CAMPUS ENVIRONMENT

Traditionally in higher education, the physical environment (campus) is important to the image of the home institution and plays a major role in building a sense of belonging for students and alumni alike. Schimek (2016) studied students' perceptions of a liberal arts college environment in relationship to its mission. She found several themes including:

- Sense of community, student focus, support, friendships
- Environment and physical space
- Well-rounded, integrative, and interdisciplinary
- Students as partners in the enterprise, not consumers

Schimek's study supports the notion of campus as place and its influence on the educational environment for students, especially in traditional institutions, but what about the virtual learning environment (VLE)?

While the physical environment plays a small role in programs that are delivered in cyberspace, some colleges and universities require periodic on-campus academic program meetings or residencies and offer special events for distance education students to experience the on-site campus. Another strategy is to provide program information materials that include pictures of the campus and campus life. This helps students identify with the physical location and landscape to form images unique to the home campus. The VLE presents challenges to teachers to develop an academic, online environment that includes faculty office hours, student and faculty meeting rooms, and learning strategies that foster a sense of community.

Jones, Stephens, Branch-Mueller, and deGroot (2016) surveyed students enrolled in a Massive Open Online Course (MOOC) for their impressions of community within the course. Concepts to guide the study were those of Wenger-Trayner and Wenger-Trayner's (2014) communities of practice and affinity spaces where students help each other, share interests, consider others' ideas, and work to meet the common goal. Jones et al. found that the 151 MOOC respondents (41% return rate) defined community as commonalities or shared experiences, including shared interests, backgrounds, and commitment.

COMPONENTS OF THE CURRICULUM

The following discussion examines each of the major components of the curriculum from the mission and/or vision statements to the philosophy statement that embraces faculty beliefs and values about liberal education and the sciences; professional values, professionalism, and nursing practice; interprofessional communication and collaboration; social justice, advocacy, diversity, and cultural competence; the health care system; prevention of disease and promotion of health; patient safety and quality health care; scholarship, research, translational science, and evidence-based practice (EBP); information systems and technology; critical thinking; and teaching and learning concepts and theories. A description follows on how the organizational framework and/or concept analysis/map, overall goal or purpose of the curriculum, end-of-program objectives/student-learning outcomes (SLOs), and level objectives guide the implementation plan that flows from the mission and philosophy statements.

THE MISSION OR VISION STATEMENT

Traditionally, higher education institutions in the United States have three major elements included in their mission, that is, teaching/learning, service, and scholarship/research. The mission statement for each institution depends on the nature of the institution and the three major elements are often divided into separate permutations. In more recent times, some organizations either replace or supplement the mission statement with a vision statement. For the purposes of this discussion, the *mission statement* is the institution's beliefs about its role and responsibilities for the preparation of its graduates (outcomes). It may discuss the classic teaching/learning, service, and scholarship functions as they relate to the purpose of the institution. A *vision statement* is outlook oriented and reflects the institution's plans and dreams about its direction for the future. It is usually short, visionary, and inspirational.

Chief administrators (presidents) of institutions of higher learning assume much of the responsibility for ensuring that the mission and vision are current and reflect the purpose of the college or university. They provide the leadership and resources for administrators, staff, faculty, and students to implement the mission and vision, to maintain its relevancy in the community, and to meet future educational needs. Developing or revising mission and vision statements is usually a part of a strategic planning process that involves all of the constituents within the institution.

The purpose/mission of the institution is examined and a vision statement is developed that looks into the future for the next decade or two. These activities foster creativity and a movement toward the future that provide the framework for planning. After consensus is reached, the mission and vision statements serve as the guiding documents for developing long-range goals and implementing them. Measures to determine if the mission is realized throughout the educational process and according to the expectations of graduates' performance in the real world give feedback as to how well the mission is met. For example, if the mission has a strong research emphasis, there should be adequate support and funding for faculty to write grants to sponsor research, and released time and facilities to conduct their studies. Leonard and Huang (2014) offer a mathematical formula for measuring SLOs according to the mission statement of the institution. While the formula may be complex, the idea to ensure that every course in the curriculum can be analyzed for its role in achieving the mission of the college/university is excellent. When evaluating, revising, and developing curricula, the courses under assessment should be analyzed according to their specific roles in meeting the mission and vision of the institution.

Unless the nursing program is a stand-alone academic entity, the mission of the major *also institution* academic division (e.g., college or school in which it resides), is examined in addition to *m+V* that of the parent institution. Both the missions of the parent institution and its academic subdivision should be congruent with each other and provide guidelines for the mission statement of the nursing program. Smaller institutions may focus on liberal arts as a basis for all disciplines and professional programs to meet societal needs, while large research-oriented universities or academic health sciences centers might espouse new knowledge breakthroughs by its faculty's and graduate students' research. In the case of the former, nursing's mission statement would reflect the graduation of well-prepared nurses to meet current and future health care demands; the latter would have an emphasis on nursing research and leadership in the profession.

As with the presidents of universities and colleges, deans and directors of nursing education programs have a leadership role in developing program missions and visions that are not only congruent with the parent institutions, but look to the future. Additionally, the mission needs to be examined frequently for its relevance to the rapidly changing health care system and the needs of society.

PHILOSOPHY *(based on m+V)*

A definition for philosophy is an analysis of the explanations for certain views or concepts as expressed into fundamental beliefs. The philosophy for a curriculum should flow from the mission and vision. It gives faculty members the opportunity to discuss their beliefs, values, and attitudes about nursing and an education that imparts a body of knowledge and skills for the next generation of care providers. Faculty members discuss their beliefs about their specific school of nursing and its role in preparing nurses for the future. Each individual member holds his or her own personal philosophy of education and nursing and thus the development of a philosophical statement can become an arduous task on which to agree. Nevertheless, the resulting statement reflects the faculty's (as an entity) rationale for the school of nursing's existence and it serves to flavor the remainder of the curriculum components, their implementation, and their outcomes.

The first task in the development of a philosophy statement is to look at those of the *1st* parent institution and the subdivision of the parent in which nursing is housed. The ideal nursing philosophy incorporates all of the components of the other two philosophies, although at times there are mismatches to some of the specific components. In those instances, a rationale as to why that incongruence exists and how the nursing program meets other components of the philosophy should be discussed. Eventually, this rationale is documented so that members of the school and external reviewers understand the fit of the nursing program within its parent institution and subdivision.

Some examples of incongruence of a nursing program's philosophy with its parent institution's philosophy occur when the program is within a traditional, liberal arts college that has no other professional programs. In this case, the nursing program's philosophy speaks to the importance of a strong liberal arts foundation for its graduates and the role of the nursing program to produce graduates who provide health care for the community. Another example is a nursing program housed within a school of engineering, along with several other professional programs such as computer science and journalism. In this case, nursing emphasizes the professional educational aspects and preparation of professionals who serve the community.

The majority of nursing education programs' philosophies include the basic theories, concepts, beliefs, and values of faculty. The statement can be brief and succinct or lengthy; however, it should offer guiding principles for the remainder of the curriculum and should be evident in the organizational framework(s), goals, objectives, and the implementation plan through its courses. The following discussion reviews many of the concepts found in nursing education program philosophies and is offered as a way for faculty to share ideas and beliefs and find consensus for developing or revising the program's philosophy.

ESSENTIALS FROM THE LIBERAL ARTS AND THE SCIENCES

The liberal arts and the sciences serve as the knowledge base for the discipline of nursing. Other health disciplines such as dietetics, medicine, and public health recognize the value of preparing professionals who can integrate the humanities, social sciences, and "the hard sciences" to provide care for those they serve (Boudreau & Fuks, 2015; Rozier & Schiff, 2013; Stein, 2014). The liberal arts and sciences provide students with the critical thinking, inquiry, philosophy, writing, communications, mathematics, science, and research skills that serve as the foundation to the professional role.

Along with the traditional requisite sciences of anatomy, chemistry, microbiology, nutrition, and physiology for nursing, genomics is now included in most programs as a separate course or integrated throughout the curriculum. The American Nurses Association (2009) published the second consensus document on the *Essentials of Genetic and Genomic Nursing: Competencies, Curricula Guidelines, and Outcome Indicators* that is useful in planning for its content in nursing education. Conley et al. (2015) discuss the integration of omics into doctoral level nursing curricula as recommended by the National Council for the Advancement of Nursing for nurse scientists to keep pace with emerging scientific findings. Omics include the sciences of genomics, transcriptomics, proteomics, epigenomics, exposomics, microbiomics, and metabolomics. The continual breakthroughs of knowledge from the national Human Genome Project (HGP) illustrate the important contributions genetics have on the health of individuals. The latest information from the HGP may be found at www.genome.gov/10001772 (National Human Genome Research Institute, 2017).

PROFESSIONAL VALUES, PROFESSIONALISM, AND NURSING PRACTICE

Nursing has the largest number of professionals in the U.S. health care system and while it has many pathways for entry into professional practice, it meets the criteria of a profession, that is, a professional discipline requiring a specific body of knowledge with members who study and practice the discipline. It includes specific ethics and theories, and it produces relevant research. Regarding ethics and professional values, Epstein and Turner (2010) provide an overview of the nursing code of ethics including the history of its development, its contribution to the profession, and its value to nurses in practice in all settings.

Fisher (2014) compared diploma, associate degree, and baccalaureate nursing students' development of professional values over the length of their programs. The students were assessed on factors contributing to professional values including caring, activism, trust, professionalism, and justice. While the study was limited to one geographical area, there were statistically significant differences found among the students in the programs particularly between the diploma students and ADN students. The author reviews Benner's (1984) novice to expert model and the idea of quantity of time as well as quality for the integration of professional values in the curriculum. She states that "personal values and morals should be molded into the ethical standards of the nursing profession while students advance along the continuum of professionalism" (p. 41).

The question of differences in the moral reasoning of various generations of students is raised by McLeod-Sordjan (2014). The author reported that according to recent studies, graduates who represent the millennial generation do not advocate for their patients or assert themselves during moral conflicts. In order to evaluate the success of a curriculum in the preparation of ethical nurses, McLeod-Sordjan recommends the integration of moral reasoning and social justice concepts into the program and the use of various assessment tools to measure learning outcomes as they progress through the program and upon graduation.

INTERPROFESSIONAL COMMUNICATION AND COLLABORATION

Nursing and other health care disciplines recognize the need for interprofessional education, and with the complexity of the current U.S. health care system, it is an important concept to include in discussions and planning for the educational program. The American Association of Colleges of Nursing (AACN, n.d.) and the NLN (2017) support the Institute of Medicine's (IOM, 2010) recommendations that call for interprofessional collaboration to meet the health care needs of the population. AACN (2008) lists one of its eight essentials of baccalaureate education as "Interprofessional Communication and Collaboration for Improving Patient Health Outcomes" and NLN lists specific recommendations for administrators and faculty for interprofessional collaboration in education and practice NLN.

Loversidge and Demb (2015) interviewed nursing and medical faculty in several Midwest universities for their perceptions on what factors influence positive interprofessional educational experiences for prelicensure medical and nursing students. Several themes came from the interviews including differences between undergraduate and graduate levels of education, the need for experiences that are authentic and facilitated by faculty, and a commitment to the concept and experiences by all faculty members (part time and full time).

Several examples from the literature exemplify the collaboration among other disciplines and serve as models for developing curricular experiences that are interdisciplinary in nature. A meta-analysis of surveys of medical and nursing students for their beliefs about interprofessional collaboration found that physicians and medical students perceived the existence of interprofessional collaboration more often than nurses and nursing students; however, nursing had a more positive attitude toward collaboration. The study also found that interprofessional education interventions help reduce the differences between nurses and physicians (Sollami, Caricati, & Srali, 2015).

J. Murphy and Nimmagadda (2015) describe an experience of interprofessional learning activities for social work and nursing students through simulation. They found that simulation is an effective strategy for meeting the core competencies of interprofessional collaboration in the curricula for both disciplines. The effectiveness of an interprofessional course for athletic training, magnetic resonance imaging, nuclear medicine, nursing, occupational therapy, and physical therapy students was studied through a content analysis of student writings (Bultas, Ruebling, Breitbach, & Carlson, 2016). The researchers identified eight themes from the analysis that included an increased self-awareness, need for a system change, need for quality care, issues of access, affordability of health care, a vision for future practice roles, the importance of disease prevention, and the value of interprofessional collaboration. The authors conclude that interprofessional courses are important to integrate into the curriculum, especially for content common to all professionals such as prevention of disease and health promotion and the health care system.

SOCIAL JUSTICE, ADVOCACY, DIVERSITY, AND CULTURAL COMPETENCE

Many of the standards for accreditation of nursing programs and requests for proposals for educational funding refer to the notion of inequality, health disparities, and lack of access to health care for some populations. Certain populations and oppressed groups suffer the consequences of discrimination and unfair treatment in the health care system. Nursing as a prime caring profession must be cognizant of these injustices and have the power and strategies to advocate for their clients and themselves to provide quality health care for all. Social justice is an important concept often found in the missions and philosophies of educational programs; however, it is sometimes difficult to find evidence of its integration into the curriculum plan and its implementation.

Wilson-Strydom (2014) makes the point that issues surrounding social justice belong in the curricula of higher education and it is advisable to review key social justice theories in order to integrate them into the curriculum and put them into practice. The author reviews three theories and supplies definitions of social justice. According to Wilson-Strydom, social justice is a complex concept that embraces the notion of the inclusion of all individuals, groups, and cultures into society and to compare the advantages and disadvantages afforded to them by society. The three theorists that Wilson-Strydom reviews are Rawls's (1999) theory of justice as that of fairness within society. The second theorist is Young (1990) who accepts the theory of fairness and adds to it the politics of difference. Young focuses on the complexities of social injustice that include exploitation, marginalization, powerlessness, cultural imperialism, and violence. Fraser (1996) talks about fairness and injustices brought about by the dominant culture's indifference or the barriers it places to other cultures' participation in society.

Integrating social justice theories and concepts into the curriculum implies not only an understanding of the concepts but also an awareness of the social injustices in society and types of actions that nurses should take to bring about change. Woodward, Smart, and Benavides-Vaello (2016) reviewed the literature to find factors that influence the participation of nurses in political participation and social action. Three themes emerged: political education in the nursing curriculum, personal interest in political knowledge, and the value of collective action through membership in professional organizations. To ensure that social justice concepts and actions are included in the nursing curriculum, theories of social justice, political action strategies, and professional responsibilities should appear not only in the philosophy but specifically integrated into courses.

Diversity, cultural competence, and the role of nursing are major concepts within the social justice system. Diversity is defined in its broadest sense not only in terms of race, ethnicity, culture, language, gender, and other differences from the dominant culture, but also, in terms of the diversity of opportunities in nursing. Thus, when faculty develops the philosophy, it must consider these factors and how the curriculum will meet society's diverse health care needs from entry-level graduates who function in all settings to those in advanced nursing roles in primary and tertiary care settings. Nursing care requires cultural sensitivity and awareness of differences among groups, while cultural competence denotes the knowledge and skills required for delivering care in cross-cultural situations.

The AACN (2016) issued a draft statement with recommendations to ensure that the concepts of diversity, inclusion, and equity are implemented in nursing programs. Recommendations include the recruitment and retention of diverse students, faculty, and staff; faculty, staff, and administrators who practice diversity, equity, and inclusion; and the concepts should be central to the mission of the educational program. Bleich, Macwilliams, and Schmidt (2015) offer organizational strategies to implement these recommendations and discuss considerations for establishing an inclusive environment that embraces diversity and equity.

Cultural competence acquisition is described by Diaz, Clarke, and Gatua (2015) who surveyed and conducted focus groups with nursing faculty, clinical educators, and graduate students in community colleges and university schools of nursing in a rural western state (94% of the participants were Caucasian). The study found that participants self-reported themselves as culturally aware; however, a review of the curricula found the concepts hard to find except in the community colleges where the concepts were more explicitly expressed. In addition, faculty members identified race and ethnicity as part of the concepts of diversity and cultural competence but did not identify marginalized groups, isolated populations, elder groups, and so forth as part of the concerns for social justice and access to health care.

THE HEALTH CARE SYSTEM

Knowledge of how the health care system is organized, financed, and regulated is essential for nurses to understand how it functions and nursing's role in it. Nurses must be prepared to provide leadership in the management of health care services and to address policy issues. The current organizational system of health care in the United States is in a state of flux owing to the enactment, implementation, and repeal of the Affordable Care Act of 2010 (ACA, U.S. Department of Health and Human Services, 2017).

Chen (2013) provides an overview of the U.S. health care system and the effect of the ACA on health care. Chen reviews two of the major health problems that currently affect and, in the future, will affect the costs and levels of care for the U.S. population. They are the 65+ population with 40.3 million in 2010 as compared to 12 million in 1950 and the growing number of health problems arising from obesity with 38% of the population obese in 2010 compared to 15% in 1960. The percent of obese children grew to 17% in 2010 compared to 4% in the mid-1960s. Health insurance coverage contributes to the rising costs of health care because of the need to distribute costs over younger, healthier populations; however, after ACA was implemented, the uninsured rates fell from 17.1% in the fourth quarter of 2013 to 12.9% in the fourth quarter of 2014. According to the Associated Press, the percent of uninsured reached an historic rate of 9% in February 2017 with more than 12.2 million people signing up for coverage at that time (Alonso-Zaldivar & Vineys, 2017). Another issue in the system is the rising costs of medical advances and technology, although the results from their use may cut costs in the long term. Two positive changes brought about by the ACA are the mandate for coverage for preexisting conditions and coverage for dependent children under 26 years.

As a result of the 2016 election, it is possible that the ACA may be repealed or revised. Nurses must keep abreast of the changes in the health care system in order to advocate for people receiving services and to ensure safe and high-quality care. Curriculum planners, looking to the preparation of knowledgeable nursing professionals, should examine the history of the system for its implications on current and future health care services and provide the tools for political action in the health care arena.

DISEASE PREVENTION AND HEALTH PROMOTION

A primary resource when planning for a curriculum that includes population health, clinical prevention, and health promotion is the Healthy People Overview website (https://www.healthypeople.gov/2020/about-healthy-people/development-healthy-people-2030) that reviews the 10-year cycle agendas of the *Healthy People* from 1990 through 2020. The goals for 2030 were under development at the time of this writing and expected to be released in 2020. The high priority health issues and actions indicated for 2030 are to promote population health, to provide access to quality health care and services for all, and to focus on individual and social determinants of health. Currently, the 2020 overarching goals provide detailed guidance for nursing educators in planning programs that prepare nurses to prevent disease and promote population health. The goals include attainment of high-quality, longer lives free of preventable disease; to achieve health equity, eliminate disparities; to create social and physical environments that promote good health; and to promote quality of life, healthy development, and healthy behaviors across life stages (Office of Disease Prevention and Health Promotion, 2017).

Implications for nursing education come from the document and include the need for knowledge of epidemiology, population health, determinants of health, and disparities to achieve health equity for all groups. Grady and Gough (2015) review the National Institute of Nursing Research's (NINR's) strategic plan to address health care challenges through nursing science and provide examples of studies in nursing that met the prevention of disease and promotion of health goals. Major topics included symptom science—promoting personalized health strategies; wellness—promoting health and preventing illness; self-management—improving quality of life for individuals with chronic illness; end-of-life care—the science of compassion; and cross-cutting areas— promoting innovation-technology to improve health. After a review of the literature, Fawcett and Ellenbecker (2015) propose a conceptual model for nursing in its role to promote population health. The authors differentiate population health from public and community health and point out the fact that the U.S. health care system emphasizes the care of individuals rather than populations. The conceptual model can serve as a guideline for nursing education, research, and practice.

PATIENT SAFETY AND QUALITY HEALTH CARE

QSEN

Patient safety and quality health care concepts are embedded in nursing knowledge and patient-centered clinical practice. Based on the recommendations of the IOM (2001) regarding patient safety, these concepts receive emphasis in the curricula of health professionals and the delivery of health care. In 2005, the AACN and the Robert Wood Johnson Foundation founded the Quality and Safety Education for Nurses (QSEN) Initiative with its goal to prepare nurses to improve patient safety and provide quality care in the health care system. The project continues to this day. Barnsteiner, Disch, Johnson, McGuinn, and Swartwout (2013) report on the goal of the nationwide project for faculty to integrate six core competencies in patient safety and quality of care. Regional institutes were held throughout the United States with more than 1,000 nursing faculty members attending. It was found that the institutes served to motivate and equip faculty with the tools needed to integrate QSEN competencies into the curriculum. For current information on the project, the QSEN website (www.qsen.org) provides information on competencies, learning modules, current conferences, and so forth.

Increased acuity levels and patients with complex physiological and psychosocial challenges add to the challenges for providing safe and quality care. In addition, all of these factors call for interdisciplinary collaboration to ensure a safe and compassionate health care environment. The Agency for Healthcare Research and Quality lists prevention quality indicators, in-patient quality indicators, patient safety indicators, and pediatric quality indicators on its website at www.qualityindicators.ahrq.gov.

AHRQ

INFORMATION SYSTEMS AND PATIENT CARE TECHNOLOGY

Information systems and patient care technology are crucial components to include in the curriculum in order to keep abreast of expanding developments in the field and their impact on the delivery of health care, research, scholarly activities, and teaching and learning modalities. The integration and use of information systems and patient care technology are included in the AACN *Essentials* document for baccalaureate, master's, and doctoral education for advanced practice education (AACN, n.d.). Carrington, Tiase, Estrada, and Shea (2014) report on their review of the nursing literature for studies related to informatics and patient care technology and their impact on the delivery of health care. In just 1 year, from 2012 to 2013, the number of articles doubled and the authors attributed the increase to the push by AACN for the integration of these concepts in its *Essentials Series*.

Lilly, Fitzpatrick, and Madigan (2015) surveyed DNP administrators and faculty for their perceptions on the integration of information technology (IT) into the DNP curriculum. Results were somewhat limited as many of the administrators responded to the survey instead of forwarding it to faculty; thus, only a few faculty responded. However, the authors found some of the following barriers to integration of IT content: lack of interest, lack of administrative vision, lack of resources, lack of time to use it, and lack of qualified faculty.

Not only do technology and informatics apply to today's nursing practice and to students to gain nursing competencies in the care of clients, they serve as platforms for the delivery of nursing education programs such as web-based, hybrid, and web-enhanced courses. In the clinical setting, professionals and students use personal digital assistants, patient information systems, computerized medical records, telemedicine/nursing, and high-tech devices for patient monitoring and care. It is important for faculty to be knowledgeable about and competent in these concepts and skills in order to integrate them into the curriculum and assist students in the application of informatics and technology. Chapter 11 discusses in more detail informatics and technology as they apply to nursing education

SCHOLARSHIP, RESEARCH, TRANSLATIONAL SCIENCE, AND EBP

Scholarship and Research

Scholarship and research provide the foundation for EBP. Both concepts appear in nursing curricula and should be addressed by faculty when developing or revising the philosophy of the educational program. Scholarship and research concepts begin at the associate degree level and continue in complexity to the PhD where new knowledge is tested and added to the body of scientific knowledge for the discipline. Faculties identify the scholarship and research competencies they expect of their graduates according to the level of the educational program and the practice areas or role functions that they expect their graduates to achieve. For example, associate degree programs expect their graduates to use EBP based on credible, research-based nursing interventions, and to challenge practices that lack data to support their use and do not result in quality patient outcomes.

Baccalaureate programs usually require a basic statistics course to support a separate nursing research course in the curriculum with expectations that graduates will understand the research process so that they can be discerning consumers of the research literature and use it to provide EBP. Writing assignments across the curriculum develop students' scholarly skills to review, analyze, and critique the literature in order to communicate professionally and apply evidence from the literature to practice. Beal and Riley (2015) surveyed chief academic officers of programs across the United States for their perspectives on the development of clinical scholars at the baccalaureate level. The majority agreed that nursing faculty need to be the stewards of the profession for preparing nurses for the future who are clinical scholars. They recommend continued faculty development to adapt to the evolving demands on nursing practice in the health care system and changing student needs.

In the document *Essentials of Master's Education for Advanced Practice Nursing* (AACN, 2011), the AACN lists factors that contribute to one of its essentials, research. Factors include review of the literature, effective communication and writing, application of new knowledge to practice, utilization of informatics and technology, and so forth. Most graduate nursing programs require graduate-level statistics and research in nursing as core courses. Depending on the nature of the institution and the degree purpose (administration, specialty advanced practice, or community health) the program usually has capstone options that include theses, scholarly projects, professional papers, or advanced practice projects. Many advanced practice programs include comprehensive examinations in addition to the written paper or sometimes as the only capstone requirement. Requiring a thesis at the master's level is decreasing; however, it can serve as a pathway to doctoral studies.

At the doctoral level, both research-intensive (PhD) and applied practice (DNP) research projects require supporting research and statistical analyses courses. The number and depth of knowledge and research contained in these courses depend on the type of doctoral program. Research-based PhD or DNS dissertations synthesize knowledge of nursing science on a selected topic and generate new knowledge through quantitative, qualitative, or mixed method processes. Until the initiation of the doctor of nursing practice (DNP), doctoral degrees in nursing in the United States carried various initials including PhD, DNS, DNSc, and DSN. Ponte and Nicholas (2015) review the literature on the use of these initials and their history pointing out that the majority of the doctorates carried research and dissertation requirements similar to the PhD and that many schools converted the DNS, DNSc, and DSNs to PhDs, some retrospectively for their alumni. The DNP clearly is an applied professional/practice degree as described in the *Essentials of Doctoral Education for Advanced Nursing Practice* (AACN, 2006). One of the first essentials listed for the DNP is the requirement of scientific underpinnings for practice and includes the conceptual foundations of nursing as a discipline. DNP programs may require culminating projects that translate existing knowledge and research on a selected topic for the development of new, evidence-based strategies for advanced practice and/or their application to leadership roles that initiate change.

Translational Science

Translational science is a relatively new discipline in health care and applies to the analyses of research and current practice in order to apply these analyses to practice. Surkis et al. (2016) reviewed the literature for studies that claimed to use translational research methods. From the review, they developed definitions of translational science and a classification system for rating studies using this type of method. M. Murphy, Staffileno, and Carlson (2015) describe the differences between DNP and PhD programs and their emphasis on research, translational science, and EBP. Their point is that there are multiple opportunities for collaboration among the students and graduates of both programs to advance the science and practice of nursing. It is a useful article for program planners who are developing curricula for doctoral-level programs in nursing.

Evidence-Based Practice

Research and translational science are the base for EBP. Therefore, it is important for all levels of nursing education from undergraduate to graduate students to understand these concepts and discern between valid and reliable evidence-based nursing interventions and interventions that have no supportive data or rationale for their use. Mackey and Bassendowski (2016) trace the history of evidence-based nursing practice from the time of Florence Nightingale to the present. They review several definitions of EBP and the literature contains many versions of it. The essential concepts of the practice include that it is research based and nursing discipline specific, reflects the entirety of nursing practice and research, applies to all levels of nursing education, is a problem-solving approach to clinical decision making, utilizes the nurse's expertise, includes the patient's perspective, and operates within the context of caring. Its purpose is to ensure patient safety and quality of care, optimize patient outcomes, and improve clinical practice.

Karnick (2016) makes an impassioned plea for nursing to recognize the differences between EBP and nursing theory and that both are essential to the delivery care. She points out that the EBP model comes from medicine (however, nursing has adapted it to nursing practice and science). She reminds nursing: "Nursing theory undergirds the foundation of the profession. It is who nursing is" (p. 284). EBP applies to all health care disciplines and its utilization has a major role in patient outcomes and quality care. As with the research process, education for EBP is leveled according to the type of nursing education program. Associate degree students should have theory and clinical experiences that demonstrate the use of EBP. Baccalaureate students further this knowledge by raising questions related to practice and seeking answers through literature review. Master's students apply EBP in advanced roles, raise questions, and investigate current research to inform their practice. Students in applied practice or professional doctoral programs synthesize this knowledge and generate new interventions for EBP. Theory-based doctoral students study the domain of EBP and develop new knowledge related to its use and value.

CRITICAL THINKING AND ITS APPLICATION TO NURSING

Development of critical thinking is essential to the preparation of nurses for clinical decision making and judgment and is part of the *Essentials of Baccalaureate Education for Professional Nursing Practice* (AACN, 2008). Interestingly, Huber and Kuncel (2016) conducted a meta-analysis of the literature about the development of critical thinking in higher education. They mention nursing as one discipline that singles out the concept as a prerequisite to professional practice. However, they did not find differences between nursing students' acquiring of critical thinking as compared to other majors. They did find that the entire college experience results in the acquisition of critical thinking skills for all students but there is a paucity of studies to find differences among majors and also, follow-up studies of graduates' critical thinking skills. Based on the findings from their study, the authors recommend that academics continue to measure the development of critical thinking skills, long-term effect, and their purported effect on program outcomes. Most philosophies for nursing curricula contain some mention of the skill and its relationship to nursing practice and thus it is useful for faculty to discuss its place in the curriculum and how it applies to its specific nursing program and outcomes.

BELIEFS ABOUT TEACHING AND LEARNING PROCESSES

Beliefs about teaching and learning form the premise for the delivery of the nursing curriculum. In the past, courses were traditionally delivered through classroom lecture, clinical laboratory sessions, and clinical experiences in the reality setting. The emphasis was on teaching and the curriculum reflected that modality. In the more recent past, with the focus on program outcomes and the advent of technology, the emphasis changed to learner-centered education. The role of the teacher, instead of transmitter of knowledge, became a role of expert, mentor, and coach. Teaching strategies fostered active student participation in learning activities instead of acting as passive receivers of knowledge. With the change in focus to the learner, theories and principles of teaching and learning served as guides for assessing the characteristics of the learners and adapting those theories and principles to the needs of the learner. Chapter 6 of this text reviews learning theories applicable to nursing education.

ORGANIZATIONAL FRAMEWORKS AND CONCEPT ANALYSIS AND MAPPING

Organizational Frameworks

ACEN, CCNE

Although accreditation is voluntary, most schools of nursing in the United States are accredited by a national organization, either the Accreditation Commission for Education in Nursing (ACEN) or the Commission on Collegiate Nursing Education (CCNE). At one time, both accrediting bodies required or implied that organizational frameworks were necessary to design the educational program's objectives, content, and instructional design. It was common for schools of nursing to use theoretical or conceptual models from nursing or other related disciplines as organizational frameworks. These frameworks served a useful purpose to place certain theories, concepts, content, and clinical learning experiences into the curriculum. While they are no longer explicitly required in the standards for accreditation, a curricular framework is implied for both the ACEN (2017) and CCNE (2017). ACEN refers to professional standards and competencies while CCNE refers to the AACN *Essentials Series*. Many of the concepts listed under the discussion of the philosophy in this text are included in the accreditation standards for the curriculum, for example, social justice, population health, cultural diversity, patient safety and quality health care.

Concept Analysis/Mapping

The process of concept analysis or mapping is useful for ensuring that essential knowledge and skills are integrated into the curriculum. Concept mapping is a detailed analysis of a concept and its relationships within the curriculum that is depicted into a map with arrows signifying relationships. It should include the expected competencies for student achievement as well as the places in the curriculum where the concept is introduced, built upon, and mastered. Goodman (2014) discusses concept-based curricula and their role in preparing nurses for practice beginning at the associate degree level to the PhD or DNP. The curriculum focuses on four domains and their related concepts including biophysical, psychosocial, professional, and the health care system. It is her contention that using these concepts and leveling them throughout the various levels of nursing education can lead to high-quality and affordable nursing education. It encourages collaboration among nursing education programs at the various levels of proficiency.

Lane and Mitchell (2015) provide an example of a curriculum development project for a school of nursing in which faculty held a retreat and used content mapping. The faculty identified where concepts were introduced and how they were threaded throughout the program from sophomore to senior level. The process helped faculty to understand the curriculum and plan for its implementation. The process of concept mapping helps identify where critical elements and concepts occur and at what level. Once the mission and philosophy for the curriculum are finalized, and faculty members identify the major theories, concepts, and skills they believe should be in the curriculum through a concept analysis and/or organizational framework, an implementation plan for the curriculum is developed. Figure 5.1 presents a sample concept map for interprofessional collaboration in a baccalaureate program.

IMPLEMENTATION OF THE CURRICULUM

Overall Purpose and Goal of the Program

After the philosophy, mission, and organizing framework/concept analysis are developed, the next logical step in curriculum development is to state the overall purpose or goal of the program. There are arguments against behavioral statements for goals as postmodernist and humanism philosophies take hold in the 21st century. The arguments

Figure 5.1 Concept map for interprofessional collaboration at the BSN level.

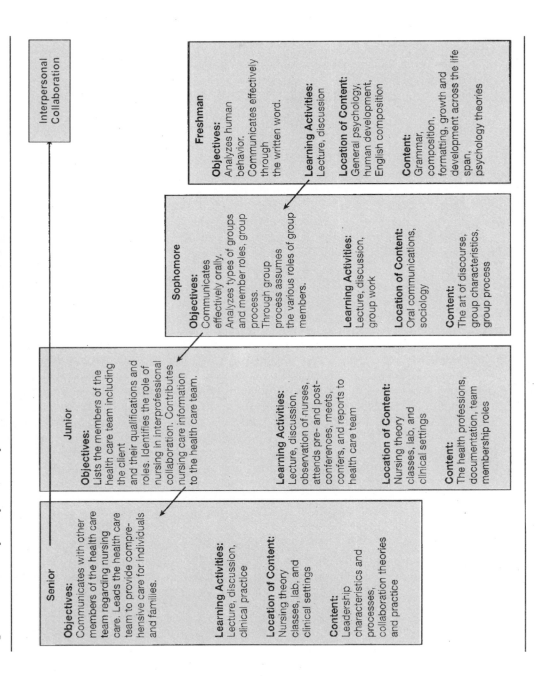

against them relate to the lack of freedom they provide for the learner and for the teacher whose role is to empower the learner. At the same time, there are accountability issues that relate to graduates' competencies in meeting the health care systems' demands and the health care needs of the people they serve. Faculty must grapple with these issues as it develops statements on the purpose of the nursing program and the overall long-term goal for graduates. Whether the statement becomes global and idealistic or specific and stated in measurable terms depends on the faculty's philosophy, values, and beliefs and subsequent statements and objectives that specify the graduates' learning outcomes.

In addition to a choice of the format of the statement of purpose or goal for a nursing program, that is, global or behavioral, there are certain components belonging to professional nursing education that faculty may wish to consider and include, if not explicitly, implicitly. Examples of concepts that might be emphasized include statements on caring, health promotion and other types of nursing interventions, client systems, professional behaviors and competencies, and the health care system. Characteristics of the graduate that are unique to the specific school of nursing can be included (e.g., "a caring, compassionate health care provider").

The type of nursing education program influences the overall program purpose or goal statement. Levels of clinical competence and knowledge acquisition will differ among licensed practical/vocational nursing, diploma, associate degree, baccalaureate, master's, and doctoral programs. Programs with multiple layers of preparation including undergraduate and graduate education usually have a global statement of purpose with each program, adapting that statement to meet its specific level of education. Although the statements of purpose and overall goal can be succinct, they act as the guides for the end-of-program objectives/SLOs.

SLOs OR END-OF-PROGRAM AND LEVEL OBJECTIVES

As reiterated throughout this chapter, nursing programs must demonstrate that they meet the overall program mission, purpose, and goal. SLOs or end-of-program objectives reflect the conceptual framework and define the specific expectations or competencies of graduates upon completion of the nursing program. In order to reach these objectives, intermediate level or semester objectives are developed in sequential order. For example, in a 2-year associate degree program, there are end-of-first-year and end-of-second-year expectations, all of which lead to the end-of-program objectives. In a baccalaureate program, there may be freshman, sophomore, junior, and senior level objectives. Some programs prefer to divide the objectives into semesters and could be titled in that fashion, that is, first semester, second semester, third semester, and so on. Graduate programs may indicate junior or senior levels, semester levels, first year and second year, doctoral candidate, and so forth.

Chapter 6 of the text provides an overview of the educational taxonomies such as the classics developed by Bloom et al. (1956). These taxonomies categorize domains of learning and provide guidelines for writing objectives related to the domains. The major domains are cognitive, affective, psychomotor, and behavioral. Furthermore, these domains are divided into levels of development and difficulty. For example, in nursing, the psychomotor skill of measuring blood pressure moves from recognition of the blood pressure measurement tools to mastery of the skill. At the same time, the student is utilizing the cognitive domain by first recalling the physiology of blood pressure and identifying the norms for blood pressure. The student continues to comprehend, apply, analyze, synthesize, and evaluate knowledge that results in nursing diagnosis and actions such as referral of clients for management of abnormal findings, teaching clients how to manage hyper- and hypotension, or in the case of the advanced practitioner, prescribing interventions to control hypertension.

The classic taxonomies assist in the development of end-of-program, level (intermediate), and course objectives. To develop or assess end-of-program objectives, the first task is to look at the program mission, purpose, and overall goal. Faculty members discuss what they expect of their graduates at the end of the program to meet the overall goal. A list of these expectations is developed into end-of-program objectives, which are analyzed for their specificity to meet the overall goal and the selected organizing or conceptual framework of the curriculum. For example, if the programs choose the AACN *Essentials of Baccalaureate Education for Professional Nursing Practice* (AACN, 2008) to guide the curriculum, the specific end-of-program outcome or SLO would state, "Apply knowledge of social and cultural factors to the care of diverse populations." From that SLO, concept analysis would take it down through the various levels of the curriculum with a junior level objective stating, "analyze the social and cultural factors affecting the care of diverse populations," and at the sophomore level, "identify the social and cultural factors that affect the care of diverse populations." Content related to these concepts would be listed under the objectives and learning activities described in order to achieve each level objective. All levels of objectives provide the guidelines for planning, implementing, and evaluating the curriculum.

Level or semester objectives follow the same pattern as the SLOs. Faculty reviews each level for the progression of objectives toward the end-of-program objectives. Some programs start from basic knowledge and skills at the first level or semester to the complex knowledge and skills expected at the senior level of the program. Other programs expect mastery of specific knowledge and skills earlier in the program that are reinforced throughout the program and practiced after graduation. Still other programs use a combination of both. Decisions on the patterns of progression will depend on the philosophy and organizational framework or concept analysis, including the developmental stage of the learner. These decisions should be documented with a rationale for their placement in the curriculum to aid in evaluation of the curriculum, total quality management of the program, and accreditation reports.

PROGRAM OF STUDY

The overall goal, SLOs, level objectives, and organizing framework serve as a master plan for placing content into the curriculum and developing a program of study. Faculty is responsible for developing the curriculum plan and revising it periodically as needed. The prerequisites for the program are examined for their logical location in the curriculum. Prerequisites for prelicensure nursing programs include the liberal arts; social, physical, and biological sciences; communications; mathematics; and other general educational requirements.

Graduate nursing programs usually require a baccalaureate in nursing, although students with associate degrees in nursing and a baccalaureate in another discipline are sometimes admitted conditionally subject to completing prescribed courses in nursing that the faculty designates as requirements for meeting the equivalent of a baccalaureate in nursing. The same principles apply to nursing or other disciplines' doctorate programs. Each doctorate program will prescribe the courses or degree work necessary to meet the equivalent of its lower degree requirements.

Once the prerequisites are completed, the nursing curriculum plan has a progressive order for sequencing nursing courses. For example, a Nursing 101 Fundamentals of Nursing course is a prerequisite for Nursing 102 Nursing Care of the Older Adult and Nursing 501 Nursing Research is the prerequisite for Nursing 502 Master's Scholarly

Project. Corequisites are courses that can be taught simultaneously and are complementary, for example, N301 Health Promotion of Children and Adolescents and N303 Nursing Care of Children and Adolescents. Again, the placement of courses depends on the curricular framework with the course objectives and content leading toward the achievement of level objectives and eventually, the program outcomes.

The numbers of units or credits are assigned to each course keeping in mind the total allotted to the major. For associate degree in nursing programs, nursing credits average 30 semester credits with total degree requirements averaging 60 to 70 semester credits. It should be noted that some programs operate on quarter credits or units that are usually 10 weeks in length as contrasted to the usual semester length of 15 weeks. In that case, one-quarter credit or unit is equivalent to two-thirds of a semester credit or unit.

Baccalaureate programs average 60 nursing credits with a total of 120 to 130 credits for the degree. The master's in nursing program ranges from 30 to 60 or more total credits depending on the nature of the program, with advanced practice roles requiring the higher number of credits. Owing to the wide range of nursing credits and the many credits required for advanced practice at the master's level, the profession is moving toward advanced practice degrees at the doctoral level. The majority of master's and doctorate degree credits are in the nursing major with only a few from other disciplines or electives.

Content experts serve as guides for nursing course placements and once the courses have been placed in logical sequence, the course descriptions are written, usually by the content expert or the person who will serve as "faculty of record" (in charge of the course). For example, the content expert for the course Nursing Care of Children and Adolescents would probably be a faculty member certified as a clinical specialist or nurse practitioner in pediatrics. Course descriptions are brief paragraphs with several comprehensive statements that provide an overview of the content of the course. They do not contain student-centered objectives.

Course objectives follow the course description, and are learner centered, based on the content of the course, their place in the curriculum plan, relationship to the level and end-of-program objectives, and relevance to the organizational framework. Finally, an outline of the course content is listed and should be tied to the objectives of the course. A course schedule is usually included and tied to the content outline. See Figure 5.2 for a classic outline for a course syllabus.

All of these components are subject to faculty approval as well as the parent institution. Once established, faculty members who are assigned to courses have the freedom to rearrange or update the content and to teach the courses in their preferred method. However, changes to the course title, credits, objectives, or descriptions must undergo the same approval processes as the original courses. Although this may appear stifling to academic freedom, it ensures the integrity of the curriculum.

Usually, new or revised course descriptions, objectives, and content outlines are presented to the program's curriculum committee for recommendations and approval, submitted to the total faculty for approval, and continue through the appropriate channels of the parent institution for final formal approval. Because of the many layers of approval, faculty members must be mindful of the initial proposals so that they will not need frequent revision, as any changes to course titles, credits, descriptions, number of credits, and objectives are subject to the same review processes.

SUMMARY

This chapter reviewed the components of the curriculum and the processes faculty members undergo in developing or revising curricula. Assessing and revising (if

Figure 5.2 The major components of a syllabus.

Parent Institution Logo
School of Nursing
Type of Program
Course # and Title
Course Description:

Credits:

Pre- or Corequisites:

Class Type: (lecture, seminar, laboratory, practicum)

Faculty Information:

Required and Recommended Texts:

Course Objectives:

Teaching and Learning Strategies: (include teacher and student expectations)

Attendance and Participation Requirements:

Evaluation Methods:

Assignments:

Course Content and Schedule:

Academic Dishonesty Statement:

Disability Statement:

necessary) each component of the curriculum in logical sequence helps maintain its integrity and ensure its quality. Faculty members are experts in their discipline and are therefore, responsible for ensuring that essential knowledge as well as the latest breakthroughs in its science are in the curriculum. Curriculum development and revision processes must be based on information from evaluation activities; the latest changes in the profession, health care, and society; and forecasts for the future. Table 5.1 provides guidelines for assessing the key components of a curriculum or educational program.

DISCUSSION QUESTIONS

- Which component(s) of the curriculum do you believe has(have) the most impact on the implementation of the curriculum?
- In which ways do you believe organizational frameworks or concept maps serve to ensure quality of the educational program? Give an example of an organizational framework that illustrates your belief.
- Why do you agree or disagree with the principle of faculty control of the curriculum?

TABLE 5.1   Guidelines for Assessing the Key Components of a Curriculum or Educational Program

Components	Questions for Data Collection	Desired Outcomes
Mission	What are the major elements of the parent institution and subdivision (if applicable) missions? Are these major elements in the nursing mission? If not, give a rationale as to why. How does the nursing mission speak to its teaching, service, and research/scholarship roles?	The nursing mission is congruent with that of its parent institution and, if applicable, the academic subdivision in which it is located. The mission reflects nursing's teaching, service, and research/scholarship role.
Philosophy	Is the nursing philosophy congruent with that of the parent institution philosophy and subdivision (if applicable)? If not, give the rationale as to why it is not. What statements in the philosophy relate to the faculty's beliefs and values about teaching and learning, critical thinking, liberal arts and the sciences, the health care system, prevention of disease and promotion of health, interprofessional collaboration, diversity and cultural competence, social justice, scholarship, research and evidence-based practice, information systems and technology, quality health care, and patient safety?	The philosophy statement is congruent with that of the parent institution and academic subdivision (if applicable). The philosophy reflects the faculty's beliefs and values on teaching and learning, critical thinking, etc.
Organizing Frameworks/Concept Analysis/Mapping	What is the organizing framework or concept map for the curriculum and how does it reflect the mission and philosophy statements? To what extent does the framework or concept map appear throughout the implementation of the curriculum? Are the concepts readily identified in all of the tracks of the programs?	The curriculum has an organizing framework or concept map that reflects its mission and philosophy. The concepts of the organizing framework or concept map are readily identified in all tracks of the nursing education program.
Overall Purpose and Goal of the Program	Does the overall goal or purpose statement reflect the mission, philosophy, and organizing framework or concept map? Is the statement broad enough to encompass all tracks of the nursing program? Does the statement lead to the measurement of program outcomes?	The overall goal or purpose statement reflects that of the mission, philosophy, and organizing framework. The overall goal or purpose includes all tracks of the nursing program. The overall goal or purpose is stated in such a way that it is a guide for measuring outcomes of the program (program review).

TABLE 5.1 Guidelines for Assessing the Key Components of a Curriculum or Educational Program (*continued*)

Components	Questions for Data Collection	Desired Outcomes
Student-Learning Outcomes or End-of-Program and Level Objectives	Are the mission, overall goal or purpose, and organizational framework reflected in the objectives? Are the objectives arranged in logical and sequential order? Is each objective learner centered and does it include the content, expected level of behavior of the learner, feasibility, and time frame?	The objectives reflect the mission, overall purpose or goal, and organizing framework. The objectives are sequential and logical. The objective statements are learner centered and include the content, expected learner behavior and at what level, feasibility, and time frame.
Implementation Plan	Does the curriculum plan reflect the organizing framework or concept map, overall goal, end-of-program, and level objectives? Is there documentation of approval of the curriculum plan in the permanent records? Does each track in the program have a curriculum plan that includes course descriptions, credits, pre- and corequisites, objectives, and content outlines?	The implementation plan for the curriculum reflects the organizing framework, overall goal or purpose, end-of-program and level objectives. The curriculum plan and its prerequisites and courses have the approval of the appropriate governing bodies. The implementation plan for each track includes all courses and credits, pre- or corequisites, descriptions, objectives, and content outlines.
Summary	Has each component of the curriculum been addressed? Is each component congruent with those of the parent institution? If not congruent, has the rationale for incongruence been addressed? Are the components of the curriculum listed and do they flow in a logical and sequential order? Does the implementation plan flow from the overall goal, SLOs, end-of-program objectives, and level objectives? Is the implementation plan congruent with the organizing framework or concept map? Is the curriculum relevant to current and future nursing practice demands and needs for nurses?	Based on an analysis of the curriculum, each component is addressed. The curriculum components are congruent with the parent institution and with each other. The components flow in a logical and sequential order. The implementation plan flows from the overall goal, SLOs, and level objectives. The implementation plan is congruent with the organizing framework or concept map. The curriculum reflects relevance to current nursing practice demands and the need for nurses and projected future changes in the health care system.

SLOs, student-learning outcomes.

LEARNING ACTIVITIES

Student-Learning Activities

1. Using the Table 5.1, assess the educational program in which you are enrolled for the components of the curriculum. Are they easily identified? What resources do you need to locate them?
2. Attend one or more Curriculum Committee meetings and identify which of the components of the curriculum are addressed. Observe faculty members' interactions, their commitment to curriculum development and evaluation, and the role they play in developing or revising the curriculum. Note evidence of the routes of approval for any changes to the curriculum.

Faculty Development Activities

1. Using Table 5.1, assess the educational program in which you teach for the components of the curriculum. Are they easily identified? What resources do you need to locate them?
2. When you attend the next Curriculum Committee meeting, identify which of the components of the curriculum are addressed. Observe faculty members' interactions, their commitment to curriculum development and evaluation, and the role they play in developing or revising the curriculum. Note evidence of the routes of approval for any changes to the curriculum.

References

Accreditation Commission for Education in Nursing. (2017). *Accreditation manual, standards and criteria*. Retrieved from http://www.acenursing.net/manuals/SC2013.pdf

Alonso-Zaldiva, R., & Viney, K. (2017, February 10). "Obama care" sees high enrollment: With health law in jeopardy, more than 12M still sign up. *The Gainesville Sun*, pp. A1, A4.

American Association of Colleges of Nursing. (n.d.). AACN essential series. Retrieved from http://www.aacnnursing.org/Education-Resources/AACN-Essentials

American Association of Colleges of Nursing. (2006). *The essentials of doctoral education for advanced nursing practice*. Retrieved from http://www.aacnnursing.org/Portals/42/Publications/DNP Essentials.pdf

American Association of Colleges of Nursing. (2008). *The essentials of baccalaureate education for professional nursing practice*. Retrieved from http://www.aacnnursing.org/Portals/42/Publica tions/BaccEssentials08.pdf

American Association of Colleges of Nursing. (2011). *The essentials of master's education for advanced practice nursing*. Retrieved from http://www.aacnnursing.org/Portals/42/Publications/Masters Essentials11.pdf

American Association of Colleges of Nursing. (2016). *Diversity, inclusion, and equity in academic nursing draft position statement*. Retrieved from http://www.aacnnursing.org/News-Information/ Position-Statements-White-Papers/Diversity-Equality

American Nurses Association. (2009). *Essentials of genetic and genomic nursing: Competencies, curricula guidelines, and outcome indicators* (2nd ed.). Retrieved from https://www.genome.gov/ pages/careers/healthprofessionaleducation/geneticscompetency.pdf

Barnsteiner, J., Disch, J., Johnson, J., McGuinn, K., Chappell, K., & Swartwout, E. (2013). Diffusing QSEN competencies across schools of nursing: The AACN/RWJF Faculty Development Institutes. *Journal of Professional Nursing, 29*(2), 68–74.

Beal, J., & Riley, J. (2015). The development of a clinical nurse scholar in baccalaureate education. *Journal of Professional Nursing, 31*(5), 379–387.

Benner, P. (1984). *From novice to expert: Excellence and power in clinical nursing practice*. Menlo Park, CA: Addison-Wesley.

Bleich, M., Macwilliams, B., & Schmidt, B. (2015). Advancing diversity through inclusive excellence in nursing education. *Journal of Professional Nursing, 31*(2), 89–94.

Bloom, B. S. (Ed.). (1956). *Taxonomy of educational objectives: Handbook I, cognitive domain*. New York, NY: D. McKay.

Boudreau, J., & Fuks, A. (2015). The humanities in medical education: Ways of knowing, doing and being. *Journal of Medical Humanities, 36*(4), 321–336.

Bultas, M., Ruebling, I., Breitbach, A., & Carlson, J. (2016). Views of the United States healthcare system: Findings from documentary analysis of an interprofessional education course. *Journal of Interprofessional Care, 30*(6), 762–768.

Carnegie Classification of Institutions of Higher Education. (2017). Basic classification description. Retrieved from http://carnegieclassifications.iu.edu/classification_descriptions/basic.php

Carrington, J., Tiase, V., Estrada, N., & Shea, K. (2014). Nursing education focus of nursing informatics research in 2013. *Nursing Administration Quarterly, 38*(2), 189–191.

Chen, Z. C. Y. (2013). A systematic review of critical thinking in nursing education. *Nurse Education Today, 30*, 236–240.

Commission on Collegiate Nursing Education. (2017). *Crosswalk table: Commission on Collegiate Nursing Education's (CCNE) Standards for Accreditation of Baccalaureate and Graduate Nursing Programs (2013) and National Task Force on Quality Nurse Practitioner Education's (NTF) Criteria for Evaluation of Nurse Practitioner Programs (2016)*. Retrieved from http://www.aacn.nche.edu/ccne-accreditation/Crosswalk-2013-Standards-2016-NTF-Criteria.pdf

Conley, Y., Heitkemper, M., Mccarthy, D., Anderson, C., Corwin, E., Daack-Hirsch, S., . . . Voss, J. (2015). Educating future nursing scientists: Recommendations for integrating omics content in PhD programs. *Nursing Outlook, 63*(4), 417–427.

Cress, C. (2008). Creating inclusive learning communities: The role of student-faculty relationships in managing negative campus climate. *Learning Inquiry, 2*(2), 95–111.

Diaz, C., Clarke, P., & Gatua, M. (2015). Cultural competence in rural nursing education: Are we there yet? *Nursing Education Perspectives, 36*(1), 22–26.

Epstein, B., & Turner, M. (2015). The nursing code of ethics: Its value, its history. *Online Journal of Issues in Nursing, 20*. doi:10.3912/OJIN.Vol20No02Man04

Fawcett, J., & Ellenbecker, C. (2015). A proposed conceptual model of nursing and population health. *Nursing Outlook, 63*(3), 288–298.

Fisher, M. (2014). A comparison of professional value development among pre-licensure nursing students in associate degree, diploma, and bachelor of science in nursing programs. *Nursing Education Perspectives, 35*(1), 37–42.

Fraser, N. (1996). *Social justice in the age of identity politics: Redistribution, recognition and participation*. Presented at the Tanner Lecturers on Human Values. Stanford University, Stanford, California.

Goodman, T. (2014). Nursing education moves to a concept-based curriculum: Association of Operating Room Nurses. *Association of periOperative Registered Nurses Journal, 99*(6), C7–C8.

Grady, P., & Gough, L. (2015). Nursing science: Claiming the future. *Journal of Nursing Scholarship, 47*(6), 512–521.

Huber, C.E., & Kuncel, N. R. (2016). Does college teach critical thinking? A meta-analysis. *Review of Educational Research, 86*(2), 431–468.

Institute of Medicine. (2001). *Crossing the quality chasm: A new health system for the 21st century*. Washington, DC: National Academies Press.

Institute of Medicine. (2010). *The future of nursing: Leading change, advancing health*. Washington, DC: National Academies Press.

Jones, K. M. L., Stephens, M., Branch-Mueller, J. & deGroot, J. (2016). Community of practice or affinity space: A case study of a professional development MOOC. *Education for Information, 32*, 101–119.

Karnick, P. (2016). Evidence-based practice and nursing theory. *Nursing Science Quarterly, 29*(4), 283–284.

Lane, A., & Mitchell, C. (2015). Two-day curriculum retreat: An innovative response to the call for reform. *Nursing Education Perspectives, 36*(4), 259–261.

Leonard, W., & Huang, C. (2014.). Linking classroom performance to the institutional mission statement. *SAGE Open, 4*(1), 1–8.

Lilly, K., Fitzpatrick, J., & Madigan, E. (2015). Barriers to integrating information technology content in doctor of nursing practice curricula. *Journal of Professional Nursing, 31*(3), 187–199.

Loversidge, J., & Demb, A. (2015). Faculty perceptions of key factors in interprofessional education. *Journal of Interprofessional Care, 29*(4), 298–304.

Mackey, A., & Bassendowski, S. (2017). The history of evidence-based practice in nursing education and practice. *Journal of Professional Nursing, 33*(1), 51–55.

McLeod-Sordjan, R. (2014). Evaluating moral reasoning in nursing education. *Nursing Ethics, 21*(4), 473–483.

Murphy, J., & Nimmagadda, J. (2015). Partnering to provide simulated learning to address Interprofessional Education Collaborative core competencies. *Journal of Interprofessional Care, 29*(3), 258–259.

Murphy, M., Staffileno, B., & Carlson, E. (2015). Collaboration among DNP- and PhD-prepared nurses: Opportunity to drive positive change. *Journal of Professional Nursing, 31*(5), 388–394.

National Human Genome Research Institute. (2017). All about the human genome project (HGP). Retrieved from http://www.genome.gov/10001772

National League for Nursing. (2014). *Annual survey of schools of nursing, 2013–2014.* Retrieved from http://www.nln.org/docs/default-source/newsroom/nursing-education-statistics/2014-survey-of-schools---executive-summary.pdf?sfvrsn=2

National League for Nursing. (2017). *Interprofessional collaboration in education and practice: A living document from the National League for nursing.* Retrieved from http://www.nln.org/docs/default-source/default-document-library/ipe-ipp-vision.pdf?sfvrsn=14

Office of Disease Prevention and Health Promotion. (2017). *Healthy people overview.* Retrieved from https://www.healthypeople.gov/sites/default/files/healthy-people-overview.pdf

Philosophy. (n.d.). In *Merriam-Webster's online dictionary.* Retrieved from https://www.merriam-webster.com/dictionary/philosophy

Ponte, P., & Nicholas, P. (2015). Addressing the confusion related to DNS, DNSc, and DSN degrees, with lessons for the nursing profession. *Journal of Nursing Scholarship, 47*(4), 347–353.

Rawls, J. (1999). *A theory of justice* (Rev. ed.). Cambridge, MA: Harvard University Press.

Rozier, M., & Scharff, D. (2013). The value of liberal arts and practice in an undergraduate public health curriculum. *Public Health Reports, 125*(5), 416–421.

Schimek, G. P. (2016). Visual expression of liberal education mission (Order No. 10137976). Available from ProQuest Dissertations & Theses Global: The Humanities and Social Sciences Collection. (1820073299). Retrieved from https://search.proquest.com/docview/1820073299?accountid=13802

Smith, W. (2015). Relational dimensions of virtual social work education: Mentoring faculty in a web-based learning environment. *Clinical Social Work Journal, 43*(2), 236–245.

Sollami, A., Caricati, L., & Sarli, L. (2015). Nurse–physician collaboration: A meta-analytical investigation of survey scores. *Journal of Interprofessional Care, 29*(3), 223–229.

Stein, K. (2014). The art and science of practice: The cross-section between liberal arts and allied health. *Journal of the Academy of Nutrition and Dietetics, 114*(8), 1157–1168.

Surkis, A., Hogle, J., DiazGranados, D., Hunt, J., Mazmanian, P., Connors, E., . . . Aphinyanaphongs, Y. (2016). Classifying publications from the clinical and translational science award program along the translational research spectrum: A machine learning approach. *Journal of Translational Medicine, 14*(1), 235. doi:10.1186/s12967-016-0992-8

Teniell, L., Trolian, T. L., Jach, E. A., Hanson, J. M., & Pascarella, E. T. (2016). Influencing academic motivation: The effects of student–faculty interaction. *Journal of College Student Development, 57*(7), 810–826.

U.S. Department of Health and Human Services. (2017). About the Affordable Care Act. Retrieved from https://www.hhs.gov/healthcare/about-the-law/index.html

Wenger-Trayner, E., & Wenger-Trayner, B. (2014). Introduction to communities of practice. A brief overview of the concept and its uses. Retrieved from http://wenger-trayner.com/introduc tion-to-communities-of-practice

Wilson-Strydom, M. (2014). University access and theories of social justice: Contributions of the capabilities approach. *Higher Education: The International Journal of Higher Education and Educational Planning, 69*(1), 143–155.

Woodward, B., Smart, D., & Benavides-Vaello, S. (2106). Modifiable factors that support political preparation by nurses. *Journal of Professional Nursing, 22*(1), 54–61.

Young, I. M. (1990). *Justice and the politics of difference.* Princeton, NJ: Princeton University Press.

CHAPTER 6

Implementation of the Curriculum

Heidi A. Mennenga

CHAPTER OBJECTIVE

Upon completion of Chapter 6, the reader will be able to:

- Analyze the application of learning theories, educational taxonomies, and critical thinking concepts to implementation of the curriculum
- Articulate the major principles of critical thinking
- Compare learner-focused instructional strategies
- Correlate student evaluation to the mission and goals of the curriculum

OVERVIEW

When planning a newly developed curriculum or a major curriculum revision, educators must address many aspects of actual implementation. When will the curriculum be implemented? How will faculty members, stakeholders, and students be informed of the plan for curriculum implementation? What are the logistics of curriculum implementation that need to be addressed? Other questions may be posed if an existing curriculum is being replaced. How will the existing curriculum be phased out? How will the change impact faculty workloads and scheduling? Beyond the logistical details of curriculum implementation, educators need to consider the foundational questions of the curriculum. What are faculty member beliefs in how students learn? What is the role of the faculty member and the student? How do faculty members best facilitate student learning? What instructional strategies will be utilized in the delivery of the curriculum? How will student learning be evaluated? How does the philosophical foundation of the curriculum impact the mission, goals, and outcomes of the program?

As faculty members consider these questions, often the task of implementing the curriculum can seem overwhelming. However, many of these decisions can be supported by having early conversations and discussions regarding the philosophical underpinnings that provide the foundation of the curriculum. Making a decision about a strong theoretical foundation for learning cannot be overemphasized as it allows faculty to provide a consistent rationale for decision making as the curriculum planning and implementation process moves forward (Dennick, 2012). The theoretical foundation provides the basis and the rationale for many other decisions, including specific instructional strategies that will be used. As educators transition from utilizing primarily teacher-centered instructional methods to more student-centered, active learning strategies, this foundation may be necessary to convince hesitant faculty members to attempt new evidence-based instructional strategies to aid in achieving the mission, goals, and outcomes of the program. Furthermore, how students are evaluated needs to be discussed and adapted to be relevant to the selected instructional strategies.

For the purpose of this chapter, the following learning theories are briefly reviewed: behaviorist learning theory, cognitive learning theory, constructivist learning theory, humanistic learning theory, adult learning theory, and brain-based learning, deep learning, multiple intelligences. Following review of the learning theories, the discussion transitions to the role of educational taxonomies and critical thinking concepts in curriculum development. This chapter concludes with an overview of learner-focused instructional strategies and student evaluation.

DEFINITION OF LEARNING

To start at the beginning, we must consider the definition of learning. Many definitions of learning exist and may vary depending on the theoretical viewpoint (Popkess & Frey, 2016). One simplified definition of learning describes it as merely "a change in behavior (knowledge, attitudes, and/or skills) that can be observed or measured and that occurs . . . as a result of exposure to environmental stimuli" (Bastable & Alt, 2014, p. 14). Some experts, such as Crow and Crow (1963), assert that learning does not occur that simply or as a result of only environment:

> Learning involves change. It is concerned with the acquisition of habits, knowledge, and attitudes. It enables the individual to make both personal and social adjustments. Since the concept of change is inherent in the concept of learning, any change in behavior implies that learning is taking place or has taken place. Learning that occurs during the process of change can be referred to as the learning process. (p. 1)

LEARNING THEORIES

Learning theories, which provide the philosophical foundation for the curriculum, attempt to describe, explain, or anticipate how learning occurs (Braungart, Braungart, & Gramet, 2014). Learning theories provide a systematic approach to curriculum planning and implementation and allow for consistency among broader program outcomes, and more narrowly, among course outcomes. Ideally, all aspects of the curriculum should be driven by an intended philosophical base that serves as the foundation of the curriculum. This decision, like many in curriculum planning, should involve all faculty members as the learning theory can provide the basis for the teaching process and direct which instructional strategies, and, therefore, which evaluation methods are utilized by faculty members. As educators see more diverse learners, additional instructional strategies and sources of evaluation may be indicated in the classroom (Hunt, 2012).

Although the select learning theories discussed in this chapter are presented separately, educators should keep in mind that they are not limited to a single learning theory, but rather may draw from several models simultaneously to inform their teaching practice. Each has its own benefits and perspectives of the teaching and learning process, which are discussed. Whichever theory or theories are selected, it/they should provide a clear reflection of viewpoints about the process of teaching, learning, and the internal and external influences of the educational environment (Iwasiw & Goldenberg, 2015).

As each learning theory is discussed, the reader is encouraged to consider the following questions:

- What influences individual learning?
- What is the educator's role in learning ("sage on the stage" or facilitator)?
- What is the learner's role in learning (passive or active)?
- How does the process of learning occur?

Behaviorist Learning Theory

Behavioral learning theories are based on the general assertion that behavior is learned and can be molded and rewarded to achieve desirable outcomes (Candela, 2016). Behaviorist learning theory emphasizes that behaviors, not thoughts or emotions of the learner, affect the consequences (Iwasiw & Goldenberg, 2015). Change in behavior occurs as a result of a stimulus or response (Warburton, Trish, & Barry, 2016). The emphasis of learning is on the environmental stimuli versus the learner's internal thinking process. The behavior (generally a desirable behavior) is repeated when reinforcement occurs and the learner begins to form associations with either positive or negative stimuli that occur in new situations (Braungart et al., 2014; Candela, 2016).

In education, behaviorism is illustrated by including behavioral student-learning outcomes that are measurable and observable. Students are aware of what they are expected to accomplish through these outcomes (Candela, 2016). In the teaching-learning process, behaviorism focuses on the faculty member as the facilitator who is responsible for designing the learning experiences and providing ongoing feedback to the student. In this theory, the role of the educator is to provide a stimulus, manipulate the environment, and merely transfer the information to the student. The student is thereby a passive recipient of the knowledge (Aliakbari, Parvin, Heidari, & Haghani, 2015).

Behaviorist learning theory focuses on the notion of simple to complex when planning a curriculum. It includes positive reinforcement and rewards for achieving behavioral outcomes (Iwasiw & Goldenberg, 2015). Continual reinforcement with positive feedback produces desirable outcomes (Candela, 2016). Critical thinking is also a key component of this learning theory, requiring the learner to sometimes practice "trial and error" to achieve the desired outcomes (Aliakbari et al., 2015).

Behaviorism occurs in the classroom or clinical settings when rewards or punishments are offered in response to desirable or undesirable behaviors. For example, the educator offering praise or positive responses may reinforce students' likelihood of answering questions in class (Braungart et al., 2014). Conversely, the educator may set up a behavioral modification contract to change behaviors for a student who is not performing well in the clinical setting. Behavioral learning theories are easy to understand and are typically used in conjunction with other learning theories. However, a main criticism is that it is a teacher-centered learning theory and may be outdated in today's student-centered learning environment.

Cognitive Learning Theory

Cognitive learning theory focuses on learning as an internal process including thinking, understanding, information organizing, and consciousness (Aliakbari et al., 2015). Cognitive learning theories explore the deeper aspect of learning, including how information is processed and the role of memory (Warburton et al., 2016). This theory proposes that behavior does not immediately change as a result of learning. Rather, students are equipped with the skills to question and problem solve, thus they are able to actively learn, solve, and search for new information. They focus on past experiences to inform better understanding (Aliakbari et al., 2015).

In education, cognitivism focuses on helping students develop the skills to think, not simply the transfer of knowledge. In the teaching-learning process, cognitivism focuses on the student as an active participant rather than a passive participant; however, the faculty member still maintains a majority of control over the learning process (Candela, 2016; Warburton et al., 2016). This learning theory supports many strategies for improving understanding and fostering memory and aligns well with the inquiry and analysis that occur in nursing classrooms.

Constructivist Learning Theory

Constructivist learning theories assert that learners create new knowledge when they base it on existing knowledge while attempting to find meaning in their experiences (Candela, 2016; Warburton et al., 2016). Social learning theory, sociocultural learning, and situated learning are examples of constructivist learning theories (Candela, 2016). In the teaching-learning process, faculty members assist students in learning how to become "expert learners." That is, faculty members provide encouragement to students to assess how their learning experiences or activities help them understand. This process of self-assessment helps students understand how they learn best (Brandon & All, 2010). Constructivism is viewed as a student-centered learning theory because of the emphasis on students' control over learning (Warburton et al., 2016). Learning is an active process in which the faculty member coaches and facilitates the learning of the student (Wittmann-Price & Price, 2015).

Specifically, social learning theory emphasizes the active information process that occurs during learning. Students learn by observing role models (Candela, 2016). In social learning theory, students are able to observe others, observe the outcomes they achieve or do not achieve, and then determine whether or not they want to emulate that behavior. This process includes four key phases: attention, retention, reproduction, and motivation. Attention requires students to identify whom they want to observe as their model; retention occurs when students observe the behavior and the outcomes; reproduction occurs when students are able to mimic the behaviors; and motivation occurs when students decide whether or not to continue the behavior based on the response they received (Warburton et al., 2016). Common teaching strategies such as simulation, clinical experiences, and role-play are often used with social learning theory as a framework (Candela, 2016).

Sociocultural learning emphasizes that learning occurs during social interaction. Students gain the ability to do some skills or tasks independently, but they must rely on others to help with other skills or tasks. As they gain knowledge, they need less and less assistance from others, eventually achieving mastery of the skill or task (Candela, 2016).

Situated learning occurs in "real-life" situations provided by educators in the academic setting, often through use of simulation or case studies. Students use these situations to enhance their learning and development of the skills needed in the real world (Candela, 2016).

Humanistic Learning Theory

Humanistic learning theory focuses on feelings and emotions with the idea that learning is an individual process (Warburton et al., 2016). Experiential learning is valued as is learning the art of "being" in nursing (Iwasiw & Goldenberg, 2015). There are several assumptions about learners in humanistic learning theory, including that they are motivated to learn, they are establishing and meeting their own set of goals, and ultimately, they will achieve self-actualization (Candela, 2016; Iwasiw & Goldenberg, 2015).

In education, humanism emphasizes the affective aspects of learning. Caring, individual worth, and autonomy are valued in the humanistic learning theory. Faculty members are facilitators in the learning process and role models, demonstrating values, such as caring and empathy (Candela, 2016; Warburton et al., 2016). Students are in control of the learning process, are accountable for their learning, and also determine their own goals and needs (Candela, 2016; Warburton et al., 2016).

Adult Learning Theory

Classified as a cognitive development theory, the adult learning theory asserts that adults are self-directed and will learn information that is useful and relevant to them. Additionally, adults bring their own knowledge based on their life experiences and generally, like to be actively involved in their learning. In the teaching-learning process, students are actively involved in the process and are accountable for their own learning. Students may also provide self-reflection regarding their progress. Educators, therefore, provide assistance to learning but work collaboratively with students in planning course information and experiences (Candela, 2016).

Brain-Based Learning, Deep Learning, Multiple Intelligences

Development of more recent learning theories focuses on the idea that the brain continues to develop and change throughout life and often, as a result of learning. These learning theories include brain-based learning, deep learning, and multiple intelligences. While it is not within the scope of this chapter to thoroughly discuss all of these, a brief overview is included. Brain-based learning asserts that learning can be enhanced by creating conditions where the brain learns best. These conditions may include relaxed alertness, where the environment is challenging yet nonthreatening; immersion in complex, multiple experiences; and actively engaging in the regular processing of experiences, which helps develop meaning. Deep learning allows students to dig deeper into complex and challenging learning situations instead of participating in surface learning only. Deep learning is intentional and creates new meaning for the learner (Candela, 2016). Multiple intelligences present the idea of seven constructs of intellects: bodily-kinesthetic, visual-spatial, verbal-linguistic, logical-mathematical, musical-rhythmic, interpersonal, and intrapersonal (Gardner, 1983). Each person has a different and unique intellect profile, some are more high functioning than others, and capitalizing on each individual's intellect "talents" may aid in the learning process (Candela, 2016).

EDUCATIONAL TAXONOMIES

Educational taxonomies, such as Bloom's taxonomy, are widely used in developing outcomes at the broader program level and, more narrowly, at course or module levels. Educational taxonomies serve to provide a framework for educators to identify, develop, and evaluate learning outcomes using a standardized system. They are helpful in identifying the level at which students need to demonstrate learning in order to achieve the expected outcomes (Scheckel, 2016).

Educational taxonomies are generally worded with the focus on what the student is expected to learn. The standardized language provides outcomes that are understandable and clear to both other educators and students. Commonly, faculty members may use educational taxonomies as a method to structure student-learning outcomes (from simple to more complex) across the curriculum.

It bears mentioning that objectives and outcomes are commonly used interchangeably. Both refer to what the student should learn or accomplish at the end of the module, course, or program. They both serve to describe the learner, the expected behavior, and the content (Wittmann-Price & Fasokla, 2010). The main difference, argued by Wittmann-Price and Fasokla (2010), is that objectives relate to the process and the goal of learning, therefore pertaining to both the student and the faculty member. Conversely, outcomes relate to the goal, or end product, therefore pertaining to the student (Wittmann-Price & Fasokla, 2010). Since education is shifting the focus of the teaching and learning environment away from the faculty member and onto the student, the term "outcomes" is more appropriate and will be used in this chapter.

Domains of Learning Within Taxonomies

Educational taxonomies provide the terminology to focus on the three main domains of learning: cognitive, psychomotor, and affective. Developed by Benjamin Bloom in the 1950s, Bloom's taxonomy is probably the most familiar and most commonly used educational taxonomy used. In the process of developing Bloom's taxonomy, the group determined that evaluation of learning must be considered through the domains of learning: cognitive—focused on knowledge; psychomotor—focused on hands-on learning and skills; and affective—focused on feelings, values, and beliefs (Halawi, McCarthy, & Pires, 2009). While this chapter briefly outlines Bloom's work, a detailed account of the work can be found in the publication of *The Taxonomy of Educational Objectives, Handbook 1: Cognitive Domain* (Bloom, 1956). Additionally, it should be noted that there are other educational taxonomies, although they are typically less commonly used.

Bloom's Taxonomy

Bloom's original taxonomy, developed in the 1950s, addressed six levels of cognitive learning including: knowledge, comprehension, application, analysis, synthesis, and evaluation. The levels were ordered from simple to complex with the idea that a learner had to master the more simple level before he or she could progress to a more complex level (Krathwohl, 2002). This thought, however, is also a criticism of the original taxonomy with many arguing that one level may not necessarily be more difficult than another (Asim, 2011). The main focus of Bloom's original taxonomy was on developing tests to evaluate students (Su & Osisek, 2011).

In 2001, Anderson, a student of Bloom's, and Krathwohl, a collaborator on the original taxonomy, substantially revised Bloom's taxonomy based on new knowledge and changes in the educational process (Bumen, 2007). The focus of the revised taxonomy was on student learning rather than only on the development of tests (Su & Osisek, 2011). Their revised taxonomy identified six levels with new terminology: remembering, understanding, applying, analyzing, evaluating, and creating (Anderson & Krathwohl, 2001).

CRITICAL THINKING CONCEPTS

The use of educational taxonomies directly relates to the role of critical thinking in nursing education. By utilizing all levels of taxonomy, educators can ensure that students develop the skills needed to critically think through situations. This requires well thought-out learning outcomes as well as structured, strategically developed activities and appropriate student evaluation of learning.

Educators are faced with the challenge of preparing graduates who are equipped with the skills necessary to care for patients in an ever-changing, highly complex environment. Patients are sicker and more complex than ever before (Finkelman & Kenner, 2012; Spector et al., 2015). While educators are constantly changing and updating content within the curriculum to keep up with the evolving demands of nurses in practice, the reality is that time with students is limited. There is only so much information that can be provided within the curriculum. Additionally, some of the content currently taught will be obsolete by the time students are practicing nurses. These challenges illustrate how important it is to teach students how to use critical thinking skills, clinical reasoning skills, and clinical judgment skills. While these terms are often used interchangeably, there are notable differences as defined here.

Critical thinking is defined by the American Association of Colleges of Nursing (2008) as, "all or part of the process of questioning, analysis, synthesis, interpretation, inference, inductive and deductive reasoning, intuition, application, and creativity. Critical thinking underlies independent and interdependent decision making" (p. 37).

Clinical reasoning is defined as the process used to acquire information, analyze data, and make decisions regarding patient care (Simmons, Lanuza, Fonteyn, & Hicks, 2003). Clinical judgment is defined as the outcomes of critical thinking in practice, a process that begins with the end in mind. Clinical judgment is based on evidence and looks at meaning and outcomes achieved (Pesut, 2001). To state another way, critical thinking and clinical reasoning are processes that occur and result in clinical judgment (Alfaro-LeFevre, 2013). The ability to critically think through situations is crucial in the provision of safe, quality care in any setting.

In a scoping review of the literature, Zuriguel Pérez and colleagues (2015) concluded that critical thinking in the nursing profession is very different than critical thinking in other professions. In the literature, critical thinking is defined as "controlled, useful thinking that requires strategies in order to obtain the desired results . . . the process of searching, obtaining, evaluating, analyzing, synthesizing and conceptualizing information . . . its attributes are reflection, context, dialogue and time" (p. 824).

While critical thinking is often an umbrella term that includes a complex list of aspects necessary for nurses to possess both in and out of the clinical setting, experts conclude that engaging students and using active learning strategies is an effective approach in teaching students to "think like a nurse" (Alfaro-LeFevre, 2013; Ward & Morris, 2016). Students must be equipped with well-developed critical thinking skills in order to gain licensure as a nurse and provide safe, quality care to patients. The National Council Licensure Examination for Registered Nurses (NCLEX-RN®) assesses the candidate's ability to critically think by utilizing higher levels of educational taxonomies. Additionally, the complexity of care required in today's nursing world mandate the ability of new nurses to critically think through situations (Alfaro-LeFevre, 2013).

STUDENT-FOCUSED INSTRUCTIONAL STRATEGIES

After identifying the learning theories that provide the foundation for the curriculum, utilizing an educational taxonomy to develop student-learning outcomes with consideration of leveling them to promote critical thinking skills, the faculty member needs to consider which instructional strategies are most appropriate to use. Faculty members must consider which learning strategy meets the goals of the curriculum as well as meets the needs of the learners.

Traditionally, lectures have been used in many nursing classrooms. Students attend class and listen to the educator speak, often following along with slides or notes. The focus has been on rote memorization with little opportunity for application or engagement in course content (Thompson, 2016). Teacher-centered learning, such as lecture, occurs when the educator focuses on pouring out information in a passive learning environment. Students are passive recipients, being provided with knowledge about facts and ideas. The focus is on "teaching" and the educator is a "sage on the stage." However, as faculty members seek out evidence-based teaching strategies and look at research surrounding student learning, a pedagogical shift occurs from teacher-focused instructional strategies to more student-focused instructional strategies. In general, these strategies focus on the educator as a facilitator of learning and students as engaged participants in learning. Students are involved in the learning process, either individually or in collaboration with peers, and are able to apply facts and ideas to actually grow their knowledge and understanding (Michaelsen & Sweet, 2008). There is research supporting this transition, stating that engaged students are more likely to meet learning outcomes (National Survey of Student Engagement, 2013).

There are several active learning strategies that can be utilized in the classroom. While it is not within the scope of this chapter to cover all of them, a select few teaching strategies are briefly discussed, including problem-based learning, team-based learning

(TBL), the "flipped" classroom, and simulation. This list is not exhaustive and other active learning strategies employed by faculty members may include discussion, case studies, concept maps, portfolios, and reflection, among others (Phillips, 2016). As with learning theories, the active learning strategies are discussed separately; however, the faculty member may utilize several different approaches or appropriately combine them to achieve student learning.

Problem-Based Learning

Problem-based learning focuses on clinical problems and professional issues that the nurse may face in practice as a mechanism for teaching students. This strategy is highly structured where students focus on real-life situations in order to learn. The faculty member acts as a facilitator of learning. Students cycle through five key steps in the process of problem-based learning. They analyze a problem, establish learning outcomes, collect information, summarize, and reflect. Problem-based learning can be done face-to-face in the classroom or in the online environment. Peer learning is a key aspect of problem-based learning (Phillips, 2016).

Advantages to using problem-based learning include the engagement of students in an active learning environment that fosters peer learning and evaluation. Dealing with real-life problems allows for information that can be translated to the clinical setting. Problem-based learning has disadvantages, particularly for the faculty member. As with many active learning instructional strategies, a significant amount of time is initially required to create meaningful problems. Additionally, students need to be oriented to their roles in the learning process. Problem-based learning can be difficult to use with large class sizes (Phillips, 2016).

The evidence surrounding problem-based learning indicates positive outcomes for students. While more research needs to be done, a systematic review by Kong, Qin, Zhou, Mou, and Gao (2014) found that problem-based learning may enhance critical thinking skills in nursing students. Problem-based learning has shown positive outcomes in clinical education and student outcomes (Shin & Kim, 2013).

Team-Based Learning

TBL is a structured, active learning strategy involving a sequence of three key phases: preclass preparation; readiness assurance process; and application. First used in business classrooms by Larry Michaelsen, TBL has now been used in a variety of classrooms including nursing. The structured TBL sequence occurs with each major unit or module of instruction. Ideally, the course is divided into five to seven major units or modules. Teams of students are formed at the beginning of the course and stay intact throughout the semester. Students complete the preclass preparation, which may include assigned readings or other assignments, before the module of instruction begins. When they physically attend class, they begin the readiness assurance process that includes completing the Individual Readiness Assurance Test (IRAT) and the Team Readiness Assurance Test (tRAT). These tests are based on the preclass preparation and consist of the same multiple-choice questions. The students first take the IRAT and then gather in their teams to take the tRAT. While not required, it is highly recommended that teams use the Immediate Feedback Assessment Technique (IF-AT) forms (available at www .epsteineducation.com/home/about/default.aspx). The IF-AT forms provide immediate feedback by allowing the teams to scratch off their answer choices (similar to scratching off a lottery ticket). If the answer is not correct, teams continue to scratch off their answer options until the correct answer is exposed. The immediate feedback provided by the forms allows for team discussion and learning to occur. Following the completion of the readiness assurance process, the educator can utilize class time to clarify any concepts and move on to the application phase. In their teams, students complete application exercises designed to engage students and allow application of key course concepts (Michaelsen & Sweet, 2008).

There are several advantages to using TBL. Students are able to achieve a deeper level of understanding because they are engaged in the course content. Because students work in teams, team skills are often improved and students gain insight into their own strengths and weaknesses. There are also benefits for struggling students who tend to perform better when TBL is used. Faulty members typically see a decrease in student absenteeism due to the reliance on teamwork and in-class activities. They are able to form more personal relationships with their students because of the increased interaction with students in class and the educational process is shared mutually between students and faculty (Michaelsen & Sweet, 2008). TBL can also be used successfully in very large classrooms, up to 400 students (Clark, Nguyen, Bray,& Levine, 2008). However, as with problem-based learning, there are challenges including student resistance and the time commitment required by faculty when preparing for class (Mennenga, 2013).

Evidence suggests positive student outcomes with the use of TBL including improved examination scores and enhanced student engagement (Chad, 2012; Della Ratta, 2015; Mennenga, 2013). Overall student satisfaction may be increased with TBL (Jafari, 2014). Additionally, a review of the literature by Haidet, Kubitz, and McCormack (2014) indicated that TBL shows evidence of positive outcomes for students regarding knowledge, engagement, and team performance.

The Flipped Classroom

Similar to TBL, the flipped classroom utilizes a reversed instruction model in which students complete preclass preparation and use in-class time for active learning activities. The idea is to "maximize the time the students and faculty have during the face-to-face time in the classroom" (Hessler, 2017, p. 12). The opportunity for students to begin learning outside of class time, independently, allows the classroom to be transformed into an engaging and interactive group learning environment. The educator acts as a facilitator of learning, guiding students as they learn to apply and critically think through concepts (Hessler, 2017).

In the flipped classroom, the typical traditional lecture is viewed by students before class time as preclass preparation. While the preparation may focus on reading assignments, many faculty members opt to use technology to capture their normal lecture content for students to view. Prerecorded video lectures, called "vodcasts," can be used to engage the student and can be viewed several times until the student gains an understanding of the material (Berndt, 2015; Hessler, 2017). Once in the classroom setting, students actively engage in learning activities focused on application of the content from the preclass preparation.

The flipped classroom offers several advantages to faculty members and students. Faculty members can use the class time more efficiently, clarify misperceptions of students, and cater to a variety of different learning styles. Students have the opportunity to be more engaged, to use technology in the educational process, and to actively participate in the learning process. There are, however, challenges that need to be addressed. Students and faculty may be initially resistant to a change in pedagogy, technology may not always work correctly, and, again, there is a time commitment required for preparation (Hessler, 2017).

Emerging evidence supports the use of the flipped classroom as an effective active learning strategy for students. In a study by McNally and colleagues (2017), student outcomes and participation were improved in a flipped classroom. While students in the study indicated the class was more difficult, it might be due to the increased student preparation required for the flipped classroom (McNally et al., 2017). Missildine, Fountain, Summers, and Gosselin's (2013) study found that student examination scores were higher with the flipped classroom strategy but students were less satisfied. A systematic review of the flipped classroom in nursing education found neutral or positive outcomes in academic performance and mixed results regarding student satisfaction. Student engagement was noted as a result of the flipped classroom strategy (Betihavas, Bridgman, Kornhaber, & Cross, 2016).

Simulation

Simulation allows students to participate in activities that mimic real-life scenarios or situations. Simulations offer students a safe place to practice and critically think through highly realistic and often complex situations they may face in the real world (Jeffries, Swoboda, & Akintade, 2016). Simulation, which may include manikins, standardized patients, role-play, or virtual simulations, has been promoted by leaders in nursing education, such as the National League for Nursing (National League for Nursing, 2015; Society for Simulation in Healthcare, 2015). In nursing education, simulation allows students to participate in experiences under the direction of a faculty member. Typically, simulation includes a debriefing that is essential to student learning. Simulation offers opportunities for interprofessional experiences and a strategic approach to structured clinical experiences in the simulation setting (Jeffries et al., 2016). Faculty members are called upon to integrate simulation with a clear idea of how it assists in achieving student-learning outcomes (National League for Nursing, 2015).

There is strong evidence supporting the use of simulation in nursing education. Benefits include active involvement of students in the learning process, effective use of faculty, improved student instruction, and opportunities for immediate feedback. One of the main challenges is ensuring faculty preparation to utilize simulation as an effective teaching strategy (Jeffries et al., 2016). Based on the conclusions of a recent National Council of State Boards of Nursing study, there is evidence that simulation can replace traditional clinical experiences for up to 50% of the time in nursing education (Hayden, Smiley, Alexander, Kardong-Edgren, & Jeffries, 2014).

When selecting instructional strategies, faculty members must also consider the most appropriate methods to meet the needs of diverse learners. Nursing students may vary in age, including traditional high school graduates who immediately entered college and older, more experienced learners, including some with a previous college degree. Learners may also vary in background, ethnicity, socioeconomic status, and academic abilities. These differences among students may impact their motivation to learn, how they learn, and their expectations (Candela, 2016). It is helpful if the faculty member can capture these differences to engage learners and enhance the learning environment.

STUDENT EVALUATION

Student evaluation determines whether or not program goals, program outcomes, and/or specific-course student-learning outcomes have been met by the learner. While often these are "end" goals for learning, educators should consider the process of how students will be evaluated early in the curriculum-planning process (Dennison, Rosselli, & Dempsey, 2015). As discussed earlier in this chapter, decisions regarding the different components of the curriculum, including student evaluation, should be based on a philosophical foundation, or learning theory.

Consistency among overall program goals, program outcomes, specific-course student-learning outcomes, and evaluation of student learning helps achieve a robust and methodologically sound curriculum plan.

On a broader scale of evaluation, curriculum planning should include alignment of overall program goals and outcomes with benchmark performance goals. These may include graduation rates, professional placement and performance of students following graduation, and performance on the NCLEX-RN. Additionally, student evaluation of learning will help guide faculty in determining whether or not the overall program goals and outcomes have been met.

In the classroom, faculty members should measure learning according to specific-course student-learning outcomes. How learning is evaluated depends on the course student-learning outcomes, the educational taxonomy level, and the instructional strategy used by the faculty member. For example, if an educator is interested in how well a learner applies information in the clinical setting, a multiple-choice exam may not be the most useful way of evaluating student learning. As the focus transitions from teacher-focused to student-focused instructional strategies, student evaluation needs to be modified. Faculty members should consider the following questions when determining how students will be evaluated:

- Do the cognitive level student-learning outcomes and the evaluation method match?
- Do the learning domain of the student-learning outcome and the evaluation method match?
- Are there various methods of evaluation included in the course?
- Are assignments group or individual?
- Are the course assignments and examinations manageable and realistic for the student to complete?
- Are the course assignment and examinations manageable and realistic for faculty? (Consider grading and providing required feedback in a timely manner.)
- Are the assignments and examinations weighted to show appropriate significance?
- Do the methods of evaluation optimize opportunity for student success?
- Do the methods of evaluation provide early signs of poor student performance (Dennison et al., 2015)?

While it is recognized that students have to pass the NCLEX-RN, which is a multiple-choice examination, it is recommended that a variety of evaluation methods be utilized in nursing education (Dennison et al., 2015). In a study with schools of nursing across the United States by Eder (2014), it was found that 95% of nursing faculty members utilize examinations as a source of evaluation. Examinations are often the preferred method of evaluation because they are relatively easy to grade and do not require large amounts of faculty time (Dennison et al., 2015).

Other alternative sources of evaluation used by faculty members may include simulations, clinical performance, demonstrations, case studies, concept maps, class discussion, role-play, games, papers, posters, presentations, portfolios, and reflections (Dennison et al., 2015; Eder, 2014; Phillips, 2016). All of these types of evaluation are appropriate for use in nursing education and may be considered by faculty members as forms of student evaluation. However, while examinations offer a straightforward, timely, objective method of evaluation, the suggested alternative sources of student evaluation may require more faculty time for planning and grading and introduce some subjectivity to the grading process. A proposed method for addressing subjectivity in the grading process is to use rubrics to evaluate students. A rubric is a tool used for scoring that clearly outlines the expectations of an assignment. Typically, a rubric includes levels of quality and the student is scored accordingly. To develop a rubric, the faculty member should use the course student-learning outcomes to determine how the specific form of student evaluation contributes to demonstrating achievement of the outcomes. Next, the criteria that are essential to the evaluation are listed with a description of the various levels of quality or performance. It should clearly describe what meets expectations and what does not meet expectations. It is recommended that the faculty member test the rubric to identify any items that may need to be edited before using it with students. Students should be educated as to how they can use the rubric to evaluate themselves before submitting assignments. Finally, the faculty member uses the rubric for student evaluation and if indicated, makes any revisions necessary based on the outcomes of evaluation (Dennison et al., 2015).

SUMMARY

As health care rapidly becomes more complex and diverse, nurses are required to know more, critically think in stressful situations, and act quickly in response to patient needs. In response, nurse educators are required to find ways to deliver the ever-increasing amounts of content, consider appropriate student-learning outcomes, experiences, and forms of evaluation. The ability of nursing educators to design a meaningful, purposeful curriculum will aid in the development of nurses who are prepared to meet today's challenges.

This chapter outlined the importance of identifying a philosophical foundation to inform decisions made in the curriculum. Beginning with an overview of select learning theories, educational taxonomies, and critical thinking concepts, the chapter illustrates the linkages considered in the process of implementing the curriculum. Education is transitioning to more learner-focused instructional strategies that are applicable to specific content, specific students, and specific environments. Appropriate use of student evaluation methods needs to be considered as well. This chapter is intended as an overview and readers who are interested in gaining a more thorough understanding of the content should seek additional specific resources.

DISCUSSION QUESTIONS

- What are the main differences and similarities among the learning theories that were presented?
- How can educational taxonomies be used to align program outcomes, program goals, and course student-learning outcomes?
- How do educational taxonomies drive the development of critical thinking skills?
- How does the use of learner-centered instructional strategies promote the development of critical thinking skills?
- How are educational taxonomies used in student evaluation?

LEARNING ACTIVITIES

Student-Learning Activities

1. Write a paper identifying your personal philosophy as an educator. Describe the faculty role and the student role related to accomplishment of learning outcomes.
2. Identify a nursing course that would interest you to teach in your future role as an educator. Develop four student course-learning outcomes and align them with Bloom's taxonomy.
3. From the activity in item #2 in the Student-Learning Activities, identify which evaluation strategies are appropriate to evaluate student learning.

Faculty Development Activities

1. Select a course you teach and plot your assignments according to Bloom's taxonomy. Compare the assignments with the course's student-learning outcomes. Share with a colleague and discuss findings.
2. Select a course you teach that is primarily teacher focused. Revise one module or activity using one of the learner-focused instructional strategies described in this chapter.
3. Develop a scoring rubric for an existing or new course assignment. Share with a colleague and ask him or her to score an assignment using the rubric. Discuss and revise as necessary.

References

Alfaro-LeFevre, R. (2013). *Critical thinking, clinical reasoning, and clinical judgment: A practical approach* (5th ed.). St. Louis, MO: Elsevier.

Aliakbari, F., Parvin, N., Heidari, M., & Haghani, F. (2015). Learning theories application in nursing education. *Journal of Education and Health Promotion, 4,* 2. doi:10.4103/2277-9531.151867

American Association of Colleges of Nursing. (2008). *The essentials of baccalaureate education for professional nursing practice.* Washington, DC: Author.

Anderson, L., & Krathwohl, D. (2001). *A taxonomy for learning, teaching and assessing: A revision of Bloom's taxonomy of educational objectives.* New York, NY: Longman.

Asim, A. (2011). Finding acceptance of Bloom's revised cognitive taxonomy on the international stage in Turkey. *Educational Sciences: Theory & Practice, 11*(2), 767–772. Retrieved from http://www.kuyeb.com/pdf/en/263fdbeb0076bbb9a65734ffeb534f82TAMEN.pdf

Bastable, S., & Alt, M. (2014). Overview of education in health care. In S. Bastable (Ed.), *Nurse educator: Principles of teaching and learning for nursing practice* (4th ed., pp. 3–30). Burlington, MA: Jones & Bartlett.

Berndt, J. (2015). Using a "flipped classroom" model to engage learners. In L. Caputi (Ed.), *Building the future of nursing* (Vol. 2, pp. 71–75). Philadelphia, PA: National League for Nursing.

Betihavas, V., Bridgman, H., Kornhaber, R., & Cross, M. (2016). The evidence for "flipping out": A systematic review of the flipped classroom in nursing education. *Nurse Education Today, 38,* 15–21. doi:10.1016/j.nedt.2015.12.010

Bloom, B. S. (1956). *Taxonomy of educational objectives, handbook 1: The cognitive domain.* New York, NY: David McKay.

Brandon, A., & All, A. (2010). Constructivism theory analysis and application to curricula. *Nursing Education Perspectives, 31*(2), 89–92. Retrieved from https://www.ncbi.nlm.nih.gov/pubmed/20455364

Braungart, M., Braungart, R., & Gramet, P. (2014). Applying learning theories to health care practice. In S. Bastable (Ed.), *Nurse educator: Principles of teaching and learning for nursing practice* (4th ed., pp. 63–110). Burlington, MA: Jones & Bartlett.

Bumen, N. T. (2007). Effects of the original versus revised Bloom's taxonomy on lesson planning skills: A Turkish study among pre-service teachers. *International Review of Education, 53*(4), 439–455. doi:10.1007/s11159-007-9052-1

Candela, L. (2016). Theoretical foundations of teaching and learning. In D. Billings & J. Halstead (Eds.), *Teaching in nursing: A guide for faculty* (5th ed., pp. 211–229). St. Louis, MO: Elsevier Saunders.

Chad, P. (2012). The use of team-based learning as an approach to increased engagement and learning for marketing students: A case study. *Journal of Marketing Education, 34*(2), 128–139. doi:10.1177/0273475312450388

Clark, M., Nguyen, H., Bray, C., & Levine, R. (2008). Team-based learning in an undergraduate nursing course. *Journal of Nursing Education, 47*(3), 111–117. doi:10.3928/01484834-20080301-02

Crow, L., & Crow, A. (1963). *Readings in human learning.* New York, NY: McKay.

Dennick, R. (2012). Twelve tips for incorporating educational theory into teaching practices. *Medical Teacher, 34*(8), 618–624. doi:10.3109/0142159X.2012.668244

Dennison, R., Rosselli, J., & Dempsey, A. (2015). *Evaluation beyond exams in nursing education: Designing assignments and evaluating with rubrics.* New York, NY: Springer Publishing.

Eder, D. (2014). Healthy assessment: What nursing schools can teach us about effective assessment of student learning. *Assessment Update, 26*(3), 3–4, 13. doi:10.1002/au.20005

Finkelman, A., & Kenner, C. (2012). *Learning IOM: Implications of the Institute of Medicine reports for nursing education.* Silver Spring, MD: American Nurses Association.

Gardner, H. (1983). *Frames of mind.* New York, NY: Basic Books.

Haidet, P., Kubitz, K., & McCormack, W. (2014). Analysis of the team-based learning literature: TBL comes of age. *Journal on Excellence in College Teaching, 25*(3–4), 303–333. Retrieved from https://www.ncbi.nlm.nih.gov/pmc/articles/PMC4643940

Halawi, L. A., McCarthy, R. V., & Pires, J. (2009). An evaluation of e-learning on the basis of Bloom's taxonomy: An exploratory study. *Journal of Education for Business, 84*(6), 274–380. Retrieved from https://eric.ed.gov/?id=EJ844509

Hayden, J. K., Smiley, R. A., Alexander, M., Kardong-Edgren, S., & Jeffries, P. R. (2014). The NCSBN National Simulation Study: A longitudinal, randomized, controlled study replacing clinical hours with simulation in prelicensure nursing education. *Journal of Nursing Regulation, 5*(2, Suppl.), S1–S64. Retrieved from https://www.ncsbn.org/JNR_Simulation_Supplement.pdf

Hessler, K. (2017). *Flipping the nursing classroom: Where active learning meets technology.* Sudbury, MA: Jones & Bartlett.

Hunt, E. (2012). Educating the developing mind: The view from cognitive psychology. *Educational Psychology Review, 24*(1), 1–7. doi:10.1007/s10648-011-9186-3

Iwasiw, C., & Goldenberg, D. (2015). *Curriculum development in nursing* (3rd ed.). Sudbury, MA: Jones & Bartlett.

Jafari, Z. (2014). A comparison of conventional lecture and team-based learning methods in terms of student learning and teaching satisfaction. *Medical Journal of the Islamic Republic of Iran, 28*(5). Retrieved from https://www.ncbi.nlm.nih.gov/pmc/articles/PMC4154282/pdf/mjiri-28 -5.pdf

Jeffries, P., Swoboda, S., & Akintade, B. (2016). Teaching and learning using simulations. In D. Billings & J. Halstead (Eds.), *Teaching in nursing: A guide for faculty* (5th ed., pp. 304–323). St. Louis, MO: Elsevier Saunders.

Kong, L., Qin, B., Zhou, Y., Mou, S., & Gao, H. (2014). The effectiveness of problem-based learning on development of nursing students' critical thinking: A systematic review and meta-analysis. *International Journal of Nursing Studies, 51*, 458–469. doi:10.1016/j.ijnurstu.2013.06.009

Krathwohl, D. R. (2002). A revision of Bloom's taxonomy: An overview. *Theory Into Practice, 41*(4), 212–218. Retrieved from http://www.depauw.edu/files/resources/krathwohl.pdf

McNally, B., Chipperfield, J., Dorsett, P., Del Fabbro, L., Frommolt, V., Goetz, S., . . . Rung, A. (2017). Flipped classroom experiences: Student preferences and flip strategy in a higher education context. *Higher Education, 73*(2), 281–298. doi:10.1007/s10734-016-0014-z

Mennenga, H. (2013). Student engagement and examination performance in a team-based learning course. *Journal of Nursing Education, 52*(8), 475–479. doi:10.3928/01484834-20130718-04

Michaelsen, L., & Sweet, M. (2008). Fundamental principles and practices of team-based learning. In L. Michaelsen, D. Parmelee, K. McMahon, & R. Levine (Eds.), *Team-based learning for health professions education* (pp. 9–34). Sterling, VA: Stylus.

Missildine, K., Fountain, R., Summers, L., & Gosselin, K. (2013). Flipping the classroom to improve student performance and satisfaction. *Journal of Nursing Education, 52*(10), 597–599. doi:10 .3928/01484834-20130919-03

National League for Nursing. (2015). *A vision for teaching with simulation: A living document from the National League for Nursing NLN Board of Governors.* Retrieved from http://www.nln.org/docs/ default-source/about/nln-vision-series-(position-statements)/vision-statement-a-vision-for-tea ching-with-simulation.pdf?sfvrsn=2

National Survey of Student Engagement. (2013). *A fresh look at student engagement: Annual results 2013*. Retrieved from http://nsse.indiana.edu/NSSE_2013_Results/pdf/NSSE_2013_Annual _Results.pdf

Phillips, J. (2016). Strategies to promote student engagement and active learning. In D. Billings & J. Halstead (Eds.), *Teaching in nursing: A guide for faculty* (5th ed., pp. 245–262). St. Louis, MO: Elsevier.

Pesut, J. (2001). Clinical judgment: Foreground/background. *Journal of Professional Nursing, 17*(5), 215. doi:10.1053/jpnu.2001.26303

Popkess, A., & Frey, J. (2016). Strategies to support diverse learning needs of students. In D. Billings & J. Halstead (Eds.), *Teaching in nursing: A guide for faculty* (5th ed., pp. 15–34). St. Louis, MO: Elsevier.

Della Ratta, C. (2015). Flipping the classroom with team-based learning in undergraduate nursing education. *Nurse Educator, 40*(2), 71–74. doi:10.1097/NNE.0000000000000112

Scheckel, M. (2016). Designing courses and learning experiences. In D. Billings & J. Halstead (Eds.), *Teaching in nursing: A guide for faculty* (5th ed., pp. 159–185). St. Louis, MO: Elsevier.

Shin, I., & Kim, J. (2013). The effect of problem-based learning in nursing education: A meta-analysis. *Advances in Health Science Education, 18*(5), 1103–1120. doi:10.1007/s10459-012-9436-2

Simmons, B., Lanuza, D., Fonteyn, M., & Hicks, F. (2003). Clinical reasoning in experienced nurses. *Western Journal of Nursing Research, 25*(6), 701–719. doi:10.1177/0193945903253092

Society for Simulation in Healthcare. (2015). About simulation. Retrieved from http://www.ssih .org/About-Simulation

Spector, N., Blegen, M., Silvestre, J., Barnsteiner, J., Lynn, M., Ulrich, B., . . . Alexander, M. (2015). Transition to practice study in hospital settings. *Journal of Nursing Regulation, 5*(4), 24–38. doi:10.1016/S2155-8256(15)30031-4

Su, W., & Osisek, P. (2011). The revised Bloom's taxonomy: Implications for educating nurses. *Journal of Continuing Education in Nursing, 42*(7), 321–327. doi:10.3928/00220124-20110621-05

Thompson, B. (2016). The connected classroom: Using digital technology to promote learning. In D. Billings & J. Halstead (Eds.), *Teaching in nursing: A guide for faculty* (5th ed., pp. 324–341). St. Louis, MO: Elsevier Saunders.

Warburton, T., Trish, H., & Barry, D. (2016). Facilitation of learning: Part 1. *Nursing Standard, 30*(32), 40–47. doi:10.7748/ns.30.32.40.s43

Ward, T., & Morris, T. (2016). Think like a nurse: A critical thinking initiative. *Association of Black Nursing Faculty in Higher Education Journal, 27*(3), 64–66. Retrieved from http://excelsior.sdstate .edu/login?url=http://search.ebscohost.com/login.aspx?direct=true&db=keh&AN=11699 0911&site=ehost-live

Wittmann-Price, R., & Fasolka, B. (2010). Objectives and outcomes: The fundamental difference. *Nursing Education Perspectives, 31*(4), 233–236. Retrieved from http://excelsior.sdstate.edu/ login?url=http://search.ebscohost.com/login.aspx?direct=true&db=keh&AN=57511435& site=ehost-live

Wittmann-Price, R., & Price, S. (2015). Educational theories, learning theories, and special concepts. In L. Wilson & R. Wittmann-Price (Eds.), *Review manual for the Certified Healthcare Simulation Educator™(CHSE™) Exam* (pp. 55–89). New York, NY: Springer Publishing.

Zuriguel Pérez, E., Lluch Canut, M., Falcó Pegueroles, A., Puig Llobet, M., Moreno Arroyo, C., & Roldán Merino, J. (2015). Critical thinking in nursing: Scoping review of the literature. *International Journal of Nursing Practice, 21*(6), 820–830. doi:10.1111/ijn.12347

CHAPTER 7

Curriculum Planning for Undergraduate Nursing Programs

Kimberly Baxter

CHAPTER OBJECTIVE

Upon completion of Chapter 7, the reader will be able to:

- Summarize current trends in prelicensure nursing education
- Analyze current regulatory, accreditation, political, and social factors that affect the development and revision of associate and baccalaureate degree pre- and postlicensure nursing education
- Describe the integration of the *Essentials of Baccalaureate Education for Professional Nursing Practice* as a foundation for developing a bachelor of science in nursing (BSN) curriculum
- Analyze the relationship between generic, accelerated bachelor of science in nursing (ABSN), and RN-to-BSN programs
- Evaluate the strengths and challenges for baccalaureate graduate residency programs that facilitate transition into practice
- Design a curriculum plan and program of study for a baccalaureate program

OVERVIEW

This chapter provides an overview of the process of curriculum development for associate degree (ADN) and baccalaureate/BSN programs. It reviews the utilization of the *Essentials of Baccalaureate Education for Professional Nursing Practice* (American Association of Colleges of Nursing [AACN], 2008) in curriculum development and discusses fast-track programs and RN-to-BSN programs. The chapter summarizes the advantages and challenges related to residency/externship programs for the new graduate.

WHEN IS IT TIME FOR CURRICULUM CHANGE?

The nature of today's complex health care environment, overwhelmed with changes in health care reform, advancing technology, and educational accountability led to an urgent call for transformation in nursing education (Institute of Medicine [IOM], 2010). The population of the United States is becoming more diverse, the income gap is widening, and baby boomers are aging. Veterans are returning from war and the prevalence of chronic illness is at an all-time high (Centers for Disease Control and Prevention, 2016). A diverse, dynamic nursing workforce is needed to fulfill these increasingly sophisticated and expanded roles in direct and indirect patient care. All of these factors affect the kinds of programs that are offered at schools of nursing, the content of the curricula, and the way that faculty teach in nursing education.

In order to prepare graduates of prelicensure nursing education programs for practice in an ever-changing health care environment, nursing curricula must be revised or updated on a regular basis. Ongoing quality improvement initiatives undertaken by nurse educators support improved learning outcomes for students (Landeen, Carr, Culver, Martin, & Matthew-Maich, 2016). Nursing schools rely on a robust evaluation plan to provide information that guides curriculum revision. In addition, there are compelling factors external to individual nursing programs that influence the need for curricular change within baccalaureate nursing programs across the country. These are reflected in the *Essentials of Baccalaureate Education for Professional Nursing Practice* (AACN, 2008).

Today's nursing workforce in the United States consists of four levels of prelicensure nursing preparation: diploma, associate degree, baccalaureate, and entry-level master's. According to the National League for Nursing (NLN; 2014), associate degree programs provide the majority of prelicensure education, 58%; baccalaureate programs provide 38%, with dwindling diploma programs at 4%. A more educated nursing workforce is needed in the current health care environment because nurses are expected to fill roles that are increasingly complex, sophisticated, and expanded (Tri-Council for Nursing, 2010). Health care organizations express concern with the quality of prelicensure nursing education and echo the need for advances in education and health technology, and educational research that identifies more effective teaching–learning strategies.

The IOM called for 80% of nurses to hold a bachelor's nursing degree by 2020 (IOM, 2010). Leaders within the nursing profession call for an increase in the number of nurses prepared at the baccalaureate level due to the need to advance the profession. The Tri-Council for Nursing (2010), a coalition of nursing organizations including the AACN, American Nurses Association (ANA), American Organization of Nurse Executives (AONE), and NLN issued a policy statement calling for a more highly educated nursing workforce as a means to meet the nation's need for safe and effective patient care. Blegen, Goode, Park, Vaughn, and Spetz (2013) identified the positive impact of BSN-prepared nurses for patients in acute care facilities with specific diseases such as heart failure, decubitus ulcers, postoperative deep vein thrombosis, and pulmonary emboli. Despite the call for an increased percentage of baccalaureate-prepared nurses and the accompanying evidence that demonstrates improved patient outcomes, the majority of prelicensure nursing programs and first time National Council Licensure Examination for Registered Nurses (NCLEX-RN®) test-takers continue to be prepared at the ADN level (National Council of State Boards of Nursing [NCSBN], 2016; NLN, 2014). Through extensive effort and support of academic progression at both associate degree and baccalaureate institutions, RN-to-BSN degree completion programs enrollment and access have increased, improving the percentage of baccalaureate-prepared nurses in many states (AACN, 2017; IOM, 2015)

COMPONENTS OF CURRICULUM DESIGN

Nursing programs exist within a context of regulation, accreditation, professional standards, and an educational milieu. Any nursing program that educates prelicensure candidates for registered nursing must adhere to regulations and standards. At the national level, the Tri-Council for Nursing (2015) developed a model nursing practice act that offers guiding principles to all state boards of nursing for regulation of education and practice. Nursing programs that exist within a public or private educational institution also meet regional accreditation standards through the parent institution, such as the Northwest Commission on Colleges and Universities or other national accrediting agencies such as the Accreditation Commission for Independent Colleges and Schools.

ASSOCIATE DEGREE PROGRAMS

The current model of ADN education providing entry into practice began after World War II when there was a nursing shortage. Haase (1990), in describing the sequence of events leading to the development of associate degree programs, states that in 1948, the Committee on the Functions of Nursing made a recommendation that nursing practice consist of two tiers of nurses, one professional and the other technical. An educational model for the community college setting was developed intended to educate a technical nurse with a more limited scope of practice than a professional nurse, but broader than that of a practical nurse. This model was piloted in an expanding number of community colleges and graduates were found to have similar knowledge and qualities as compared with university and diploma nursing graduates (Haase, 1990). Although the model was subsequently implemented, the practice issue of technical versus professional nurse was not addressed. The model did, however, provide an evolutionary educational step by moving nursing education from the type of apprentice program (diploma) that was controlled by hospitals and physicians to the college and university system (Orsilini-Hain & Waters, 2009).

Part of the attraction of ADN programs is that they are affordable and provide streamlined access to the nursing profession. The Urban Institute (2009) emphasized that many rural and underserved communities rely on community colleges for their nursing workforce. These programs have the largest number of minorities and preparation of rural nurses in underserved areas (Organization for Associate Degree Nursing & ANA, 2017). The NLN (2014) states that there continues to be a substantial increase in the percentage of associate degree students who are over 30 years old, highlighting the maturity and second-degree nature of many ADN students.

Health care reform is driving the need for a changed nursing education model as care moved from the hospital to different practice settings (IOM, 2010). These changes demand that nursing students be competent in such areas as health policy, financing, leadership, quality improvement, and systems thinking since graduates are called on to work within teams and lead care coordination efforts. No longer can nurses learn everything they need to know about the content areas of maternity, mental health, pediatrics, and medical–surgical nursing. Associate degree programs, however, are being forced to reduce credit requirements for the degree. In an era pushing for increased education, these combined forces could result in a "perfect storm," threatening ADN education itself, according to Sportsman and Allen (2011).

ADN programs receive accreditation status through the Accreditation Commission for Education in Nursing (ACEN) or the NLN Commission for Nursing Accreditation (CNEA).

The five NLN CNEA standards for accreditation are

1. Culture of Excellence—Program Outcomes
2. Culture of Integrity and Accountability—Mission, Governance, and Resources
3. Culture of Excellence and Caring—Faculty
4. Culture of Excellence and Caring—Students
5. Culture of Learning and Diversity—Curriculum and Evaluation Processes (NLN CNEA, 2016)

ACEN (2017) has six standard categories:

1. Mission and Administrative Capacity
2. Faculty and Staff
3. Students
4. Curriculum
5. Resources
6. Outcomes

Mission or Vision and Philosophy Statements

ACEN (2017) accreditation standards for ADN programs require that the nursing program's mission and/or philosophy reflect the governing organization's core values and be congruent with the outcomes, strategic goals, and objectives. When developing or revising the mission and philosophy statements, the faculty and leaders of the nursing program should develop the program's mission in relation to those of the institution. Recommended sources of guidance are other programs within a system or programs that are similar or have good reputations. An ongoing program evaluation process ensures that the mission statement is continuously evaluated, both for congruence and currency. The philosophy flows from the mission statement and reflects the beliefs of the program's faculty and staff about nursing, nursing education, students, teaching and learning, critical thinking, and evidence-based practice. These are generally longer statements that help guide curricular development and content.

Student-Learning Outcomes

Establishing learner outcomes and assessing whether students achieve those outcomes are required by all accrediting agencies. According to ACEN (2017), student-learning outcomes (SLOs) are used to organize the curriculum, guide the delivery of instruction, direct learning activities, and evaluate student progress. SLO statements are broad and describe desired and expected behaviors of the program's graduates and differ from program outcomes such as first-time NCLEX-RN® graduate pass rates, retention rates, employment rates, and program satisfaction. The SLOs should be reflected in level and course objectives.

Quality and Safety Education for Nurses (QSEN) provides an example of competencies that can be used to embed safety and quality outcomes within a curriculum for nurses (Pauly-O'Neill, Cooper, & Prion, 2016). QSEN developed a comprehensive listing of the knowledge, skills, and attitudes (KSAs) necessary to continuously improve the quality and safety of the care that nurses provide (QSEN, 2014).

Program of Study

There are many practical matters to consider in developing and revising nursing programs of study. Course sequencing, program length, prerequisite and corequisite courses, and admission criteria should be based on national and regional standards, as well as any respective state board of nursing regulations. ACEN (2017) standards require that the nursing program length must meet state and national standards and best practices. The parent college or university establishes requirements for corequisite and general education courses that must be included within the program of study.

ADN programs were designed at inception to require only 2 years of instruction (Orsilini-Hain & Waters, 2009). However, additive curricula and the increasing complexity of nursing practice expanded the curricula, which now must be reevaluated in order to serve graduates. In revising curriculum, each program needs to determine what students need in order to be successful in their program's nursing curriculum, and course SLOs need to flow from the program SLOs.

MAGERS & QUINN
BOOKSELLERS

Minneapolis, Mn
est 1994

Assessment

The achievement of SLOs must be evaluated by the faculty as a means of determining the quality of instruction and overall improvement needs (ACEN, 2017). Through regular and systematic assessment, each program must demonstrate that students who complete their programs, no matter where or how they are offered, achieved these outcomes. For nursing programs, this means that each course within a nursing curriculum must have course and content learning outcomes or objectives that guide the delivery of content. These are the important and measureable behaviors or competencies for students in the course.

Level objectives for each semester or year are developed to assess the expected performance at specific points. All objectives and program learning outcomes are measurable so that they can be assessed at each step within the program. If results are less than expected, curriculum and instructional changes should be made that are based on evidence. ACEN (2017) or NLN CNEA (2016) standards and criteria can be used to establish a method of curriculum review that offers evaluation of both student learning and the curriculum itself.

BACCALAUREATE PROGRAMS

There is significant concern with the preparedness of entry-level nurses to provide quality care within the complex and changing health care environments in which they practice. In addition, the shortage of nursing faculty and reduced capacity of clinical sites compel nursing educators to reconsider more traditional models of prelicensure clinical education. The IOM (2001, 2010) clearly recommends a mandate for change in health care education, compelling schools of nursing to focus on patient-centered quality and safety in the health care system. Benner, Sutphen, Leonard, and Day (2010) describe a practice–education gap, which must be addressed by improving the quality of nursing education. The AONE (2010) took the position that the nurse of the future will need different skills, baccalaureate preparation will be necessary to meet the demands of practice, and BSN education must be "reframed" in order for graduates to be prepared.

Baccalaureate Essentials

The *Essentials* (AACN, 2008) reflect current priorities in:

- Health care, including expanded emphasis on safety and quality, patient technology, patient-centered care, population health, health care regulation, and globalization
- Nursing education, with a focus on the liberal arts and information management
- Professional nursing practice, which is grounded in evidence-based practice, interprofessional communication and collaboration, and enduring social values (See Table 7.1 for a list of the AACN *Essentials*.)

The *Essentials* (AACN, 2008) are supported by landmark documents such as IOM reports (2001, 2003, 2010) and related QSEN competencies that include indicators for patient-centered care, teamwork and collaboration, evidence-based practice, quality improvement, safety, and informatics (QSEN, 2014). Other compelling and influential documents that impact nursing curricula include *Healthy People 2020* (U.S. Department of Health and Human Services, 2014), the professional nursing study supported by the Carnegie Foundation for the Advancement of Teaching (Benner et al., 2010), and numerous research and position papers authored by a variety of key health care and educational organizations. The *Essentials* (AACN) are the foundation for BSN curriculum development and are referenced frequently throughout the discussion in this chapter.

TABLE 7.1   The *Essentials of Baccalaureate Education for Professional Nursing Practice*

Essential I: Liberal Education for Baccalaureate Generalist Nursing Practice
- A solid base in liberal education provides the cornerstone for the practice and education of nurses.

Essential II: Basic Organizational and Systems Leadership for Quality Care and Patient Safety
- Knowledge and skills in leadership, quality improvement, and patient safety are necessary to provide high-quality health care.

Essential III: Scholarship for Evidence-Based Practice
- Professional nursing practice is grounded in the translation of current evidence into one's practice.

Essential IV: Information Management and Application of Patient Care Technology
- Knowledge and skills in information management and patient care technology are critical in the delivery of quality patient care.

Essential V: Health Care Policy, Finance, and Regulatory Environments
- Health care policies, including financial and regulatory, directly and indirectly influence the nature and functioning of the health care system and thereby are important considerations in professional nursing practice.

Essential VI: Interprofessional Communication and Collaboration for Improving Patient Health Outcomes
- Communication and collaboration among health care professionals are critical to delivering high-quality and safe patient care.

Essential VII: Clinical Prevention and Population Health
- Health promotion and disease prevention at the individual and population level are necessary to improve population health and are important components of baccalaureate generalist nursing practice.

Essential VIII: Professionalism and Professional Values
- Professionalism and the inherent values of altruism, autonomy, human dignity, integrity, and social justice are fundamental to the discipline of nursing.

Essential IX: Baccalaureate Generalist Nursing Practice
- The baccalaureate graduate nurse is prepared to practice with patients, including individuals, families, groups, communities, and populations across the life span and across the continuum of health care environments.
- The baccalaureate graduate understands and respects the variations of care, the increased complexity, and the increased use of health care resources inherent in caring for patients.

Source: AACN (2008).

Curriculum Development

The curriculum reflects the heart and soul of a nursing faculty member. For each school, at least some of the current faculty members were most likely involved in developing the existing curriculum and are invested in its success. The curriculum expresses the faculty members' values and beliefs about nursing and education, and reflects their professional identities. In most schools of nursing, the curriculum is familiar and comforting. These factors mean that curriculum change is one of the most challenging undertakings. It may prove difficult to build consensus about a new program based on different values and priorities among a diverse group of faculty members. Some faculty members keep up with best practices and innovation in nursing education, while others are content with the status quo. Ideally, curriculum revision is driven by the faculty and begins with an agreement by the faculty as a whole to enter into the process.

Once a decision has been made to revise an existing curriculum or develop a new curriculum, next steps include selecting a work group or committee, developing a plan, and exploring best practices in nursing education. The composition of the group that will be leading the work is of primary importance to the success of the endeavor, and the members should be selected with intention. A strong team includes a diverse group of tenured and untenured faculty members with various areas of expertise and backgrounds who are committed to the goal, motivated to do the difficult work of curriculum development, and able to work collaboratively through the process of change (Robert Wood Johnson Foundation, 2014). In addition to faculty with passion for curriculum, a balanced group includes both faculty members with current practice experience and those with expertise by virtue of their long teaching careers. Nursing students bring a unique and practical perspective to the work and their participation enriches the curriculum development process. As the group organizes, a discussion about roles within the committee and ground rules facilitates the process. An early discussion of bias, territoriality concerns, and "sacred cows" contributes to the process. Other suggestions include a tentative plan and timeline to help the group to stay on schedule; a plan for communicating the progress of the curriculum revision; and points for feedback from the faculty as a whole.

The initial preparatory work of the curriculum development group is to review program evaluation data and plan a variety of strategies to identify best practices in nursing education. The extent of this effort will depend on the time elapsed since the last curriculum revision and the extent of the planned revision. The following information and documents will inform the committee and provide data for difficult discussions and decision making.

- The *Essentials* (AACN, 2008) document is foundational and should be made available to all members from the beginning. The document includes rationale, performance indicators, and sample content for each essential that are helpful in understanding the scope of each statement for application to a particular program of study.
- A comprehensive search of the literature identifies best practices and innovation in nursing education; synthesizing the information for the faculty as a whole facilitates shared understanding.
- A review of professional standards such as the ANA *Code of Ethics* (2015) and various published competencies for BSN graduates is important. Based on current issues and priorities in nursing practice, specific baccalaureate level competencies have been developed for quality and safety (QSEN, 2014); cultural competency (AACN, 2008, NLN, 2015); genetics and genomics (Greco, Tinley, & Seibert, 2011); geriatric nursing care (AACN & John A. Hartford Foundation, 2010); and palliative and end-of-life care (AACN, 2016).
- A survey of other regional and national programs provides examples of model programs of study. Programs that have been recently updated and incorporate innovation, have similar missions, and have been recently accredited may be of most value.
- Focus groups or surveys of stakeholders including students, faculty, and clinical or community partners provide invaluable information regarding expectations and priorities and create an inclusive process. These surveys provide meaningful local information about what was working and not working in the old curriculum, suggested changes or direction, new information and trends to be aware of, and priority knowledge and skills to include in the new curriculum.

Information in this chapter is relevant to the development or revision of curricula for several types of baccalaureate programs that are addressed, including 4-year traditional collegiate nursing programs, transfer programs in which students complete prerequisites and general education courses before entering the nursing program, accelerated (or fast-track) bachelor's degree programs, and RN completion programs. If a school has more than one type of program, there must be consistency and congruency among programs. The suggested approach is to start with the development of the generic prelicensure program and then develop modifications based on the core curriculum model.

Concept-Based Curriculum Development

The concept-based model for curriculum development is one strategy to reduce content saturation brought about by faculty's penchant for overloading courses with "need to know" content. The conceptual framework (theoretical or organizational model) guides the development of the program of study and makes it unique; it unifies the curriculum and creates a coherent approach across courses and levels (Ervin, Bickes, & Schim, 2006). In this approach, nursing faculty identifies, classifies, and defines concepts that subsequently provide the organizational framework for the curriculum and are threaded through courses (J. F. Giddens, Wright, & Gray, 2012; Hendricks & Wangerin, 2017). While nursing faculty members are using many active learning strategies in their content delivery, lengthy lectures continue to be a mainstay in prelicensure nursing education (Hendricks & Wangerin, 2017). Faculty barriers to implementation of the concept-based model include lack of administrative buy-in, lack of knowledge, role identify struggles, and resistance to change (Hendricks & Wangerin, 2017). Strategies to support faculty and program success in the implementation of a concept-based curriculum include detailed planning, training, and availability of resources with supportive feedback (Patterson, Crager, Farmer, Epps, & Schuessler, 2016). Nielsen (2016) demonstrated that structured concept-based learning in the clinical setting fosters deep learning and promotes clinical judgment in prelicensure nursing students.

Curriculum Outcomes

The next step in the BSN curriculum development process is to identify level and terminal or end-of-program outcomes/SLOs (or objectives or competencies), which must be directly related to the *Essentials* (AACN, 2008) in the context of the school's philosophy. Mapping is a strategy for ensuring that all elements of the *Essentials* (AACN) are included (see Chapter 5). Whether a school uses outcomes, objectives, or competencies to create the curricular structure, the term must be defined, used consistently, and leveled across the program. The outcomes form the backbone of the curriculum and will be the foundation for program evaluation. SLOs (end-of-program outcomes) are developed by reviewing each essential and writing outcome statements that address the key concepts. This task can be completed either by the curriculum development group or can be more inclusive and involve the faculty as a whole by assigning a small group of individuals to write outcomes for specific *Essentials* (AACN). When all outcome statements are reviewed and analyzed as a package, there will most likely be overlap and areas that need to be strengthened in preparing the final document. As the outcomes statements are combined and synthesized, some may address more than one essential, but all *Essentials* (AACN) must be addressed. When the terminal outcomes are identified, the level outcomes are developed and spiraled to show students' progression through the program.

ADVANCES IN EDUCATIONAL TECHNOLOGY

Advances in educational technology and web-based learning radically altered the process of prelicensure nursing education delivery and impacted the structure of the curriculum and how nurses are taught (NLN, 2015). Online education is considered commonplace in nursing education today. Skiba (2016a) describes student expectations from technology and it has been integrated into most learning situations. Institutions are increasingly examining ethical issues associated with the use of these modalities. As digital natives, students are often more technologically competent than faculty and expect current learning technology to be incorporated into the curriculum for interactive learning (Clark, Glazer, Edwards, & Pryse, 2017; Skiba, 2016a). Computer-based simulations such as the virtual neighborhood or community (Foronda & Bauman, 2014; Risling, 2017; Schaffer, Tiffany, Kantack, & Anderson, 2016) and interactive avatars (Kidd, Knisley, & Morgan, 2012; Skiba, 2016a) are examples of innovations that are woven throughout the structure of the curriculum. Applications are available for teaching students to use electronic health records (Foronda et al., 2017). Distance education and high-fidelity simulation learning strategies have been expanded and integrated into BSN programs. Exciting new technologies are under development, with the potential to identify how students best learn and adapt accordingly (Foronda et al., 2017; Skiba, 2016b).

Distance Education

Online learning is increasingly integrated into nursing education, although application of web-based approaches varies widely between nursing programs. Quality standards, such as Quality Matters (www.qualitymatters.org), have been developed for online education and faculty development and instructional design support are essential to ensure the effective delivery of online coursework. While specific nonclinical courses may be taught online or offered as an alternative method of delivery, most prelicensure programs continue to be offered in a face-to-face format. Distance education is increasingly becoming the primary pedagogy for baccalaureate completion programs (Skiba, 2016a). Distance applications include electronic classrooms and videoconferencing that facilitate inclusion of rural students and teaching across college campuses, or facilitate supervision for students involved in off-site practicum experiences. New software applications are proliferating and significantly expand the resources available for educators. The availability of distance education technologies and the related philosophy of an academic institution toward their use as a teaching–learning methodology have significant implications for curriculum development. As with all technology use in nursing education, the expertise and support of educators using these modalities are vital to student success.

High-Fidelity Simulation

Nursing education focuses on integrating theoretical knowledge with experiential learning. In the traditional nursing education model, the opportunities to apply knowledge may be limited. Even in an optimal clinical setting, lack of predictable experiences and potential risk to patients impacted the ability to provide consistent, guaranteed experiences. While nursing educators have long employed low- and mid-fidelity simulation in nursing skills labs, high-fidelity simulation has become the "gold standard" as schools of nursing incorporate this teaching strategy into curricula to prepare students for clinical experiences and to supplement or replace clinical hours. Simulated learning experiences can be developed to support the progressive achievement of curriculum outcomes by intentionally spiraling core concepts and skills throughout the curriculum in increasingly more complex scenarios (Blodgett, Blodgett, & Bleza, 2016; Bussard, 2016). Interprofessional simulations can provide an opportunity for students to learn about teamwork and collaboration and the roles of other health care professions (Buckley et al., 2012; Foronda, MacWilliams, McArthur, 2016; Scherer, Myers, O'Connor, & Haskins, 2013). Bussard (2016) found that self-reflection on video-recorded high-fidelity simulation supported the development of clinical judgment. Although students routinely report high stress in the simulated learning environment, the human patient simulation experiences were found to be a valuable learning tool (Cantrell, Meyer, & Mosack, 2017). Cantey, Randolph, Molloy, Carter, and Cary (2017) recognized the role of simulation as a teaching strategy for improving cultural awareness and understanding social determinants of health. Zinsmaster and Vliem (2015) found high-fidelity simulation to have a significant impact on knowledge acquisition; however, they did not find a significant influence on knowledge retention.

According to Hayden, Smiley, Alexander, Kardong-Edgren, and Jeffries (2014), the landmark NCSBN National Simulation Study of 2014 highlighted the positive role of simulation as a substantive clinical opportunity. This landmark, national, multisite randomized control trial concluded that simulation could be substituted for up to 50% of traditional clinical experiences. Faculty supporting these simulation experiences should be formally trained with subject matter experts conducting any debriefing experiences (Hayden et al., 2014). Depending on the goal of instruction, lower fidelity simulation can be an effective alternative (Sharpnack & Madigan, 2012). Simulation using live actors as standardized patients is also a powerful strategy with the potential to change attitudes, beliefs, and behaviors among student participants (Bornais, Raiger, Krah, & El-Masri, 2012; Luctkar-Flude, Wilson-Keates, & Larocque, 2012; Noone, Sideras, Gubrud-Howe, Voss, & Mathews, 2012; Ward, Cody, Schaal, & Hojat, 2012).

The focus in simulation in nursing education has been primarily on learning, including prebriefing and debriefing, with less emphasis on more high-stakes summative evaluation (Cantrell et al., 2017). In planning for use of simulation in a curriculum, schools are advised to check with their state boards of nursing regarding regulations for percentage or replacement of clinical hours with high-fidelity simulation. The importance of evidence-based faculty training and support cannot be underestimated and supports positive student and program outcomes (Jeffries, Dreifuerst, Dardong-Edgren, & Hayden, 2015). In order to make the best use of this technology, simulation must be approached with vision and intention in the curriculum development process. All aspects of simulation within a given curriculum should be guided by evidence-based approaches, such as the Standards of Best Practice: Simulation (International Nursing Association for Clinical Simulation and Learning, 2013).

TRANSFORMATIVE APPROACHES TO CLINICAL EDUCATION

One of the most challenging aspects of curriculum revision is designing an approach to students' clinical experiences that reflects the school's theoretical model and integrates new learning pedagogies in the context of local realities regarding the availability of qualified clinical faculty and clinical sites. While clinical experience is essential in preparation for practice, what constitutes clinical experience? What kinds of clinical learning activities and how much time in what kind of health care settings are most effective for BSN students to meet generalist competencies and transition successfully into practice? The NLN Think Tank on Transforming Clinical Nursing Education (2008) made recommendations for the ideal clinical educational model that described integrative experiences, including cross-disciplinary experiences; new relationships within learning communities, including innovative relationships with clinical partners; and reconceptualized learning experiences in which all students do not have clinical experiences in traditional rotations.

According to Hayden et al., (2014) the landmark NCSBN National Simulation Study of 2014 highlighted the positive role of simulation as a substantive clinical opportunity. These researchers broke through barriers and changed the landscape in what learning experiences can constitute nursing clinical experiences. While there are scarce data about the effectiveness of either traditional or other new clinical models, it is incumbent on nurse educators to develop and test models and approaches and contribute to the database. Each school of nursing needs to develop an approach that best utilizes its resources and fits its theoretical model. Jessee and Tanner (2016) discuss the vital role of discourse and clinical supervisor–student relationship and coaching in clinical reasoning development. Frameworks and tools support clinical faculty and preceptors in providing feedback and evaluating clinical development (Jessee & Tanner, 2016; Nielsen, Lasater, & Stock, 2016).

COMPLETING THE CURRICULUM DEVELOPMENT PROCESS

Concurrent with the development of the program of study, additional work must be completed as part of the comprehensive curriculum package. A glossary defines terms that have special meaning within the mission, vision, and philosophy; theoretical model; and curriculum plan, including concepts that provide the organizational framework for the curriculum. Prerequisites including humanities, science, and social science courses that serve as the foundation for the nursing coursework must be identified and negotiated with various other departments. These include college-wide requirements such as general education. Progression issues must be considered, including minimum grade point average for admission into the school of nursing, a description of how students will progress from semester to semester, and prerequisites and corequisites for each course. The curriculum development group will need to work with the administrative team to cost out the curriculum, including faculty and other resources that will be needed to manage the new curriculum. Often old and new curricula will be offered simultaneously for a period of time until the students in the old program graduate, which may require additional resources. The curriculum package must be approved by the nursing faculty and be directed through academic channels for approval. The new curriculum must be submitted to the state board of nursing and the national accrediting body.

THE INCLUSIVE CURRICULUM: PAYING ATTENTION TO DIVERSITY

There is a national call to increase the enrollment of students from underrepresented populations in schools of nursing, and recent reports show that some progress is being made (AACU, 2013; Budden, Zhong, Moulton, & Cimiotti, 2013). Relf (2016) described the need for academic nursing to increase its efforts to ensure the nursing workforce matches the demographics of the U.S. population. The uniqueness of each individual includes recognition of differences in race, ethnicity, gender, sexual orientation, gender identify, socioeconomic status, age, physical abilities, religious beliefs, political beliefs, and other attributes (NLN, 2016b). Schools of nursing typically have not considered the needs of students who are minorities, low-income students, first in family to attend college, or multilingual, nonnative English speakers, or disabled in developing the plan of study or the curriculum structure. Further complicating the goal of meaningful inclusion is the lack of nursing educators from underrepresented and diverse populations (NLN, 2016b).

It is logical to assume that diversity and inclusion should be threaded throughout the curriculum, including the mission statement, and course, level, and program outcomes (AACU, 2013). Ideally, the curriculum should be creative, flexible, and reflect the multicultural perspectives of the pluralistic society (Moore & Clark, 2016). The American Association of Colleges and Universities (2013) promotes *inclusive excellence*, a commitment to diversity and equity based on the understanding that becoming an educated person in a pluralistic society includes developing the ability to communicate and interact with individuals and populations that are different from ourselves. This philosophy presupposes a broad definition of diversity, and compels faculty members to facilitate the success of all students, including those with diverse backgrounds and learning styles.

Faculty may not be aware of how programmatic organization affects students differentially. These learners best achieve academically in a curriculum model that more closely integrated theory and clinical experience. Kellett and Fitton (2016) recommend a foundation of inclusive information systems and the creation of gender-neutral safe places to promote a culture of inclusion for the transgender student.

Other ways of demonstrating inclusiveness in curriculum planning include preentry nursing courses, parallel academic support courses, culture-focused or special interest general education courses or electives, and international experiences as part of the program of study. The cocurriculum can play an important role in supporting and validating underrepresented students on the campus. Other ideas include development of clinical models that facilitate clinical experiences with diverse populations and intentionally threading exemplars throughout the curriculum that address health care issues experienced by particular ethnic, cultural, or minority groups. And finally, admission and progression requirements for incoming students that support or, conversely, disadvantage those who were educated in another country or are multilingual nonnative English speakers will shape the student body and affect the quality of learning for all the students. A diverse student body has been shown to be associated with improved outcomes among all students (AACU, 2013; Murray, Pole, Ciarlo, & Holmes 2016).

INTERPROFESSIONAL EDUCATION: PREPARING FOR COLLABORATIVE PRACTICE

In response to safety and quality standards in health care and a vision for accessible, patient-centered care, AACN collaborated with leadership from other professional organizations to develop competencies for interprofessional practice (Interprofessional Education Collaborative Expert Panel, 2011), which were integrated into the *Baccalaureate Essentials* (AACN, 2008). The World Health Organization (2010, p. 7) stated that interprofessional education (IPE) "occurs when students from two or more professions learn about, from and with each other to enable effective collaboration and improve health." Health professions schools are developing models for IPE in classroom, simulation, and, more recently, clinical and community settings. IPE models have been studied in undergraduate nursing programs (Hudson, Sanders, & Pepper, 2013). Gannon et al. (2017) developed an interprofessional activity with nursing and pharmacy students exploring end-of-life care beliefs.

At Oregon Health and Sciences University (OHSU), interprofessional student groups work with a nursing faculty in residence and collaborate with community partners to address social determinants of health for some of the most vulnerable and marginalized clients, families, and populations in target neighborhoods. Details can be found at www.ohsu.edu/i-can. Friend, Friend, Ford, and Ewell (2016) provided a semester-long interprofessional activity that allowed nursing and medical students to explore the occurrence and impact of interprofessional conflict in high acuity areas and address resolution techniques.

Although there are significant logistical, cultural, and historical barriers to IPE and practice, the benefits of IPE for prelicensure students are many, including greater understanding of roles and contributions of other health care professionals and dynamics within the health care team; development of professional pride and identity; importance of effective interprofessional communication and reflective practice; knowledge of patient conditions and increased comfort with targeted patient populations; improved cultural sensitivity; building of professional networks; and an improved sense of collaboration and cooperation (Buckley et al., 2012; Kostoff, Brukhardt, Winter, & Shrader, 2016; Mellor, Cottrell, & Moran, 2013; Moradi, Najarkolai, & Keshmiri, 2016). Each school has unique opportunities and, moving forward, IPE/interprofessional collaborative practice must be considered as an integral element of every baccalaureate curriculum.

TRANSITION TO PRACTICE

Transition of new BSN graduates into clinical practice is recognized as an issue since *Reality Shock* was first published (Kramer, 1974). Internships or integrative clinical experiences prior to beginning work in the professional role have been shown as one curriculum strategy that contributes to the socialization of graduate nurses into practice (Adams, Alexander, Chisari, Gaurdia, & McAuley, 2015). Recommendations from national reports about transition from the academic environment to the nursing practice environment showed significant support for the formation of academic and service partnerships to develop standardized residency programs (Benner et al., 2010; Commission on Collegiate Nursing Education [CCNE], 2008; IOM, 2010). The Commission on Collegiate Nursing Education (2008) implemented accreditation for postbaccalaureate nurse residency programs (NRPs). The standards for accreditation focus on NRP course faculty, institutional commitment and resources, NRP program curriculum, and program effectiveness (CCNE, 2008).

The goal of transition programs is primarily to facilitate professional formation and socialization into the culture of the health care organization, assist the new graduate to develop clinical competency, improve recruitment retention, and reduce orientation costs for the employer. Programs may be situated prior to graduation or following, and include educational and psychosocial support strategies such as mentoring, preceptor training, clinical coaching, expanded orientation, clinical and professional skill development, classes, and other learning and support activities targeted at the needs of the developing professional (Hopkins & Bromley, 2016; Olson-Sitki, Wendler, & Forbes, 2012).

A model residency program that promotes point-of-care leadership was developed and evaluated by the University Health System Consortium and AACN. This curriculum focuses on three content areas: leadership, patient safety, and professional role. Among other findings, an evaluation demonstrated that the residents' perceptions of confidence and competence, capacity to organize and prioritize, and ability to communicate and provide leadership improved significantly. In addition, retention rates of new graduates improved (Goode, Lynn, & McElroy, 2013).

One major challenge in residency program management is preparing and maintaining committed and effective mentor/preceptors. The literature notes positive reports from clinical managers on new graduate performance as well as enhanced new graduate satisfaction and retention (Letourneau & Fater, 2015). In the current climate of scarce resources, evaluation should include not only the cost–benefit analysis related to retention of new graduates but factors such as quality indicators of professional achievement of nurse residents and the relationship to patient outcomes (Adams, et. al., 2015; Mallory & Franqueiro, 2017).

ALTERNATIVE BACCALAUREATE PATHWAYS

Accelerated Bachelor of Science in Nursing Programs

The first accelerated bachelor of science in nursing (ABSN) programs were initiated in the early 1970s and grew rapidly in number since the 1990s. In 2013, there were 293 established ABSN programs in 46 states with 13 new programs in development and 62 entry-level master's programs (AACN, 2015). The continuing development of these programs has been in response to the projected shortage of nurses and is viewed as a viable option to help meet the future need for more nurses (AACN, 2013). Accelerated programs are generally offered as intensive full-time courses of study with no breaks between semesters or terms. Most programs are 11 to 18 months in length (AACN, 2015). Graduates from ABSN programs are highly valued by employers because of their maturity, ability to learn quickly, and clinical skills (AACN, 2015).

Priority for admission to ABSN programs is often given to second-degree–seeking students. Having successfully completed a prior baccalaureate, students in accelerated programs are experienced learners who understand the challenges of college and have learned how to effectively navigate the system. These skills, grounded in their previous college experiences, help them cope with the rigors of a professional program. As mature and motivated as ABSN students might be, they have reported high levels of stress when challenged by the expectations of the student role and balancing the demands of family, work, and finances (Payne, Glaspie, & Rosser, 2014). Brandt, Boellaard, and Wilberding (2017) found that ABSN graduates were motivated to find a job and felt the rigor of the accelerated program prepared them well for professional practice.

Weathers and Hunt Raleigh (2013) compared retention rates and performance evaluation ratings by nurse managers of traditional and ABSN graduates after 1 year of practice and found that the retention rate was higher for ABSN graduates, as were the performance ratings. Findings such as these demonstrate that ABSN programs are producing graduates who remain in the workplace and also pursue advanced degrees soon after graduation. As engaged and motivated adult learners, ABSN students and graduates can offer important insights as part of the planning group during curriculum redesign initiatives.

Baccalaureate Completion Programs

Baccalaureate completion programs, also called "RN-to-BSN" programs, are designed for RNs who are graduates of accredited associate degree or hospital-based diploma programs and who seek a BSN degree. Based on research demonstrating improved performance on quality and safety outcomes when nurses are educated at the baccalaureate level or higher, AACN maintains that the BSN degree should be the minimum educational requirement for professional nursing practice (Tri-Council for Nursing, 2010). The BSN has become the preferred preparation for practice in health care settings, including Magnet hospitals and organizations that require the baccalaureate for specific nursing roles (Wojner & Whelan, 2016). Nurses who seek positions in case management, public health and community-based settings, and leadership find that the BSN is an essential requirement for employment.

Nurses who enroll in RN-to-BSN programs have a variety of life and work experiences, in addition to experiences in previous educational programs. They are often motivated to enroll in RN-to-BSN programs and achieve the higher degree in order to secure employment, advance their careers, or fulfill their personal goals (Wojner & Whelan, 2016). The BSN degree is the gateway to graduate education and subsequent roles in advanced practice, nursing education, and research. The purpose of the completion program is to assist students to develop higher level critical thinking skills, broaden their scope of practice, and understand the social, cultural, economic, and geopolitical context of health care in order to assume expanded professional roles (AACN, 2017). Clinical partnerships prove to be a valuable partner identifying and implementing rich didactic content and securing diverse clinical opportunities for this population of students (Wojner & Whelan, 2016).

Academic Progression for Nurses

Based on increasing demands in health care and the need for high-quality health outcomes across all care settings, the IOM (2010) recommended that the nursing education system be improved to support nurses' achievement of higher levels of education. Subsequently, the IOM challenged nurse leaders to work together to increase the number of baccalaureate-prepared nurses from 50% to 80% by the year 2020. As a result, academic nurse leaders recognized the need to develop collaborative relationships between community colleges and higher degree programs (J. L. Giddens & Meyer, 2016; Zittel, Moss, O'Sullivan, & Siek, 2016). Certain states have mandated articulation agreement requirements that facilitate academic progression for nurses. For example, the Administrative Rule Division 21 requires that all prelicensure programs in Oregon have an articulation agreement in place to facilitate progression to a baccalaureate or higher degree nursing program (Ingwerson, 2012).

Articulation agreements are renewable agreements negotiated to ensure equivalency between college and university courses, support educational mobility, and facilitate the seamless transfer of academic credit between ADN and BSN programs (AACN, 2014). Articulation agreements address the needs of students and programs by facilitating a more streamlined progression experience. Students benefit from transferring credit between institutions, making informed decisions about course selection, and experiencing the collaboration across nursing programs (AACN, 2014; Ingwerson, 2012; Wojner & Whelan, 2016). Some agreements have been as specific as offering dual enrollment in the associate and baccalaureate programs upon admission to the associate degree program (Gorski, Farmer, Sroczynski, Close & Wortlock, 2015; Ingwerson, 2012). Dual enrollment provides students with additional benefits such as academic advising and support as well as more diverse course offerings.

Other models for academic progression for the ADN-prepared nurse include conferral of BSN degrees at the community college level (Farmer et al., 2017). Researchers found potential in the use of a competency-based curriculum that allows the RN-to-BSN student to demonstrate competency in program-designated clinical and professional outcomes (Gorski et al., 2015). This model has the potential to reduce redundancy and identify significant content; however, it is challenged by the lack of a unified set of competencies for BSN degree completion. Master's or graduate entry programs are a popular option that allow progression and expedite the journey to advanced degrees (Gorski et al., 2015).

Well-known major barriers to BSN degree completion are time and cost. More recently, absence of mentoring/guidance and lack of exposure to evidence supporting the importance of a BSN or higher degree have been identified (Zittel et al., 2016). Academic partnerships with clinical agencies that employ ADN-prepared nurses, coupled with regulatory support, have the potential to address these important issues.

RN-to-BSN Program of Study

The mission, vision, philosophy, theoretical model, and SLOs for an RN-to-BSN program are often the same as the generic BSN program at a particular school, although the program of study may look very different. Program credits and length are variable between schools, and the design of the curriculum often offers part-time and online options in order to meet the needs of working nurses.

Credit for Prior Learning

As the nursing workforce is challenged to meet the increasingly complex needs of the current and future health care system, nursing programs across the country are challenged to encourage RNs to return to school for BSN completion. Nursing programs responded to this challenge by acknowledging that the RN holds knowledge, skills, and abilities related to prior work experience that can be applied to the current degree they are seeking. It is typical for RN-to-BSN completion programs to require introductory courses that are designed to validate this prior knowledge and to "bridge" or "transition" the RN from diploma or associate degree preparation. In addition to providing an opportunity to validate prior knowledge and skills, these introductory courses offer learning experiences, such as professional portfolio activities, that assist with the role transition and socialization to the BSN level of preparation. The nurse is granted credit for selected prelicensure courses offered at the upper division level once the transition course is successfully completed.

Curriculum Strategies

The RN-to-BSN curriculum addresses nurses' need for socialization, preparation for graduate study, career growth, and leadership development (Wojner & Whelan, 2016). In the typical RN-to-BSN curriculum, the nurse is prepared for an expanded professional role through coursework focused on enhancing professional communication, theoretical perspectives, community and population-based nursing care, health promotion, and leadership. The senior practicum hours are spent working with nurse preceptors in acute care settings as well as in community-based settings where the nurses build on previous knowledge and enhance their effectiveness across the continuum of care. Many programs incorporate professional projects designed to meet the needs of the clinical agency from an evidence-based perspective, while other activities include projects related to nursing leadership, health promotion, disease prevention, and the care of vulnerable populations.

With a growing awareness about the positive outcomes associated with advancing to higher levels of education and increasing encouragement from employers who provide tuition support for RN-to-BSN programs, more and more nurses are returning to school to complete a baccalaureate degree (Zittel et al., 2016). In order to meet the demand for BSN completion, nursing programs responded by offering curricula delivered through online and distance learning, the traditional classroom setting, or by using combined methods such as hybrid or web-enhanced approaches (AACN, 2012; Robert Wood Johnson, 2014). Distance education provides RN-to-BSN students, who are usually employed and juggling multiple roles, with greater accessibility to attend class at times of the day that meet their needs. Nurses attending online completion programs also benefit from geographic flexibility, self-directed learning and motivation, professional socialization, and peer support.

Clinical Experiences

The increasing enrollment in RN-to-BSN programs creates additional strain on scarce clinical practicum sites and faculty. However, the fact that RN-to-BSN students are licensed, as compared to the BSN student, allows for placement of licensed nurses in a variety of traditional and nontraditional clinical sites. This ability generates opportunities for students to provide nursing care in settings in which they can begin to view caring in new ways, awakening a sense of advocacy, civic responsibility, and concern for political action (Zittel et al., 2016). A sense of responsibility is gained from various types of experiential and service learning experiences that extend beyond the singular nurse–client relationship to embrace the client's family, community, and society. Clinical experiences designed for service in community-based settings assist the nurse in adopting a broader, global view of nursing practice (NLN, 2015).

RN-to-BSN students benefit from being able to explore areas of interest for their clinical experiences as well as collaborating with faculty to identify creative ways to meet their goals for learning. There is the potential for deep engagement and mutuality for preceptors and staff in clinical sites within the student's community. RN-to-BSN students often choose experiences in public and community health, school-based health settings, correctional nursing, mental and behavioral health centers, addiction treatment and homeless shelters, geriatric settings, and home health and hospice settings. In addition, RN-to-BSN students are uniquely suited for participation in global health care delivery when interested in opportunities for international travel and meeting the needs of the vulnerable and underserved.

International clinical placements and studies abroad are recognized as broadening students' cultural understanding and preparing them for authentic relationships in the professional clinical setting (Edgecombe, Jennings, & Bowden, 2013). Students have the opportunity to explore diverse cultures and communities as well as gain knowledge of different health care systems. RN-to-BSN students who complete international clinical experiences have described meaningful learning that took place related to awareness of diversity and cultural competence in nursing, enhanced skills in intercultural communication, an increased awareness of social and political injustices, and a greater understanding of poverty.

Inexperienced RN-to-BSN Students

As the trend toward hiring "BSN preferred" nurses continues, it is anticipated that more nurses will enter RN-to-BSN completion programs immediately following graduation from associate degree and diploma programs. In order to meet admission requirements for RN-to-BSN completion programs, applicants must pass the NCLEX examination for licensure and obtain an RN license. Since the RN-to-BSN curriculum builds upon the prior work experience of the RN, nurses just beginning nursing practice require special consideration related to their relative lack of clinical experience. There may be new graduate nurses who have not found nursing jobs following completion of their initial degree and have no work experience, which challenges some of the assumptions of many RN-to-BSN programs. Depending on the structure of the curriculum, inexperienced RN-to-BSN students may have difficulty engaging in classroom activities designed for experienced RNs to apply new knowledge and insights to their current practice. In the clinical setting, the less experienced RN requires additional oversight and support by faculty and preceptors, beyond what is usually provided for licensed students.

Despite some of the challenges for new graduate nurses who enter completion programs, RN-to-BSN programs provide valuable experiences for students. Students benefit from learning collaboratively with nurses who have varied years and types of clinical experiences. Research suggests that RN students, in their quest for higher education, seek to attain professional credibility, career mobility, personal achievement, and longevity in nursing (Gorski et al., 2015; Zittel et al., 2016). The RN-to-BSN completion programs provide a rich and supportive environment for nurses returning to school. Nursing faculty members have the opportunity to mentor and role-model professional behaviors that assist in building positive connections and influence the learning of their students.

SUMMARY

Robust baccalaureate nursing education programs are foundational to the health of the profession and the population and as preparation for graduate nursing education. Curriculum development and revision are both a challenge and an opportunity to shape the future. Collaboration with stakeholders including other health care professionals, consumers of health care, and health care service organizations is essential in order to innovate and find local solutions in a new age of health care reform. It is incumbent upon nursing educators to try new curricular approaches, evaluate their efficacy, and share the results with the professional community.

This author would like to thank the authors of this content in the previous editions of this book for their hard work and excellent foundation.

DISCUSSION QUESTIONS

- Identify your primary partners in service or education. What is the nature of those relationships and how could they be expanded to create innovative clinical experiences for nursing students?
- What are the most common groups of underrepresented students in your region? How could your admission process and curriculum be changed to be more inclusive of these groups?
- What are the barriers to prelicensure graduates' successful transition into practice? Describe strategies in your curriculum that help mediate "reality shock." What are some new ideas that could be developed? Do any clinical agencies in your area have a new graduate residency program?
- How will health care reform affect your prelicensure program? Interview the chair of the undergraduate curriculum committee at your school to determine if there is a plan for curriculum revision.
- Create an innovative clinical educational model and describe how this would integrate and meet learning outcomes within a given curriculum.
- Describe IPE activities that could be integrated into the curriculum at each of the various levels at your college or university. Think about different professions with whom you could partner.

LEARNING ACTIVITIES

Faculty Development Activities

1. Map your curriculum outcomes according to the AACN *Essentials* (2008). What changes need to be made to update your program?
2. Create a visual representation of your school's theoretical/conceptual model.
3. Invite a colleague to coffee and discuss the "sacred cows" at your institution that could be barriers to innovative curriculum revision.

References

Accreditation Commission for Education in Nursing. (2017). *ACEN 2017 standards and criteria associate.* Retrieved from http://www.acenursing.net/manuals/SC2017.pdf

Adams, J. M., Alexander, G. A., Chisari, R. G., Banister, G., McAuley, M. E., Whitney, K. B., & Erickson, J. I. (2015). Strengthening new graduate nurse residency programs in critical care: Recommendations from nurse residents and organizational stakeholders. *Journal of Continuing Education in Nursing, 46*(1), 41–48.

American Association of Colleges and Universities. (2003). Board statement on diversity, equity, and inclusive excellence. Retrieved from http://www.aacu.org/about/statements/2013/inclusive excellence.cfm

American Association of Colleges of Nursing. (2008). *The essentials of baccalaureate education for professional nursing practice.* Retrieved from http://www.aacnnursing.org/Portals/42/Publications/ BaccEssentials08.pdf

American Association of Colleges of Nursing. (2012). AACN-AONE Task Force on Academic-Practice Partnerships: Guiding principles. Retrieved from http://www.aacnnursing.org/ Academic-Practice-Partnerships/The-Guiding-Principles

American Association of Colleges of Nursing. (2013). Accelerated programs: The fast-track to careers in nursing. Washington, DC: Author. Retrieved from http://www.aacnnursing.org/ Nursing-Education/Accelerated-Programs/Fast-Track

American Association of Colleges of Nursing. (2014). Articulation agreements among nursing education programs. Washington, DC: Author. Retrieved from http://www.aacnnursing.org/News-Information/Fact-Sheets/Articulation-Agreements

American Association of Colleges of Nursing. (2015). Fact sheet: Accelerated baccalaureate and master's degrees in nursing. Retrieved from http://www.aacnnursing.org/Students/Accelerated-Nursing-Programs

American Association of Colleges of Nursing. (2016). *Competencies and recommendations for educating undergraduate nursing students*. Retrieved from http://www.aacnnursing.org/Portals/42/ELNEC/PDF/New-Palliative-Care-Competencies.pdf?ver=2017-07-27-151036-973

American Association of Colleges of Nursing. (2017). Fact sheet: The impact of education on nursing practice. Retrieved from http://www.aacnnursing.org/Portals/42/News/Factsheets/Education-Impact-Fact-Sheet.pdf

American Association of Colleges of Nursing & the John A. Hartford Foundation Institute for Geriatric Nursing. (2010). *Recommended baccalaureate competencies and curricular guidelines for the nursing care of older adults*. Washington, DC: Author. Retrieved from www.aacnnursing.org/Portals/42/AcademicNursing/CurriculumGuidelines/AACN-Gero-Competencies-2010.pdf

American Nurses Association. (2015). *Code of ethics for nurses with interpretive statements*. Silver Spring, MD: Author.

American Organization of Nurse Executives. (2010). *AONE guiding principles for future patient care delivery*. Retrieved from http://www.aone.org/resources/future-patient-care.pdf

Benner, P., Sutphen, M., Leonard, V., & Day, L. (2010). *Educating nurses: A call for radical transformation*. San Francisco, CA: Jossey-Bass.

Blegen, M. A., Goode, C. J., Park, S. H., Vaughn, T., & Spetz, J. (2013). Baccalaureate education in nursing and patient outcomes. *Journal of Nursing Administration, 43*(2), 89–94.

Blodgett, T. J., Blodgett, N. P., & Bleza, S. (2016). Simultaneous multiple patient simulation in undergraduate nursing education: A focused literature review. *Clinical Simulation in Nursing, 12*(8), 346–355.

Bornais, J. A. K., Raiger, J. E., Krahn, R. E., & El-Masri, M. M. (2012). Evaluating undergraduate nursing students' learning using standardized patients. *Journal of Professional Nursing, 28*(5), 291–296.

Brandt, C. L., Boellaard, M. R., & Wilberding, K. M. (2017). Accelerated second-degree bachelor of science in nursing graduates' transition to professional practice. *Journal of Continuing Education in Nursing, 48*(1), 14–19.

Buckley, S., Hensman, M., Thomas, S., Dudley, R., Nevin, G., & Coleman, J. (2012). Developing interprofessional simulation in the undergraduate setting: Experience with five different professional groups. *Journal of Interprofessional Care, 26*, 362–369.

Budden, J. S., Zhong, E. H., Moulton, P., & Cimiotti, J. P. (2013). Highlights of the national workforce survey of registered nurses. *Journal of Nursing Regulation, 4*(2), 5–13.

Bussard, M. E. (2016). Self-reflection of video-recorded high-fidelity simulations and development of clinical judgment. *Journal of Nursing Education, 55*(9), 522–527.

Cantey, D. S., Randolph, S. D., Molloy, M. A., Carter, B., & Cary, M. P. (2017). Student-developed simulations: Enhancing cultural awareness and understanding social determinants of health. *Journal of Nursing Education, 56*(4), 243–246.

Cantrell, M. L., Meyer, S. L., & Mosack, V. (2017). Effects of simulation on nursing student stress: An integrative review. *Journal of Nursing Education, 56*(3), 139–144.

Centers for Disease Control and Prevention. (2016). Chronic disease prevention and health promotion. Retrieved from https://www.cdc.gov/chronicdisease/index.htm

Clark, A., Glazer, G., Edwards, C. & Pryse, Y. (2017). Transforming nursing education with apple technology. *Nurse Educator, 42*(2), 91–94.

Commission on Collegiate Nursing Education. (2008). *Nurse residency programs*. Washington, DC: Author. Retrieved from www.aacn.nche.edu/Accreditation/PubsRes.htm

Edgecombe, K., Jennings, M., & Bowden, M. (2013). International nursing students and what impacts their clinical learning: Literature review. *Nurse Education Today, 33*(2), 138–142.

Ervin, N. E., Bickes, J. T., & Schim, S. M. (2006). Environments of care: A curriculum model for preparing a new generation of nurses. *Journal of Nursing Education, 45*(2), 75–80.

Farmer, P., Meyer, D., Sroczynski, Close, L, Gorski, M. S., & Wortock, J. (2017). RN to BSN at the community college: A promising practice for nursing education transformation. *Teaching and Learning in Nursing, 12*(2), 103–108.

Foronda, C., & Bauman, E. (2014). Strategies to incorporate virtual simulation in nurse education. *Clinical Simulation in Nursing, 10*(8), 412–418.

Foronda, C., MacWilliams, B., & McArthur, E. (2016). Interprofessional communication in healthcare: An integrative review. *Nurse Education in Practice, 19,* 36–40.

Foronda, C., Alfes, C. M., Dev, P., Kleinheksel, A. J., Nelson, D. A., O'Donnell, J. M., & Samosky, J. T. (2017). Virtually nursing: Emerging technologies in Nursing. *Nurse Educator, 42*(1), 14–17.

Friend, M. L., Friend, R. D., Ford, C., & Ewell, P. J. (2016). Critical care interprofessional education: Exploring conflict and power-lessons learned. *Journal of Nursing Education, 55*(12), 696–700.

Gannon, J., Motycka C., Egelund E., Kraemer D., Smith W., & Solomon K. (2017). Teaching end-of-life care using interprofessional simulation. *Journal of Nursing Education, 56*(4), 205–210.

Giddens, J., & Meyer, D. (2016). Foundational courses for the baccalaureate nursing degree: Enhancing efficiency for academic progression. *Journal of Nursing Education, 55*(7), 373–378.

Giddens, J., Wright, M., & Gray, I. (2012). Selecting concepts for a concept-based curriculum: Application of a benchmark approach. *Journal of Nursing Education, 51*(9), 511–515.

Goode, C. J., Lynn, M. R., & McElroy, D. (2013). Lessons learned from 10 years of research on a post-baccalaureate nurse residency program. *Journal of Nursing Administration, 43*(2), 73–79.

Gorski, M. S., Farmer, P. D., Sroczynski, M., Close, L., & Wortock, J. M. (2015). Nursing education transformation: Promising practices in academic progression. *Journal of Nursing Education, 54*(9), 509–515.

Greco, K. E., Tinley, S., & Seibert, D. (2011). *Essential genetic and genomic competencies for nurses with graduation degrees.* Retrieved from http://www.aacnnursing.org/Portals/42/AcademicNursing/CurriculumGuidelines/Essenetials-Genetic-Genomic-Competencies-2011.pdf?ver=2017-05-18-101520-227

Haase, P. T. (1990). *The origins and rise of associate degree nursing education.* Durham, NC: Duke University Press.

Hayden, J. K., Smiley, R. A., Alexander, M., Kardong-Edgren, S., & Jeffries, P. R. (2014). The NCSBN National Simulation Study: A longitudinal, randomized, controlled study replacing clinical hours with simulation in prelicensure nursing education. *Journal of Nursing Regulation, 5*(2, Suppl.), S1–S64.

Hendricks, S. M. & Wangerin, V. (2017). Concept-based curriculum: Changing attitudes and overcoming barriers, *Nurse Educator, 42*(3), 138–142.

Hopkins, J. L., & Bromley, G. E. (2016). Preparing new graduates for interprofessional teamwork: Effectiveness of a nurse residency program. *Journal of Continuing Education in Nursing, 47*(3), 140–148.

Hudson, C. E., Sanders, M. K., & Pepper, C. (2013). Interprofessional education and prelicensure baccalaureate nursing students: An integrative review. *Nurse Educator, 38*(2), 76–80.

Ingwerson, J. (2012). Articulation agreements support moving forward. *Oregon State Board of Nursing Sentinel, 31*(2), 8–9.

Institute of Medicine. (2001). *Crossing the quality chasm.* Washington, DC: National Academies Press.

Institute of Medicine. (2003). *Health professions education: A bridge to quality.* Washington, DC: National Academies Press.

Institute of Medicine. (2010). *The future of nursing: Leading change, advancing health.* Washington, DC: National Academies Press.

Institute of Medicine. (2015). *Assessing progress on the IOM report. The future of nursing.* Retrieved from http://nationalacademies.org/hmd/reports/2015/assessing-progress-on-the-iom-report-the-future-of-nursing.aspx

International Nursing Association for Clinical Simulation and Learning. (2013). Standards of best practice: Simulation. *Clinical Simulation in Nursing, 9*(6S), S3–S11.

Interprofessional Education Collaborative Expert Panel. (2011). *Core competencies for interprofessional collaborative practice: Report of an expert panel.* Washington, DC: Interprofessional Education Collaborative. Retrieved from http://www.aacn.nche.edu/education-resources/ipec report.pdf

Jeffries, P. R., Dreifuerst, K. T., Dardong-Edgren, S., & Hayden, J. (2015). Faculty development when initiating simulation programs: Lessons learned from the National Simulation Study. *Journal of Nursing Regulation, 5*(4), 17–23.

Jessee, M. A., & Tanner, C. A. (2016). Pursuing improvement in clinical reasoning: Development of the clinical coaching interactions inventory. *Journal of Nursing Education, 55*(9), 495–504.

Kellett, P., & Fitton, C. (2016). Supporting transvisibility and gender diversity in nursing practice and education: Embracing cultural safety. *Nursing Inquiry, 24*(1), e121–e146.

Kidd, L. I., Knisley, S. J., & Morgan, K. I. (2012). Effectiveness of a second life simulation as a teaching strategy for undergraduate mental health nursing students. *Journal of Psychosocial Nursing, 50*(7), 28–37.

Kostoff, M., Burkhardt, C., Winter, A., & Shrader, S., (2016). An interprofessional simulation using the SBAR communication tool. *American Journal of Pharmaceutical Education, 80*(9), 1–8.

Kramer, M. (1974). *Reality shock: Why nurses leave nursing.* St. Louis, MO: Mosby.

Landeen, J., Carr, D., Culver, K., Martin, L., Matthew-Maich, N., Noesgaard, C., & Beney-Gadsby, L. (2016). The impact of curricular changes on BSN students' clinical learning outcomes. *Nurse Education in Practice, 21*(2), 51–58.

Letourneau, R. M., & Fater, K. H. (2015). Nurse residency programs: An integrative review of the literature. *Nursing Education Perspectives, 36*(2), 96–101.

Luctkar-Flude, M., Wilson-Keates, B., & Larocque, M. (2012). Evaluating high-fidelity human simulators and standardized patients in an undergraduate nursing health assessment course. *Nurse Education Today, 32,* 448–452.

Mallory, C., & Franqueiro, T. (2017). Attributes of effective transition to practice program leaders. *The Journal of Continuing Education in Nursing, 48*(2), 57–59.

Mellor, R., Cottrell, N., & Moran, M. (2013). "Just working in a team was a great experience . . .": Student perspectives on the learning experiences of an interprofessional education program. *Journal of Interprofessional Care, 27,* 292–297.

Moore, B. S., & Clark, M. C. (2016). The role of linguistic modification in nursing education. *Journal of Nursing Education, 55*(6), 309–315.

Moradi, K., Najarkolai, A. R., & Keshmiri, F. (2016). Interprofessional teamwork education: Moving toward the patient-centered approach. *Journal of Continuing Education in Nursing, 47*(10), 449–460.

Murray, T. A., Pole, D. C., Ciarlo, E. M., & Holmes, S. (2016). A nursing workforce diversity project: Strategies for recruitment, retention, graduation, and NCLEX-RN success. *Nursing Education Perspectives, 37*(3), 138–144.

National Council of State Boards of Nursing. (2016). *2015 nurse license volume and NCLEX examination statistics.* Retrieved from https://www.ncsbn.org/16_2015_NCLEXExamStats_vol68.pdf

National League for Nursing. (2014). *Annual survey of schools of nursing, 2014.* Retrieved from http://www.nln.org/docs/default-source/newsroom/nursing-education-statistics/percentage -of-basic-rn-programs-by-program-type-1994-to-1995-and-2003-to-2012-and-2014-(pdf).pdf ?sfvrsn=0

National League for Nursing (2015). *A vision for the changing faculty role: Preparing students for the technological world of health care.* Retrieved from http://nln.org/docs/default-source/about/nln -vision-series-%28position-statements%29/nlnvision_8.pdf?sfvrsn=4

National League for Nursing (2016). Achieving diversity and meaningful inclusion in nursing education. Retrieved from http://www.nln.org/docs/default-source/about/vision-statement -achieving-diversity.pdf?sfvrsn=2

National League for Nursing Commission for Nursing Education Accreditation (2016). *Accreditation standards for nursing education programs.* Retrieved from http://nln.org/docs/default-source/accreditation-services/cnea-standards-final-february-201613f2bf5c78366c709642ff00005f0421.pdf?sfvrsn=10

National League for Nursing Think Tank on Transforming Clinical Nursing Education. (2008). *Final report of the 2008 NLN think tank on transforming clinical nursing education.* Retrieved from http://www.nln.org/facultydevelopment/pdf/think_tank.pdf

Nielsen, A. (2016). Concept-based learning in clinical experiences: Bringing theory to clinical education for deep learning. *Journal of Nursing Education, 55*(7), 365–371.

Nielsen, A., Lasater, K., & Stock, M. (2016). A framework to support preceptors' evaluation and development of new nurses' clinical judgment. *Nurse Education in Practice, 19,* 84–90.

Noone, J., Sideras, S., Gubrud-Howe, P., Voss, H., & Mathews, L. R. (2012). Influence of a poverty simulation on nursing student attitudes toward poverty. *Journal of Nursing Education, 51*(11), 617–622.

Organization for Associate Degree Nursing & American Nurses Association. (2017). Joint position statement on academic progression to meet the needs of the registered nurse, the health care consumer, and the U.S. health care system. Retrieved from https://www.oadn.org/images/pdf/Position%20Statements/160113_OADN_ANA_PositionStatement_Academic_Progression_150602.pdf

Olson-Sitki, K., Wendler, M. C., & Forbes, G. (2012). Evaluating the impact of a nurse residency program for newly graduated registered nurses. *Journal for Nurses in Staff Development, 28*(4), 156–162.

Orsilini-Hain, L., & Waters, V. (2009). Education evolution: A historical perspective of associate degree nursing. *Journal of Nursing Education, 48*(5), 266–271.

Patterson, L. D., Crager, J. M., Farmer, A., Epps, C. D., & Schuessler, J. B. (2016). A strategy to ensure faculty engagement when assessing a concept-based curriculum. *Journal of Nursing Education, 55*(8), 467–470.

Pauly-O'Neill, S., Cooper, E., & Prion, S. (2016). Student QSEN participation during an adult medical–surgical rotation. *Nursing Education Perspectives, 37*(3), 165–172.

Payne, L. K., Glaspie, T., & Rosser, C. (2014). Comparison of select outcomes between traditional and accelerated BSN programs: a pilot study. *Nursing Education Perspectives, 35*(5), 332–334.

Quality and Safety Education for Nurses. (2014). QSEN Competencies. Retrieved from http://qsen.org/competencies/pre-licensure-ksas

Relf, M. V. (2016). Advancing diversity in academic nursing. *Journal of Professional Nursing, 32*(5), S42–S47.

Risling, T. (2017). Educating the nurses of 2025: Technology trends of the next decade. *Nurse Education in Practice, 22,* 89–92.

Robert Wood Johnson Foundation. (2014). Progress and barriers towards innovation in clinical nursing education. Retrieved from http://www.rwjf.org/en/library/articles-and-news/2014/10/progress-and-barriers-toward-innovation-in-clinical-nursing-educ.html

Schaffer, M. A., Tiffany, J. M., Kantack, K., & Anderson, L. J. W. (2016). Second life® virtual learning in public health nursing. *Journal of Nursing Education, 55*(9), 536–540.

Scherer, Y. K., Myers, J., O'Connor, T. D., & Haskins, M. (2013). Interprofessional simulation to foster collaboration between nursing and medical students. *Clinical-Simulation in Nursing, 9,* e497–e505. doi:10.1016/j.ecns.2013.03.001

Sharpnack, P. A., & Madigan, E. A. (2012). Using low-fidelity simulation with sophomore nursing students in a baccalaureate nursing program. *Nursing Education Perspectives, 33*(4), 264–268.

Skiba, D. J. (2016a). On the horizon: Trends, challenges, and educational technologies in higher education. *Nursing Education Perspectives, 37*(3), 183–189.

Skiba, D. J. (2016b). The state of online education. *Nursing Education Perspectives, 37*(4), 244–247.

Sportsman, S., & Allen, P. (2011). Transitioning associate degree in nursing students to the bachelor of science in nursing and beyond: A mandate for academic partnerships. *Journal of Professional Nursing, 6,* e20–e27.

Tri-Council for Nursing. (2010). *Tri-Council for Nursing issues new consensus policy statement on the educational advancement of registered nurses.* Retrieved from http://www.aacn.nche.edu/education-resources/TricouncilEdStatement.pdf

Tri-Council for Nursing. (2015). Scope of practice decision making framework. Retrieved from https://www.ncsbn.org/decision-making-framework.htm

Urban Institute. (2009). The nursing workforce challenge: Public policy for a dynamic and complex market. Retrieved from http://www.urban.org/publications/411933.html

U.S. Department of Health and Human Services. (2014). *Healthy People 2020.* Washington, DC: U.S. Government Printing Office. Retrieved from http://www.healthypeople.gov/2020/default.aspx

U.S. Department of Health and Human Services, Health Resources and Services Administration, Bureau of Health Workforce, & National Center for Health Workforce Analysis. (2014). *Sex, race, and ethnic diversity of U.S. health occupations (2010–2012).* Rockville, MD: Author.

Ward, J., Cody, J., Schaal, M., & Hojat, M. (2012). The empathy enigma: An empirical study of decline in empathy among undergraduate nursing students. *Journal of Professional Nursing, 28*(1), 34–40.

Weathers, S. M., & Hunt Raleigh, E. D. (2013). 1-year retention rates and performance ratings: Comparing associate degree, baccalaureate, and accelerated baccalaureate degree nurses. *Journal of Nursing Administration, 43*(9), 468–474.

Wojner, D. M., & Whelan, W. M. (2016). Preparing nursing students for enhanced roles in primary care: The current state of prelicensure and RN-to-BSN education. *Nursing Outlook, 65*(2), 222–232.

World Health Organization. (2010). *WHO framework for action on interprofessional education and collaborative practice.* Geneva, Switzerland: WHO Press.

Zinsmaster, J., & Vliem, S. (2016). The influence of high-fidelity simulation on knowledge gain and retention. *Nursing Education Perspectives, 37*(5), 289–297.

Zittel, B., Moss, E., O'Sullivan, A., & Siek, T. (2016). Registered nurses as professionals: Accountability for education and practice. *Online Journal of Issues in Nursing, 21*(3), 8–10.

CHAPTER 8

Curriculum Planning for Specialty Master's Nursing Degrees and Entry-Level Graduate Degrees

Stephanie S. DeBoor

Sarah B. Keating

CHAPTER OBJECTIVE

Upon completion of Chapter 8, the reader will be able to:

- Discuss the process of curriculum development for master's programs in nursing including the:
  - RN-to-master of science in nursing (MSN) programs
  - Entry-level MSN
  - Clinical nurse leader (CNL)
  - Advanced practice programs
  - Functional roles, for example, case management, nursing administration/leadership, and nurse educator
- Review recommendations from accrediting, professional specialty and educational organizations, and certification agencies for master's degrees in nursing
- Analyze issues surrounding graduate-level nursing at the master's level:
  - Entry into practice
  - Terminal degrees and advanced practice
  - Postmaster's certificates
  - Certification, licensure, and regulation

OVERVIEW

In the 20th century, as nursing education matured in the academic world and the profession grappled with the issue of defining itself as a discipline, graduate education in nursing evolved. Nursing leaders recognized the need for additional education to be prepared for faculty and administrator roles. Since there was a dearth of graduate nursing programs, nurses often sought degrees in other disciplines such as education, business, and health care administration. Nurses in practice focused their services on clinical specialties such as pediatrics, obstetrics, psychiatric/mental health, medical/surgical nursing, and intensive care, and they too, felt the need for additional specialty training, many seeking nondegree certification. In community settings, it was recognized that public health nurses (PHNs) needed knowledge in epidemiology and the public health sciences, and the specialty roles of nurse midwives and nurse anesthetists required advanced educational preparation and clinical practice. Many of these programs were first offered in baccalaureate programs or as certificate programs to expand on knowledge and skills from basic nursing programs; however, all eventually moved into the graduate level.

The first master's degree in a clinical nursing specialty was awarded in 1956 from Columbia University School of Nursing (Columbia University School of Nursing, 2016). In the 1970s, schools of nursing in higher degree institutions developed master's degree programs that focused on the preparation of nursing faculty, administrators, and some of the classic specialties such as pediatrics, maternity, community health, and psychiatric/mental health nursing. These latter specialties became clinical specialties and as they were developing, the advent of the nursing role in primary care began with the introduction of nurse practitioners. With acute care rising in complexity, it became apparent that nurses with blended specialty role preparation were needed, such as the acute care nurse practitioner. More recently, with the implementation of the Affordable Care Act (ACA; U.S. Department of Health and Human Services, 2017) and the Institute of Medicine's (IOM's, 2015) *Assessing Progress on the Institute of Medicine Report, The Future of Nursing*, the demand for advanced practice nurses has increased exponentially.

See Chapter 1 for a history of graduate nursing education to gain an appreciation for how nursing evolved in its role in health care to match the needs of the health care system with its growing demands for well-educated providers of care. Out of all of these changes and demands came master's degrees that focused on the specialties, primary care, management/administration, and education. More recently, nursing is moving away from the master's for advanced clinical practice and toward the practice doctorate (doctor of nursing practice [DNP]) with the master's programs emphasizing the need for systems management for the delivery of health care. Nursing's history as well as that of the other health care professions traditionally took place in silos of education such as schools of medicine, nursing, physical therapy, psychology, and so forth with few opportunities for combined theory courses and clinical practice; yet, the complex health care system calls for interprofessional collaboration to meet the needs of the population and improve outcomes of care. Recently, many academic medical centers are promoting and developing interprofessional educational programs to meet these challenges (Gerard, Kazer, Babington, & Quell, 2015).

This chapter discusses the various types of master's-level programs offered in today's nursing educational system. In 2017, there were approximately 537 master's-level nursing programs in the United States accredited by the Accreditation Commission for Education in Nursing (2017) and the Commission on Collegiate Nursing Education (2017). The chapter breaks the various master's-level programs into groups from the RN to MSN, entry-level master's (generic), advanced generalist (CNL), and finally, to the advanced practice specialty and functional roles that are available in today's graduate programs. Each group is reviewed and its role in graduate nursing and the profession is discussed. Some of the major issues related to master's-level nursing education are discussed throughout.

RN-TO-MSN PROGRAMS

With the call for higher education for nurses by the IOM's recommendations on *The Future of Nursing* (2010) and the *Assessing Progress on the Institute of Medicine Report on the Future of Nursing* (2015) to meet the needs of the U.S. health care system, there is renewed interest in accelerated RN-to-MSN programs. The shortage of nursing faculty adds to this need for nurses with clinical work experience to gain higher education in order to assume faculty roles. According to the American Association of Colleges of Nursing (AACN, 2017a; American Association of Community Colleges, 2014) in 2016, there were, then, 230 RN-to-MSN programs available across the United States.

There are several permutations of curricula for accelerating RNs who have a diploma or associate degree to the master's degree. One format awards the baccalaureate along the way as the RN completes courses equivalent to the upper division–level bachelor of science in nursing (BSN). The other format is to not award the BSN but, rather, have the RN complete both upper division baccalaureate and master's-level courses and receive the MSN upon completion of the program. Sometimes, both the BSN and MSN are awarded upon completion of the program. Factors that determine the type of program of study include regional accreditation issues, parent institution standards, and the faculty's philosophy. For example, awarding the BSN along the way of the program gives students a baccalaureate whose circumstances prohibit them from completing the master's portion of the program.

The typical patterns for the curricula consist of 1-year accelerated study to complete the baccalaureate upper division–level equivalent courses. Following completion of these courses, students enter graduate-level courses and, depending on the program, may take another 1½ to 3 years of master's-level courses depending on the type of master's degree, with advanced practice degrees spending more theory courses and clinical hours specific to that branch of advanced practice. Some courses are developed to match the experience of the RNs to the level of education indicated and double count toward both the higher level of the baccalaureate and the introductory-level master's courses. Since the large majority of RN students are working, the usual platforms for delivery of the programs are web-based, online, evenings, and/or weekend classes to accommodate their needs.

There are few, if any, studies to compare RN-to-MSN graduates to post-BSN and entry-level master's programs, thus research is called for. The types of master's program (advanced practice or functional role) and the platform for delivery of the program (online, nontraditional, or traditional) should be studied for their effectiveness and student, faculty, and employer satisfaction.

ENTRY-LEVEL MASTER'S DEGREE PROGRAMS IN NURSING (AKA: GENERIC, ACCELERATED MASTER'S FOR NONNURSES, SECOND-DEGREE MASTER'S)

When planning an entry-level master's program, it is wise to consult with the regional accrediting body and the state board of nursing to identify any possible barriers to offering the degree. For example, some regional or state accrediting bodies and boards of nursing may require a baccalaureate in nursing prior to earning a master's degree in the same discipline, even if the person has a baccalaureate in another discipline. There are two major pathways or programs of study for nonnursing college graduates to reach licensure (RN) requirements and a graduate degree in nursing. They are described as follows.

The first program provides basic nursing knowledge and skills courses specifically designed for college graduates and taught at the postbaccalaureate level. Included in the program or required as prerequisites are the usual sciences, social sciences, and liberal arts courses. Examples of classic prerequisites for any entry-level nursing program (associate degree, baccalaureate, and master's) are anatomy, chemistry, English, genetics, human development, mathematics/statistics, microbiology, nutrition, physiology, psychology, sociology, and speech/communications. Students in the entry-level master's complete nursing theory and clinical courses at the upper division level, advanced nursing theory and clinical courses at the graduate level, and a capstone experience that can be a thesis, project, and/or comprehensive examination. (Fewer master's programs are requiring a thesis because of the increase in research-focused/translational science doctoral-level education.) Schools of nursing differ in their preparation of these graduates by offering either an advanced generalist master's degree for entry into practice or a specialist track to prepare graduates for advanced levels of nursing practice or roles.

The other entry-level curriculum requires students to complete courses equivalent to or the same as existing courses in baccalaureate-level nursing programs. They are not necessarily specifically revised for college graduates. As with the first program, students either must have the prerequisite sciences and liberal arts courses or complete them in the program. After completion of the baccalaureate-level courses, students enter into the master's program to complete either an advanced generalist role such as the CNL or a specialty, such as clinical specialist, nurse anesthetist, nurse midwife, or nurse practitioner; acute care practitioner; or a role specialty such as case management, nursing educator, or administrator. The track record for the graduates of entry-level master's programs is excellent. Students in the programs bring life experience, a previously earned higher degree, and academic achievement as most programs require at least a 3.0 grade point average (GPA) in the undergraduate program for admission.

According to the AACN (2017b), there were 69 entry-level master's programs in the United States. Descriptions of the programs and the student and graduate characteristics may be found in the accelerated BSN and MSN programs AACN website (www.aacn.nche.edu/media-relations/fact-sheets/accelerated-programs). Downey and Assein (2015) conducted an integrative literature review pertaining to the students' and faculty members' perceptions regarding accelerated master's programs for non-nursing graduates of baccalaureate or higher degree programs. They found that students entering the programs did so based on their beliefs about nursing as a caring profession. The majority were female, older, and above average academically. The students were surprised at the rigor of the nursing education program. The authors noted the lack of studies and the need for investigation related to the perceptions of students and faculty as they experience the educational program.

THE CNL

The CNL program was developed by the AACN in response to the need for health care providers to manage clients or groups of clients at the point of care. AACN (2007, 2017c) provides the following description of the role of the CNL: "The Clinical Nurse Leader[SM] or CNL® is a master's educated nurse, prepared for practice across the continuum of care within any health care setting. The CNL was developed by AACN in collaboration with leaders from health care practice and education to address the critical need to improve the quality of patient care outcomes. The CNL is a clinical leader—at the point of care—who focuses on: Care Coordination, Outcomes Measurement, Transitions of Care, Interprofessional Communication & Team Leadership, Risk Assessment, Implementation of Best Practices Based on Evidence, and Quality Improvement." In 2017, there were 109 accredited nursing programs that provided the CNL major at the master's level (AACN, 2017d). The AACN (2013) document on the *Competencies and Curricular Expectations for CNL Education and Practice* provides specific information for curricular planning for programs wishing to offer this degree. Certification for the CNL is overseen and awarded by an autonomous branch of AACN, the Commission on Nurse Certification (CNC; AACN, 2017e).

Bender (2014) conducted a review of the literature on the CNL role, job analysis, and outcomes of care toward quality improvement. Based on the review, the author recommends further research on the role in practice in comparison to the specific CNL curriculum developed by the AACN and its influence on the quality of care. Hicks and Rosenberg (2016) describe the phasing out of a baccalaureate in nursing program and the development of an entry-level master's program for the preparation of CNLs. A 2016 job analysis was conducted by the CNC and Schroeder Measurement Technologies, Inc., to examine the relationship between the knowledge, skills and abilities of the CNL and the content of the certification examination (Commission on Collegiate Nursing Education, 2016). Based on this analysis, content specifications are reflected in the certification examination that began in April 2017. This examination blueprint is a supportive guide in curriculum development and evaluation. Establishment of practice partners or academic partnerships is one strategy for arranging clinical experiences for the CNL. The U.S. Department of Veterans Affairs (VA) hospitals are frequent sites of these academic partnerships. VA medical centers have been participants of the CNL Initiative since 2013 (U.S. Department of Veterans Affairs, 2016).

ADVANCED PRACTICE MASTER'S DEGREE PROGRAMS IN NURSING

The classic advanced practice roles encompass the clinical specialist, nurse anesthetist, nurse midwife, and nurse practitioner. As discussed in Chapter 1 on the history of master's education, the advanced practice roles emerged in the 1960s and 1970s. Nurse anesthetists (certified registered nurse anesthetists [CRNAs]) and nurse midwives predated these programs by many years (centuries for midwives and 150+ years for CRNAs); however, their move into higher education/graduate education occurred about the same time period as did the clinical specialist and nurse practitioner roles. A few advanced practice nurses still have a certificate to practice depending on state licensure laws, although most states now require the master's degree for entry into advanced practice. With the advent of the DNP degree, many of these nurses are continuing their education to earn a DNP. See Chapter 9 for discussion of the DNP. The AACN in 2004 issued a statement that the DNP should be the entry level for advanced practice in nursing by 2015 and according to its website in 2017, there were approximately 277 DNP programs with another 100 considering opening a program (AACN, 2017f).

All master's degree programs that prepare advanced practice nurses require a baccalaureate in nursing or in rare cases, its equivalent, and some have additional prerequisites, for example, CRNA programs often require more than one or two chemistry courses. Both the clinical specialist and nurse practitioner programs have subspecialties, for example, adult, cardiovascular, family, geriatric, pediatrics, psychiatric/mental health, women's health, and so on.

The 2008 Consensus Report for APRN Regulation (AACN, 2008) limits the blended role of primary and acute care foci to adult-geriatric and pediatric roles only and specifies that graduates must be nationally certified for both the primary (practitioner) and acute care (clinical specialist) roles. The consensus model was a product of meetings with the leading professional nursing organizations, specialty organizations, accrediting bodies, nursing education organizations, certification agencies, and the National Council of State Boards. It was the intention of the group to clarify advanced practice roles for the profession and the public and to begin an initiative for consistent regulation encompassing licensing, accreditation, certification, and education (LACE) across the various states in the nation. The APRN Regulatory Model depicting the advanced practice registered nurse (APRN) roles, population foci, and specialties can be accessed at www.aacn.nche.edu/education-resources/APRNReport.pdf (p. 10).

Recently, the National Council of State Boards presented an update on the Consensus Report for APRN Regulation (Cahill, Alexander, & Gross, 2014). It lists the major elements of APRN regulations as:

- Title is advanced practice registered nurse (APRN).
- Roles of APRNs and recognition of each follow: certified nurse practitioner (CNP), clinical nurse specialist (CNS), CRNA, certified nurse midwife (CNM).
- Licensure: APRNs hold both an RN and APRN license.

- Education: Graduate education is required for APRNs regardless of role.
- Certification: Every APRN is required to meet advanced certification requirements.
- Independent practice: The APRN shall be granted full authority to practice independently without physician oversight or a written collaborative agreement.
- Full prescriptive authority. The APRN shall be granted full prescriptive author without physician oversight or a written collaborative agreement. (p. 5)

Cahill et al. (2014) list the progress toward meeting the elements of the consensus report state by state with some forward progress. As the health care system evolves in the United States, it is expected that the consensus model will continue to move forward in response to increased demands for well-qualified and educated APRNs. As of August 2016, there were 29 states and the District of Columbia that allowed for full-practice authority for APRNs (National Council of State Boards of Nursing, 2016).

Advanced practice nurses have a key role in the delivery of quality care. With the ever-growing shortages in providers and reform of health care, Murphy (2011) identified that APRNs were poised to provide primary care. The American Nurses Association published a white paper in 2012 describing the value of the APRN in improving the delivery of health care through care coordination (American Nurses Association, 2012). It is estimated that 32 million adults in the United States visit an advanced practice clinician (APC) yearly and yet insurers reimburse APCs at lower rates than physicians (Davis, Guo, Titler, & Friese, 2017). To provide further evidence of the impact the APRN has on the health care delivery system, the following reports from the literature verify this statement. Stanik-Hutt et al. (2013) performed a systematic review comparing health care quality, safety, and effectiveness outcomes between nurse practitioners (NPs) and MDs. Results indicated that NPs are comparable or better than MDs for all outcomes (lipid screening, satisfaction of care, health status, functional status, emergency visits/hospitalizations, blood glucose, blood pressure, and mortality) reviewed. Kurtzman et al. (2017) examined whether state-granted APRN independence had an effect on patient-level quality, service utilization, and referrals. Data were analyzed using propensity score matching and multivariate regression for each outcome. Results identified that outcomes were unaffected by states' APRN independence status.

Irvin, Sedlak, Walton, Collier, and Bernhofer (2017) reported on the use of NPs as wound care consultants (WCCs) and their impact on the rate of hospital-acquired pressure injuries (HAPIs) within a community hospital setting. A retrospective, comparison design was used for this study. The researchers compared 48 months of HAPI data: 24 months before and after the hiring of NPs as WCCs. They found that HAPI rates were considerably lower during the time the NPs provided care than were noted in the previous years. It was Irvin et al.'s conclusion that using NPs as WCCs to assess and provide interventions during hospital admissions may be helpful in reducing the rates of HAPIs.

Lutfiyya et al. (2016) compared outcomes of diabetes care management for Medicare patients by provider types (physician or nurse practitioner). A cross-section retrospective study examined a random sampling of the 2012 U.S. Medicare National Claims History. Utilizing a medical productivity index, patients who were cared for by either an NP or MD were classified as healthiest to least healthy. Also analyzed were health service utilization, health outcomes, and health care cost variables. The authors concluded that NPs are effective providers of diabetes care management. Their patients had significantly improved outcomes when compared with primary care physician providers in relation to service utilization, health outcomes, and costs.

To further ensure patient safety and quality care, the scope of practice decision-making framework was developed by the Tri-Council for Nursing in collaboration with the National Council of State Boards of Nursing in 2015. After reviewing the literature for algorithms related to decision making, a tool was developed to assist the nurses in identifying what safely falls within their role based on each nurse's level of education, licensure, certification, and state board regulations (Ballard et al., 2016; National Council of State Boards of Nursing, 2017).

In summary, the traditional role for advanced practice continues to play an important role in the delivery of high-quality, safe, and cost-effective care. Nursing continues to find it necessary to illustrate this to not only the health care industry but the public as well. As advanced practice roles become more delineated, knowledge of one's scope is more important than ever in ensuring best patient outcomes.

COMMUNITY/PUBLIC HEALTH NURSING

Community/public health nursing master's programs prepare nurses for advanced practice roles in community settings. There are some schools of nursing that offer a joint degree awarding both the MSN and the master of public health (MPH). Others have community health nursing as a clinical specialty. The American Nurses Credentialing Center (ANCC, 2017a) offers a PHN—Advanced specialty certification by portfolio for graduates of master's, postgraduate certificate, or doctoral degree in nursing or hold a master's, postgraduate, or doctorate in public health with a BSN.

Transformation of health care legislated by the ACA has required the relationship between public health and health care systems to strengthen their collaborative efforts in order to meet the changes in our national health care landscape. Edmonds, Campbell, and Gilder (2016) explored the knowledge, perceptions, and practices of PHNs under the ACA. Participants were recruited via e-mail lists, flyers, and announcements at the 2014 American Public Health Association 142nd Annual Meeting along with listservs of four of the Quad Council of Public Health Nursing Organizations. A web-based survey was utilized. Over 1,100 responded to the survey. Almost half of the respondents reported changes in their current jobs following the institution of the ACA. They identified being somewhat or very actively involved in: integration of primary care and public health, provision of clinical preventive services, care coordination, patient navigation, establishment of private-public partnerships, population health strategies, population health data assessment and analysis, community health assessments, involvement in medical homes, provision of maternal and child health home visiting services, and involvement in Accountable Care Organizations (p. 54). The authors of this study concluded that PHNs are making significant contributions based on their reported areas of involvement.

The dual MSN and MPH has been in existence for quite some time and continues to be offered at universities throughout the United States. The launch of the ACA in 2010 resulted in a complex health care environment requiring a higher level of skills, knowledge, and expertise to ensure quality care. Shaw, Harpin, Steinke, Stember, and Krajicek (2016) discuss the DNP/MPH dual degree as an educational option to better prepare PHNs.

MASTER'S DEGREES IN NURSING FOR FUNCTIONAL ROLES

There are other roles and specialties for nurses with master's degrees not included in the advanced practice and advanced generalist roles. They include case management, nursing administration, nurse educator, staff development/patient education, and other leadership roles. Nurses prepared for these roles usually have nursing theory, health care policy, and research as core courses along with the courses that focus them into a specific function within the health care system. The following discussion presents a few examples of the programs that prepare nurses for specific roles.

Case Management

The educational preparation for roles in case management in nursing usually requires at least a baccalaureate in nursing, with a master's preferred. Case managers provide coordination of services for aggregates in many health care settings. They work closely with other health care professionals. The role began in the 1970s with its purpose to work with patients to individualize care, avoid duplication of services, enhance the quality of care, and promote cost-effectiveness (White & Hall, 2006). There are approximately 20 schools of nursing that offer case management master's degrees. The ANCC (2017b) offers certification, which requires 2,000 hours of clinical practice in case management, RN licensure, practice as an RN for 2 years, and 30 hours of continuing education in case management in the past 3 years.

Nursing Administration

The most common master's degrees in nursing to prepare nurse leaders are the master's in nursing administration or leadership. Some programs offer joint master's degrees with nursing such as business administration (MBA) or health care administration. The graduates of these programs are not prepared for advanced practice roles such as clinical specialists and nurse practitioners, but rather have education in the management of health care systems including staffing, human resources, finances, budgeting, and administration. There are several ways for nurse administrators to receive national certification through the American Organization of Nurse Executives (2017) for executive nursing or as a nurse manager and leader. The latter requires only a baccalaureate in nursing, while the executive certification requires a master's. ANCC (2017c) also has a national certification exam for nurse executives. In addition to these roles in management and administration, there are other leadership certifications for infection control nurses, legal nurse consultants, quality control nurses, and risk managers. These certifications occur through specialty organizations and for the most part require or prefer that nurses have a master's degree as well as continuing education and experience for the specific role.

Nursing Educator

The role of the nursing educator in health care agencies includes staff development and patient education. There are programs in schools of nursing that specifically prepare nurses for this role at the master's level. The Association for Nursing Professional Development (2017) recommends that staff developers become credentialed by ANCC for the nursing clinical specialty in which they are prepared.

With the recent growth of nursing education programs to help relieve the shortage of nursing faculty, many of the programs offer a track for nurse educators in schools of nursing and some offer postmaster's certificates in nursing education. According to the AACN (2015) 2014–2015 report on enrollments, 68,938 qualified applicants to nursing schools were turned away in 2014 due to lack of faculty, clinical sites to support practicums, classroom space, and budgetary issues. Nearly two-thirds of the schools reported that faculty shortages contributed to the rejection of seating students in nursing programs. Owing to the shortage, there has been a surge of master's programs that prepare nurses for faculty roles. In addition, there are many postmaster's certificate programs in education.

It is recommended that faculty members have at least the same degree level for the type of program in which they teach and it is highly recommended that they have one degree higher. Therefore, faculty teaching in associate degree programs should have at the very least a baccalaureate, but most boards of nursing require the master's degree for program approval, while those teaching in baccalaureate and higher degree programs should have a doctorate. However, with the shortage in nursing, it is not uncommon for master's-prepared nurses to teach clinical courses in specialties that match their expertise, and in some states, boards of nursing allow nurses with baccalaureates in nursing to teach under the supervision of an experienced educator.

There is continuing debate about whether nursing faculty need to have special courses in education since they are specialists in their fields. There is no question that there is a separate body of knowledge related to curriculum development, instructional design and strategies, instructional technology, and program and student evaluation. Without this knowledge, many instructors in nursing do not have the background in learning theories that support best practices in education for meeting the needs of learners, nor do they have the curriculum planning and evaluation background to connect the program to the actual implementation (teaching) of the program. Such knowledge ensures the quality of the program so that learning experiences are linked to the mission and goals of the program. The same is true for evaluation for program review to measure outcomes and student evaluation to measure students' progress in the program. At the same time, it is equally important that nursing faculty members have the content knowledge and theory on the material that they are teaching. To further support these statements the National League for Nursing (2017a) offers national certification for nurse educators. Eligibility qualifications require a master's or doctorate in nursing, with a major emphasis on nursing education, or nine or more credit hours obtained in graduate-level education courses (e.g., curriculum development and evaluation; instructional design; principles of adult learning; assessment/measurement & evaluation; principles of teaching and learning, instructional technology; National League for Nursing, 2017b).

SUMMARY

Chapter 12 reviewed common master's degree programs in nursing and the differences among the majors available in nursing at that level. Roles for master's degree–prepared nurses were discussed and postgraduate certification possibilities were reviewed. Some issues were raised such as the advent of the DNP and its impact on advanced practice master's programs, entry into practice at the master's level, expectations of the educational preparation for nursing faculty, and the place for the advanced generalist master's degree graduate in the health care system.

DISCUSSION QUESTIONS

- Debate the pros and cons of entry into practice at the master's level versus the second baccalaureate for college graduates.
- How should nursing differentiate between advanced practice roles and advanced knowledge roles such as administrators, case managers, risk managers, and so on?
- Is it important for nursing educators in the practice setting and in schools of nursing to have graduate degrees and what levels of advanced education are necessary? Why or why not?

LEARNING ACTIVITIES

Student-Learning Activities

1. Review the literature and websites for nursing education to identify how many possible majors there are for master's degrees in nursing. Compare the majors to the job market for these specialties in your region. Discuss the pros and cons for the continuation or discontinuation of some of the programs.

2. Go to the websites of various credentialing and certification organizations for nursing and identify how many require at least a master's degree in nursing. Discuss why or why not certification for advanced roles should continue.

Faculty Development Activities

1. Review the latest follow-up survey of the graduates of your master's program for data on the employment of the graduates in settings where they use the focus of their graduate degrees. Determine if your program prepared graduates for the needs of the health care system and why or why not. Consider the effect of your findings on curriculum revision, or possibly, discontinuance of a program or development of new programs.
2. Discuss among yourselves your beliefs about master's education for advanced practice or roles in leadership and, if the master's degree serves your graduates as a terminal degree and/or pathway to doctoral studies.

References

Accreditation Commission for Education in Nursing. (2017). Accredited programs. Retrieved from http://www.acenursing.us/accreditedprograms/programSearch.htm

American Association of Colleges of Nursing. (2007). *White paper on the education and role of the clinical nurse leader.* Washington, DC: Author.

American Association of Colleges of Nursing. (2008). *Consensus model for APRN regulation: Licensure, accreditation, certification, & education.* Retrieved from https://www.aacn.org/~/media/aacn-website/nursing-excellence/standards/aprnregulation.pdf?la=en

American Association of Colleges of Nursing. (2013). *Competencies and curricular expectations for clinical nurse leader education and practice.* Retrieved from http://www.aacnnursing.org/Portals/42/AcademicNursing/CurriculumGuidelines/CNL-Competencies-October-2013.pdf

American Association of Colleges of Nursing. (2015). Nursing faculty shortage. Retrieved from http://www.aacnnursing.org/Portals/42/News/Factsheets/Nursing-Shortage-Factsheet-2017.pdf?ver=2017-10-18-144118-163

American Association of Colleges of Nursing. (2017a). Schools offering RN to Master's Programs, Fall 2016 (N = 230). Retrieved from http://www.aacnnursing.org/News-Information/Fact-Sheets/Degree-Completion-Programs

American Association of Colleges of Nursing. (2017b). Schools offering entry-level or 2nd degree master's programs, Fall 2016 (N = 68). Retrieved from http://www.aacnnursing.org/Nursing-Education

American Association of Colleges of Nursing. (2017c). CNL. Clinical nurse leader. Retrieved from http://www.aacnnursing.org/News-Information/Fact-Sheets/Degree-Completion-Programs

American Association of Colleges of Nursing. (2017d). CNL programs. Retrieved from http://www.aacnnursing.org/CNL-Certification/Apply-for-the-Exam/Eligible-CNL-Programs

American Association of Colleges of Nursing. (2017e). CNL certification. Retrieved from http://www.aacnnursing.org/cnl-certification

American Association of Colleges of Nursing. (2017f). Program directory. Retrieved from http://www.aacnnursing.org/dnp

American Association of Community Colleges. (2014). RN to MSN program information. Retrieved from http://www.aacc.nche.edu/Resources/aaccprograms/health/cap/Pages/rn-msn.aspx

American Nurses Association. (2012). *The value of nursing care coordination: A white paper of the American Nurses Association.* Retrieved from http://www.nursingworld.org/carecoordinationwhitepaper

American Nurses Credentialing Center. (2017a). Advanced public health nursing portfolio. Retrieved from http://nursecredentialing.org/AdvancedPublicHealthNurse-Portfolio

American Nurses Credentialing Center. (2017b). Nursing case management. Retrieved from http://nursecredentialing.org/NursingCaseManagement

American Nurses Credentialing Center. (2017c). Nurse executive. Retrieved from http://nursecre dentialing.org/NurseExecutive

American Organization of Nurse Executives. (2017). AONE credentialing center certification programs. Retrieved from http://www.aone.org/initiatives/certification.shtml

Association for Nursing Professional Development. (2017). Become a staff educator. Retrieved from http://www.anpd.org

Ballard, K., Haagenson, D., Christiansen, L., Damgaard, G., Halstead, J. A., Jason, R. R., . . . Alexander, M. (2016). *Scope of nursing practice decision-making framework*. Retrieved from https://www.ncsbn.org/2016JNR_Decision-Making-Framework.pdf

Bender, M. (2014). The current evidence base for the clinical nurse leader: A narrative review of the literature. *Journal of Professional Nursing, 30*(2), 110–123.

Cahill, M., Alexander, M., & Gross, L. (2014). The 2014 NCBSN report on APRN regulation. *Journal of Nursing Regulation, 4*(3), 3–12.

Columbia University School of Nursing. (2016). History of the school. Retrieved from nursing.columbia.edu/about-us/history-school

Commission on Collegiate Nursing Education. (2016). *Clinical Nurse Leader (CNL®) 2016 job analysis summary & certification examination blueprint*. Retrieved from http://www.aacnnursing.org/Portals/42/CNL/2016-CNL-Job-Analysis-Final-Report.pdf

Commission on Collegiate Nursing Education. (2017). CCNE-accredited master's nursing degree programs. Retrieved from http://directory.ccnecommunity.org/reports/rptAccreditedPrograms_New.asp?sort=state&sProgramType=2

Davis, M. A., Guo, C., Titler, M. G., & Friese, C. R. (2017). Advanced practice clinicians as a usual source of care for adults in the United States. *Nursing Outlook, 65*(1), 41–49.

Downey, K., & Assein, M. (2015). Accelerated master's programs in nursing for non-nurses: An integrative review of students' and faculty's perceptions. *Journal of Professional Nursing, 3*(3), 215–225.

Edmonds, J. K., Campbell, L. A., & Gilder, R. E. (2016). Public health nursing practice in the Affordable Care Act era: A national survey. *Public Health Nursing, 34*(1), 50–58.

Gerard, S., Kazer, M., Babington, L., & Quell, T. (2015). Past, present, and future trends in master's education in nursing. *Journal of Professional Nursing, 30*(4), 326–332.

Hicks, F., & Rosenberg, L. (2016). Enacting a vision for a master's entry clinical nurse leader program: Rethinking nursing education. *Journal of Professional Nursing, 32*(1), 41–47.

Institute of Medicine. (2010). *The future of nursing. Leading change, advancing health*. Retrieved from http://nacns.org/wp-content/uploads/2016/11/5-IOM-Report.pdf

Institute of Medicine. (2015). *Assessing progress of the Institute of Medicine Report: The future of nursing*. Retrieved from http://www.jonascenter.org/docs/Assessing-Progress-on-the-Institute-of-Medicine-Report-The-Future-of-Nursing_Dec2015.pdf

Irvin, C., Sedlak, E., Walton, C., Collier, S., & Bernhofer, E. I. (2017). Hospital-acquired pressure injuries: The significance of the advanced practice registered nurse's role in a community hospital. *Journal of the American Association of Nurse Practitioners, 29*(4), 203–208.

Kurtzman, E. T., Barnow, B. S., Johnson, J. E., Simmens, S. J., Lind Infeld, D., &Mullan, F. (2017). Does the regulatory environment affect nurse practitioner's patters of practice or quality of care in health centers? *Health Services Research, 52*(51), 437–458.

Lutfiyya, M. N., Tomai, L., Frogner, B., Cerra, F., Zismer, D., & Parente, S. (2016). Does primary care diabetes management provided to Medicare patients differ between primary care physicians and nurse practitioners? *Journal of Advanced Nursing, 73*(1), 240–252.

Murphy, K. (2011). Advanced practice nurses: Prime candidates to become primary caregivers in relation to increasing physician shortages due to health care reform. *Journal of Nursing Law, 14*(3–4), 117–119.

National Council of State Boards of Nursing. (2016). CNP independent practice map. Retrieved from https://www.ncsbn.org/5407.htm

National Council of State Boards of Nursing. (2017). Scope of practice decision-making framework. Retrieved from https://www.ncsbn.org/decision-making-framework.htm

National League for Nursing. (2017a). Certification for nurse educators. Retrieved from http://www.nln.org/facultycertification/index.htm

National League for Nursing. (2017b). Eligibility. Retrieved from http://www.nln.org/profes sional-development-programs/Certification-for-Nurse-Educators/eligibility

Shaw, K., Harpin, S., Steinke, G., Stember, M., & Krijicek, M. (2016). The DNP/MPH dual degree: An innovative graduate education program for advanced public health nursing. *Public Health Nursing, 34*(2), 185–193.

Stanik-Hutt, J., Newhouse, R. P., White, K. M., Johantgen, M., Bass, E. B., Zangara, G., . . . Weiner, J. P. (2013). The quality and effectiveness of care provided by nurse practitioners. *The Journal for Nurse Practitioners, 9*(8), 492–500.

U.S. Department of Health and Human Services. (2017). About the Affordable Care Act. Retrieved from http://www.hhs.gov/healthcare/facts/timeline

U.S. Department of Veterans Affairs. (2016). Clinical nurse leader (CNL). Retrieved from https://www.va.gov/NURSING/practice/cnl.asp

White, P., & Hall, M. E. (2006). Managing the literature of case management nursing. *Journal of the Medical Library Association, 94*(2), 99–106.

CHAPTER 9

Planning for Doctoral Education

Stephanie S. DeBoor
Felicia Lowenstein-Moffett

CHAPTER OBJECTIVES

Upon completion of Chapter 9, the reader will be able to:

- Differentiate between applied practice/professional doctorates and research-focused degrees
- Describe the role(s) of the doctor of nursing practice (DNP) and PhD in practice, the health care system, and education
- Analyze the components of the research-focused doctoral programs as recommended by the American Association of Colleges of Nursing (AACN)
- Analyze the educational preparation necessary for the DNP and PhD
- Review program evaluation and accreditation requirements for DNP programs

OVERVIEW

In 2010, the Institute of Medicine (IOM) published *The Future of Nursing* report that called for doubling the number of nurses with doctorates by 2020. Many initiatives were developed to support that mission of growth. According to the AACN, as of Fall 2016 there were 353 programs offering doctoral degrees in the United States (AACN, 2015a). In the *2014–2015 AACN Enrollment and Graduations in Baccalaureate and Graduate Programs in Nursing* report, enrollments in doctoral programs continued to grow with DNP programs showing a 26.2% increase and PhD programs increasing 3.2% (AACN, 2015a). The DNP is the highest level of advanced nursing practice and one of the fastest growing doctorates in the United States (AACN, 2014).

This chapter reviews the purpose of the research-focused doctoral programs in nursing and addresses the curriculum and evaluation of its quality. Issues common to research-focused programs are discussed. In addition, this section reviews the DNP, the nature of the professional doctorate, and differences from research-focused degrees; its role in practice, health care, and education; the essentials of a curriculum for the degree as recommended by AACN; and the standards for accreditation by the Accreditation Commission for Education in Nursing (ACEN) and the Commission on Collegiate Nursing Education (CCNE).

THE ROLE OF THE RESEARCH-FOCUSED DOCTORAL PROGRAM IN NURSING

Research-focused doctoral programs prepare students to pursue intellectual inquiry and conduct independent research that results in extension of knowledge (AACN, 2010; National League for Nursing [NLN], 2013; Rice, 2016). From a theoretical perspective, PhD programs are theory based and focus on testing theory, while doctor of nursing science (DNS) programs are oriented more toward clinical practice research (Ponte & Nicholas, 2015). However, AACN does not differentiate the PhD from DNS programs and it is often difficult to tell the difference in the programs based on their curricula. Clearly the commonality in the program designations is the focus on original research that has potential to contribute to the body of knowledge in the discipline. The PhD in the scientific world is the entry-level preparation needed to develop an independent program of research (AACN, 2010). Graduates are scholars (Melnyk, 2013), although the nature of the knowledge and how it contributes to the field is unique to each candidate and may reflect the explicit foci within the various schools.

In reality, the designation as a PhD or DNS program often is determined by the school's specific mission and philosophy, as well as by institutional criteria for research doctoral program approval. While holding the highest academic degree in the field, nurses from research-focused institutions are prepared and expected to be leaders in nursing as demonstrated by their role in knowledge generation and dissemination, professional organizations, and policy. In fact, graduates of research doctoral programs have been called the stewards of the discipline, those entrusted with preserving the past as the basis for the future of the discipline (AACN, 2010).

In the United States, there are 131 research-focused programs that offer a nursing PhD/DNS; 88 schools are offering baccalaureate to PhD as of Fall 2016 (AACN, 2017). In 2015, there were 4,330 students enrolled in research-focused doctoral programs, 743 graduated, male students constituting 9.6% of the student body, and 69% of the students were White, indicating that one in three is non-White (AACN, 2015b, 2016a). As of Fall 2016, 44 states, the District of Columbia and Puerto Rico have research-focused doctoral programs in nursing (AACN, 2016b). The number of research-focused programs as well as enrollment is stable and growing slowly. Neither the number of programs nor enrollments have increased as rapidly as those of the DNP programs (AACN, 2015a).

Li, Kennedy, and Fang (2017) in a *Special Survey on Vacant Faculty Positions for Academic Year 2016–2017* report the following data. There remains a shortage of faculty, illustrated by the fact that 7.9% of full-time budgeted nursing faculty positions are vacant in the United States. Vacancies in schools vary from 1 to 36 with the average being 1.8 per school. In addition, 16.1% of schools report no full-time vacancies but need additional faculty. In the schools that responded to the AACN survey, barriers to hiring for 2016 through 2017 included lack of funds for salaries (63.9%), unwillingness of administration to commit to full-time positions (49.6%), inability to recruit due to marketplace competition (38.3%), and lack of qualified applicants (24.1%; Li et al., 2017). Furthermore, the top faculty recruitment–related issues identified were the limited number of doctorally prepared faculty (65.8%), noncompetitive salaries (63.0%), finding faculty willing/able to teach in practicum settings, and having faculty with the right specialty mix (65.3%; Li et al., 2017).

Lack of faculty impacts student enrollment. In 2014 AACN reported that 68,938 qualified undergraduate and graduate applicants were denied admission due to faculty shortages (AACN, 2015c). In addition, the faculty in nursing education is aging. Across the various levels of nursing programs, the mean age of professors is 61.6 years, associate professors is 57.6 years, and assistant professors is 51.4 years (AACN, 2015c). This same report identified many statewide initiatives to address the educator and nursing shortages.

Most graduates from research-focused programs work in academia where scholarly activity/research, service to the university and profession, professional competence, and teaching are core criteria for tenure and promotion. Recognizing responsibilities across these various areas, there is no question that research is the focus of research-intensive doctoral education. Pedagogical preparation requires additional course work and practice that focuses on teaching to develop skills and knowledge commensurate with role expectations (Oermann, 2017). Similarly, preparation in health policy may require additional coursework and practice.

PhD/DNS graduates work in research-intensive or teaching-intensive universities. In the research-intensive university, the most highly rewarded activity is research and scholarship. New PhD/DNS faculty members are expected to develop a program of research that is externally funded, publish in peer-reviewed journals, develop a national and, eventually, international reputation as a scholar, provide scientific critique and review for journal articles and grants, and influence policy (Beck, 2016; Smeltzer et al., 2016). The expectation is that they will mentor and teach PhD/DNS students who subsequently will become faculty members who are research scientists. Leadership in the profession, a national reputation (and eventually international), and service to their institution are markers of a successful faculty member at a research-intensive university.

In teaching-intensive programs, PhD/DNS faculty members teach and mentor prelicensure students as well as graduate students. Scholarly activity is required but may be more broadly defined than in the research-intensive university and may include writing textbooks, conducting externally funded quality assurance or education-focused studies, and publishing clinically focused papers. Committee service in the university and leadership in professional organizations and the community are also usual expectations in these schools.

Some PhD/DNS graduates work in industry, government, and policy. While their roles vary, they are hired for their expertise and leadership capacity, much of which is the product of their doctoral education. In industry, they may work in clinical research and direct or monitor research studies. In government, they may assume a role in the National Institute of Nursing Research as well as various other agencies (e.g., Veterans Administration or a branch of the military). Doctorally prepared nurses may work in policy to affect public, industry, or government opinion on health-related issues (e.g., smoking). Some research-focused doctoral graduates seek postdoctoral study. Postdoctoral study focuses on increasing depth in research expertise to help develop a robust program of research. Activities during postdoctoral study may include learning a new method, extending expertise in substantive content, publication of papers from the dissertation, and writing research grants to fund future research.

THE ROLE OF THE DNP IN PRACTICE

The concept of an applied practice doctoral degree in nursing was first introduced in the late 1990s and early 2000s. The launch of the DNP was met with much controversy from inside and outside of the profession related to the role of nurses with doctorates. An issue raised by nursing was the many different nursing doctoral degree programs and titles that confused the public and the profession itself. In October 2004, the members of AACN endorsed the *Position Statement on the Practice Doctorate in Nursing*. This position identified the need for entry level to practice for advanced practice registered nurses (APRNs) to move from the master's level to the doctorate level by 2015 (AACN, 2016c). The IOM issued a recommendation in 2010, *The Future of Nursing: Leading Change, Improving Health* to double the amount of doctorally prepared nurses by 2020.

There are several major roles for DNP-prepared nurses. The DNP-prepared nurse is prepared to work in diverse areas of health care such as direct patient care, academia, clinical research, or administration throughout the health care system. The following present a few of the current roles where DNP graduates are employed:

- Advanced clinician who is dedicated to a practice career such as clinical specialists, nurse anesthetists, nurse midwives, and nurse practitioners in primary care and specialty practices
- Health care leader in public health and community health centers
- Health care policy leader to improve health care for the populations
- Interdisciplinary leader in health care systems, national organizations, and specialty groups
- Nursing educator (While the focus of the DNP is not to prepare nursing educators, graduates of DNP programs are involved in the clinical education of nurses and DNP students.)
- Leader in applied and translational nursing research

Redman (2015) conducted a literature review to determine the impact DNP-prepared nurses are making in health care. This review revealed that the scholarly work being done is exponentially increasing for DNP-prepared nurses with a rapid increase in scholarly publications related primarily to clinical practice. A pivotal finding of this research was that as of 2014, the goal set forth by the IOM in 2010 to increase doctorally prepared nurses is much closer to becoming reality. Recommendations are made to embrace both the DNP and the PhD as crucial roles in the nursing profession.

THE PhD CURRICULUM

The curriculum of each research-focused doctoral program is unique and is based on the school's mission and philosophy as interpreted and implemented by the faculty. Usual core coursework includes the history and philosophy of nursing science, theories that guide the discipline and practice, research methods, advanced statistics, substantive nursing in a specific area of expertise, and role-related content (e.g., pedagogy). Depending on the program, required content may include mentoring, leadership, interdisciplinary research teamwork, and health policy. Cognates from supporting disciplines, such as sociology or physiology, are often required. Dreifuerst et al. (2016) found that those who are exploring doctoral education take into consideration the type of program and its delivery, time to complete, faculty expertise and research interests, and the overall cost. Students report that mentors, funding opportunities, and teaching preparation are important in PhD education (Nehls, Barber, & Rice, 2015). The variability in the curriculum among programs is seen in the requirements of research-focused doctoral programs. Surveys of research-focused doctoral programs show that a research practicum was required by 77.1%, attendance at a professional meeting by 36.8%, presentation at a professional meeting by 21.1%, and submitting a paper for publication by 31.6%. Dissertation format was also quite variable whereas traditional format was utilized by the majority of schools (61.4%), while the publication of at least one paper was required by a few schools (6.9%); and some schools (30.7%) allowed either approach (Minnick, Norman, & Donaghey, 2013).

EDUCATIONAL PREPARATION FOR THE DNP

DNP programs continue to grow across the country and according to AACN, enrollment in DNP programs increased substantially across the nation (AACN, 2015a). AACN reports that from 2014 to 2015 the number of students enrolled in DNP programs increased from 18,352 to 21,995 and the number of graduates from DNP programs increased from

3,065 to 4,100 (AACN, 2016c). DNP curricula are based on *The Essentials of Doctoral Education for Advanced Nursing Practice* (2006).

These eight *Essentials* are as follows:

1. Scientific Underpinnings for Practice
2. Organizational and Systems Leadership for Quality Improvement and Systems Thinking
3. Clinical Scholarship and Analytical Methods for Evidence-Based Practice
4. Information Systems/Technology and Patient Care Technology for the Improvement and Transformation of Health Care
5. Health Care Policy for Advocacy in Health Care
6. Interprofessional Collaboration for Improving Patient and Population Health Outcomes
7. Clinical Prevention and Population Health for Improving the Nation's Health
8. Advanced Nursing Practice

Each of these *Essentials* is described in detail by AACN and specific learning objectives are listed. AACN discusses the incorporation of specialty competencies for programs that prepare DNPs for advanced practice roles such as clinical specialists, nurse practitioners, nurse midwives, nurse anesthetists, clinical nurse leaders, and others. The National Organization of Nurse Practitioner Faculty (2014) lists expected competencies for all advanced practice nurses and nurse practitioners completing the nursing practice doctorate. Academic program developers are directed to specialty organizations for the lists of competencies required for national certification in advanced nursing roles.

There are two entry levels to the DNP program of study. The first is the postmaster's DNP program that admits nurses with master's degrees who are nationally certified as an APRN (nurse anesthetists, midwives, practitioners, and clinical nurse specialists). Additionally, nursing administrators, managers, and other nurse leaders with or without national certification enroll in DNP programs to gain additional education and experiences for leadership roles in the health care system. These include administration, informatics, health care systems analysis, development of policies, and academic leadership roles. Many of these programs were first initiated to meet the needs of master's-prepared nurses wishing to earn a doctorate to advance their practice, act as change agents in the health care system, and increase interprofessional collaboration. While it is expected that advanced practice nurses currently in practice who do not have the DNP will be "grandparented in" for licensure to practice in the states in which they are licensed and recognized, it is anticipated that many will wish to further their education with the DNP degree.

The second entry to DNP education is directly from the postbaccalaureate nursing program (BSN) to the DNP program. These programs prepare BSNs for advanced practice roles similar to the programs for advanced practice nurses at the master's level, for example, certified registered nurse anesthetists (CRNAs), clinical specialists, nurse midwives, and nurse practitioners. Additional course work related to health care systems management, population health care, and leadership at the doctorate level is included. In addition to the traditional advanced practice courses and roles, some BSN to DNP programs offer other options for roles in informatics and technology, health care management, public health, and/or administration. Supervised clinical experiences are included in the programs to meet professional accreditation and/or certification standards and account for at least 1,000 hours of clinical practice.

Students have courses that include the content of the eight *Essentials* recommended by AACN (2006), as well as completion of the specialty role in which they are enrolled.

Graduates are eligible for national certification depending on the program of study's specialization and meeting of eligibility requirements for specific certifications. While many schools (65%) want to adopt this plan of study, there are barriers (costs, faculty, securing clinical sites, preceptors, management of capstone projects, and most importantly, obtaining approval from leadership, regional accreditors, and boards; Auerbach et al., 2014). Dennison, Payne, and Farrell (2012) reviewed the history of DNP programs by tracing them from research-focused doctoral degrees to the nursing practice doctorate (DNP). The authors focused on the advanced practice roles of the DNP and linked them to the AACN *Essentials* (AACN, 2006). This article provides a model for curriculum planners for both the postmaster's and the BSN to DNP programs with a table that ties the AACN *Essentials* to program competencies.

Frantz (2013) provides an overview of the resources needed when planning, implementing, and sustaining a DNP program. Identified are the necessary faculty members and their qualifications; resources such as classrooms and simulation facilities; the infrastructure for delivering courses online and on campus; potential collaboration between the PhD and DNP programs' course faculty and, possibly, other academic institutions; faculty and student practice opportunities; health care agencies' resources for clinical experiences (both advanced practice and administrative); and administrative and staff support specific to the DNP program.

The final project for DNP education is often a topic of concern. Questions regarding the differentiation between an MSN and DNP project are often posed at national conferences. The intent of the DNP project is to be focused as an application of practice as opposed to a knowledge-generating research effort (AACN, 2006). Current recommendations and clarifications for the DNP project can be found in the AACN Task Force report on the implementation of the DNP (AACN, 2015d). Understanding these issues is important when considering the development of DNP curricula.

PhD PROGRAM EVALUATION

There is no professional accreditation for research-focused doctoral programs. However, quality indicators are provided by AACN (2010) to guide the evaluation of these programs. The quality of research-focused doctoral nursing programs is established and maintained by the individual programs. AACN (2010) provides evaluation criteria that are divided into categories of faculty and administration, students, resources and infrastructure, and evaluation plan. Programs often supplement these measures with their own indicators. For example, for a state-supported program, one rubric might be the proportion of state residents in the student body and/or the number of international students enrolled. However, to date, little comparative data exist about quality of programs other than objective measures of enrollment, race/ethnicity and gender of students, length of program, number of grants, and the amount of funding awarded from federal and private grants to nursing faculty.

DNP PROGRAM EVALUATION AND ACCREDITATION

Program evaluation and accreditation are essential to the quality of DNP programs. Each school of nursing that has a DNP program usually has a master plan of evaluation for all programs and the DNP is included. DNP programs, in addition to the usual layers of approval within the home institution, are subject to the institution's governing board's approval, and if they are preparing entry-level advanced practice nurses, depending on state regulations, they must undergo program approval by their state board of nursing. Program evaluation provides the data for assessing the effectiveness and quality of the program. Developing evaluation plans that incorporate all of the parameters of the program for assessment are important but it is also essential that plans are in place to implement the assessment. The methods for collecting and analyzing the data, the persons responsible, and when and how the findings from the analysis are used for program improvements are key factors to include.

Specific to DNP program accreditation are the roles of the ACEN (2013) and the CCNE (2017). The *Standards for Accreditation of Clinical Doctorate Programs* by the ACEN (2013) can be found at www.acenursing.net/manuals/SC2013.pdf.[1] There are six categories of standards:

1. Mission and Administrative Capacity
2. Faculty and Staff
3. Students
4. Curriculum
5. Resources
6. Outcomes

Details concerning these standards are found at the ACEN website.

CCNE (2009) determined that it would accredit doctoral degrees that reflected the terminal practice degree in the profession, not research-focused degrees. This is in line with other professional or applied practice doctoral degrees in other disciplines. To be eligible for CCNE accreditation, programs are required to base their curricula on the AACN *Essentials of Doctoral Education for Advanced Practice* (2006). In addition, programs must have students enrolled for at least 1 year before hosting an on-site evaluation with a self-study submitted prior to the visit (CCNE, 2015). Action on accreditation takes place after a site visit and during the next scheduled CCNE Board of Commissioners meeting. This usually means that students enrolled in the program will graduate from a CCNE-accredited program. Since the DNP is a relatively new degree, most programs must also have regional accreditation, as a new degree is considered a substantive change. See Chapter 12 for more details on program evaluation and accreditation.

DIFFERENCES BETWEEN PROFESSIONAL AND RESEARCH-BASED DOCTORATES

The movement toward a doctorate in nursing for advanced practice and leadership roles grew tremendously over the past decade. According to the AACN, the DNP is the highest level of advanced nursing practice (AACN, 2015a). DNP programs are continuing to flourish across the nation as graduate nursing programs move graduate advanced practice and clinical leader degrees from master's preparation to the terminal DNP degree. AACN (2016c) reports a total of 289 existing DNP programs in 49 states, with another 128 new programs that are currently in various planning stages.

The ever-changing landscape of doctoral education identifies the need for collaborative relationships between the research-focused and practice doctorates. There is ongoing debate concerning the role of DNP and the differences in the PhD degree as it pertains to the profession of nursing, advanced practice, and health care. Murphy, Staffileno, and Carlson (2015) describe the roles of the PhD and the DNP degree programs and their specific purposes and differences with implication for collaboration of practice and research. Historically, nursing recognized several doctoral degrees and titles; academe currently recognizes only two of them as terminal degrees of the profession. The first is the research-focused PhD, and its equivalent counterpart the DNS.

---

1. The 2013 Standards and Criteria for Clinical Doctorate as presented will be replaced by the 2017 Standards and Criteria for Clinical Doctorate, effective 01/01/2017, mandatory 01/01/2018

Research-focused doctorates foster the development of new knowledge in nursing. The DNP is necessary to the vision of nursing, scholarly clinical practice, and leadership within the nursing profession and health care system. During this complex time in health care, the impetus behind the growing surge of DNP-prepared nurses includes: rapid expansion of knowledge that informs clinical practice, doctorally prepared faculty shortages, increased complexity and acuity of patient care, concerns over quality and safety in health care, and innovative leadership needs in all aspects of health care (AACN, 2016c).

Historically, PhD-prepared faculty members were the sole tenure-track professors in institutions of higher education. The rationale for this was that research-focused institutions prefer faculty members who are prepared to develop new knowledge and theories in their respective disciplines and bring recognition to the university through their scholarly activities. The clinical scholar with an applied practice doctorate DNP prepares graduates for analysis and application of evidence-based research directly into health care and clinical practices. Currently, some DNP-prepared faculty hold tenure-track positions in universities across the nation, yet there are still universities in the United States that limit tenure-track positions to only those PhD-prepared candidates (Auerbach et al., 2014).

Nursing education programs vary in their hiring practices. Oermann, Lynn, and Agger (2016) examined the aims of nursing program directors as they apply to hiring DNP- and PhD-prepared faculty. They found that baccalaureate and higher degree programs have a preference for hiring PhD-prepared faculty. Additionally, they reported that the hiring of DNP faculty was largely due to the university's interest in adding a DNP program. If the intent of the student is to teach in academia, then both the research-focused (PhD, DNS) and the practice focused (DNP) doctoral students are strongly encouraged to take courses in education. Finally, Oermann et al. (2016) found that there was variance regarding tenure or nontenure-track appointments for DNP faculty among those surveyed.

Tenure is the guarantee of employment based on past and ongoing scientific contributions to a profession and was designed for the research doctorate. The process of promotion and tenure is based on research, scholarship, and service (Nicholes & Dyer, 2012). Some colleges and universities promote DNP clinicians into tenure-track positions recognizing that the DNP focus is on applied research, practice, and translational science practice. The profession of nursing and its educators recognize the role of DNP graduates for providing instruction and clinical-focused education in undergraduate and graduate nursing programs owing to their expertise in evidence-based clinical practice. Many DNP graduates demonstrate extensive scholarly work and research in clinical practice and scholarship that contribute to the science of nursing. DNP graduates who desire to teach in schools of nursing should compare tenure-track policies in potential employing institutions to other types of positions such as clinical faculty that are not research focused, but still offer academic ranks from instructor to full professor.

SUMMARY

This chapter reviewed the growth of doctoral programs in the nation, educational preparation, curriculum, roles of both research-focused (PhD, DNS) and practice (DNP) doctorates, program evaluation, and differences between the two. Research-focused doctoral programs produce scientists. Most work in academia after graduation and balance research with the other dimensions of their work (teaching, service). The DNP prepares nurses to translate the science developed by nurse researchers into practice. All nursing doctorates play an important role in the changing and challenging components of health care within the United States. Collaboration between PhD/DNS graduates and DNP graduates contribute to the success of meeting these health care needs of our nation.

- Propose how interdisciplinary research might be supported and developed as part of a PhD/DNS program.
- What are the strengths and limitations of having students admitted to a PhD/DNS with a baccalaureate degree in nursing, a master's degree in nursing, and a DNP degree?
- To what extent do you believe the DNP as the terminal degree for advanced practice resulted in consensus within the nursing profession?
- Debate research-focused degrees as contrasted to professional degrees and how research activities differ or are the same. What effect do you believe this debate has on the profession of nursing as a discipline?

Student-Learning Activities

1. Compare and contrast the PhD and DNP programs. What are the similarities and differences in course work, research training, and available faculty mentorship in your area of expertise?
2. Review the latest research and literature (the past 2 years) to identify the state of debate on the DNP and its role in research and academe.

Nurse Educator/Faculty Development Activities

1. Compare one online and one in-person PhD or DNP program. What are the strengths of each? Consider how you can make the best use of these data in your program.
2. If the student population in your program does not reflect the racial–ethnic or gender mix of the general population, what three things might you consider to rectify this disparity?
3. If your school of nursing has a DNP program, analyze its curriculum for its congruence with the AACN *Essentials* document. If your school does not have a DNP program, find a school that does and review its program of study to compare to the *Essentials*.

References

Accreditation Commission for Education in Nursing. (2013). *ACEN accreditation manual: Section III standards and criteria glossary*. Retrieved from http://www.acenursing.net/manuals/SC2013.pdf

American Association of Colleges of Nursing. (2006). *The essentials of doctoral education for advanced nursing practice*. Retrieved from http://www.aacnnursing.org/Portals/42/Publications/DNP Essentials.pdf

American Association of Colleges of Nursing. (2010). *The research-focused doctoral program in nursing: Pathways to excellence*. Retrieved from http://www.aacnnursing.org/Portals/42/Publica tions/PhDPosition.pdf

American Association of Colleges of Nursing. (2014). DNP fact sheet. Retrieved from http://www .aacnnursing.org/News-Information/Fact-Sheets/DNP-Fact-Sheet

American Association of Colleges of Nursing. (2015a). New AACN data confirm enrollment surge in schools of nursing. Retrieved from http://www.jonascenter.org/news/post/amid -calls-for-a-more-highly-educated-rn-workforce-new-aacn-data-confirm-enrollment-surge-in -schools-of-nursing

American Association of Colleges of Nursing. (2015b). *Leading excellence and innovation in academic nursing. Annual report 2015*. Retrieved from http://www.aacnnursing.org/Portals/42/Publi cations/Annual-Reports/AnnualReport15.pdf

American Association of Colleges of Nursing. (2015c). Nursing faculty shortage fact sheet. Retrieved from http://www.aacnnursing.org/Portals/42/News/Factsheets/Faculty-Shortage-Factsheet-2017.pdf

American Association of Colleges of Nursing. (2015d). *The doctor of nursing practice: Current issues and clarifying recommendations: Report from the task force on the implementation of the DNP.* Retrieved from http://www.professionalnursing.org/article/S8755-7223(15)00100-3/pdf

American Association of Colleges of Nursing. (2016a). Table 11a. *Race/ethnicity of students enrolled in generic (entry-level) baccalaureate, master's, and doctoral (research-focused) programs in nursing, 2006–2015.* Retrieved from http://www.aacnnursing.org/Portals/42/News/Surveys-Data/EthnicityTbl.pdf

American Association of Colleges of Nursing. (2016b). DNP education. Retrieved from http://www.aacnnursing.org/Nursing-Education-Programs/DNP-Education

American Association of Colleges of Nursing. (2016c). DNP fact sheet. Retrieved from http://www.aacnnursing.org/News-Information/Fact-Sheets/DNP-Fact-Sheet

American Association of Colleges of Nursing. (2017). Nursing education programs. Retrieved from http://www.aacnnursing.org/Nursing-Education

Auerbach, D. I., Martsolf, G., Pearson, M. L., Taylor, E. A., Zaydman, M., Muchow, A., . . . Dower, C. (2014). *The DNP by 2015: A study of the institutional, political, and professional issues that facilitate or impede establishing a post-baccalaureate doctor of nursing practice program.* Retrieved from http://www.aacn.nche.edu/dnp/DNP-Study.pdf

Beck, C. (2016). *Developing a program of research in nursing.* New York, NY: Springer Publishing.

Commission on Collegiate Nursing Education. (2009). *Achieving excellence in nursing education: The first 10 years of CCNE.* Washington, DC: Author.

Commission on Collegiate Nursing Education. (2015). Overview of the CCNE accreditation process. Retrieved from http://www.aacn.nche.edu/ccne-accreditation/Checklist.pdf

Commission on Collegiate Nursing Education. (2017). CCNE accreditation. Retrieved from http://www.aacn.nche.edu/ccne-accreditation

Dennison, R. D., Payne, C., & Farrell, K. (2012). The doctorate in nursing practice: Moving advanced practice in nursing even closer to excellence. *Nursing Clinics of North America, 47,* 225–240.

Dreifuerst, K. T., McNelis, A. M., Weaver, M. T., Broome, M. E., Draucker, C. B., & Fedko, A. S. (2016). Exploring the pursuit of doctoral education by nurses seeking or intending to stay in faculty roles. *Journal of Professional Nursing, 32*(3), 202–212.

Frantz, R. A. (2013). Resource requirements for a quality doctor of nursing practice program. *Journal of Nursing Education, 52*(8), 449–452.

Institute of Medicine. (2010). *The future of nursing: Leading change, advancing health.* Washington, DC: National Academies Press.

Li, Y., Kennedy, K. A., & Fang, D. (2017). *Special survey on vacant faculty positions for academic year 2016–2017.* Retrieved from http://www.aacn.nche.edu/leading-initiatives/research-data/vacancy16.pdf

Melnyk, B. M. (2013). Distinguishing the preparation and roles of doctor of philosophy and doctor of nursing practice graduates: National implications for academic curricula and health care systems. *Journal of Nursing Education, 52*(8), 442–448.

Minnick, A. F., Norman, L. D., & Donaghey, B. (2013). Defining and describing capacity issues in U.S. doctor of nursing practice programs. *Nursing Outlook, 61*(2), 93–101.

Murphy, M. P., Staffileno, B. A., & Carlson, E. (2015). Collaboration among DNP- and PhD-prepared nurses: Opportunity to drive positive change. *Journal of Professional Nursing, 31,* 388–394.

National League for Nursing. (2013). *A vision for doctoral preparation for nurse educators: A living document from the National League for Nursing.* Retrieved from http://www.nln.org/docs/default-source/about/nln-vision-series-%28position-statements%29/nlnvision_6.pdf

National Organization of Nurse Practitioner Faculty. (2014). *Nurse practitioner core competencies content.* Retrieved from https://c.ymcdn.com/sites/nonpf.site-ym.com/resource/resmgr/competencies/20170516_NPCoreCompsContentF.pdf

Nehls, N., Barber, G., & Rice, E. (2015). Pathways to the PhD in nursing: An analysis of similarities and differences. *Journal of Professional Nursing, 32*(3), 163–172.

Nicholes, R., & Dyer, J. (2012). Is eligibility for tenure possible for the doctor of nursing practice prepared faculty? *Journal of Professional Nursing, 28*(1), 13–17. doi:10.1016/j.profnurs.2011.10.001

Oermann, M. H. (2017). Preparing nurse faculty. It's for everyone [Editorial]. *Nurse Educator, 42*(1), 1.

Oermann, M. H., Lynn, M. R., & Agger, C. A. (2016). Hiring intentions of directors of nursing programs related to DNP- and PhD-prepared faculty and roles of faculty. *Journal of Professional Nursing, 32*(3), 173–179.

Ponte, P. R., & Nicholas, P. K. (2015). Addressing the confusion related to DNS, DNSc, and DSN degrees with lessons for the nursing profession. *Journal of Nursing Scholarship, 47*(4), 347–353.

Redman, R. (2015). Nurses in the United States with a practice doctorate: Implications for leading in the current context of healthcare. *Nursing Outlook, 63*(2), 124–129.

Rice, D. (2016). The research doctorate in nursing: The PhD. *Leadership & Professional Development, 43*(2), 146–148.

Smeltzer, S. C., Cantrell, M. A., Sharts-Hopko, N. C., Heverly, M. A., Jenkinson, A., & Nthenge, S. (2016). Assessment of the impact of teaching demands on research productivity among doctoral nursing program faculty. *Journal of Professional Nursing, 32*(3), 180–192.

CHAPTER 10

A Proposed Unified Nursing Curriculum

Sarah B. Keating

CHAPTER OBJECTIVES

Upon completion of Chapter 10, the reader will be able to:

- Review the issues in nursing education that led to numerous points of entry into the practice of nursing
- Differentiate among the various levels of nursing education and their role in preparing nurses for practice in the current and future health care systems
- Consider a proposed unified nursing curriculum that could streamline nursing education, verify its position as a profession, and ensure well-prepared health care providers (nurses) to meet the health care needs of the population

OVERVIEW

As reviewed in Chapter 1, nursing education in the United States has a long history of preparing health care professionals through various pathways leading to professional practice and licensure (whose purpose is to ensure the safety of patients through the testing of professionals for their knowledge and competence). Diploma schools that were hospital and training based started in the late 19th century, while early in the 20th century, higher education, university-based programs began to appear. In the mid-20th century, additional baccalaureate programs appeared along with the recommendation from professional organizations that they serve as the entry point into the profession. However, at about the same time, associate degree, community college-based programs came on the scene that prepared nurses at the technical level in accordance with the purpose of community colleges, and at the same time prepared them for licensure. To meet professional standards, these programs increased requirements for the associate degree to include core courses in the sciences and liberal arts. Moving on to the later 20th and early 21st centuries, nursing started to respond to the increasing complexity of the health care system and population heath care needs by developing entry level master's programs such as the clinical nurse leader (CNL) role for nonnursing college graduates and also the advanced practice doctorate, previously found at the master's level.

Philosophically and realized in current nursing curricula, the profession believes in a strong foundation in liberal arts and sciences and, at the same time, prescribes the nursing major to constitute at least half of the total major. Following the usual pattern for lower and upper division majors in higher education, the usual number of units for associate degrees is 65 to 70 and bachelor's degrees range from 120 to 130 units/credits. Classically, the prerequisite courses required by nursing and usually counted toward general education requirements include

English composition, speech (communications), sociology, human development, psychology, anatomy, physiology, microbiology, chemistry, nutrition, and statistics. There are other courses that nursing values as foundations for practice such as the arts, language, philosophy, genetics, economics, political science, computer science, and business. And yet, there is little or no room for these courses in the 70- or 125-unit undergraduate nursing degree programs. As one begins to add up the credits, it becomes apparent that nursing as a profession and like other professions, must be at the higher degree level. The Institute of Medicine's report (2011) validates the assumption that nursing needs to move toward the goal of requiring a higher education degree for entry into professional practice as illustrated by the recent tremendous growth of the doctor of nursing practice (DNP) programs and the decline of diploma programs over the past decade. A review of the Accreditation Commission for Education in Nursing (ACEN, 2017) and Commission for Collegiate Nursing Education (CCNE, 2017) websites revealed 36 accredited diploma programs in 2017 and about 285 doctoral programs with 100 more considering the start of a DNP.

LEVELS OF NURSING EDUCATION AND THEIR ROLE IN PREPARING NURSES FOR PRACTICE

Diploma, Associate Degree, and Baccalaureate Levels

Existing levels of nursing education to prepare nurses for licensure in the United States remain at the diploma, associate degree (ADN), bachelor's (BSN), and master's levels. As noted previously, the numbers of diploma programs have decreased rapidly and the number of associate degree programs has remained steady although more programs that seamlessly move the associate degree graduate into the baccalaureate are increasing. Masters (2015) describes a partnership between community college and university programs that facilitates access for ADN graduates into the baccalaureate. Giddens, Keller, and Liesveld (2015) describe a statewide program that provides direct access for students in associate degree programs into the baccalaureate, while at the same time allowing a step-out option for those wishing to complete the ADN. To gain some verification of the differences between the ADN and BSN outcomes and therefore, levels of practice, Kumm, Godfrey, Tucci, Muenks, and Spaeth (2014) analyzed one state's accredited ADN programs for a comparison of ADN outcomes to BSN outcomes. They found that 42 of 109 BSN outcomes were met that included generalist nursing practice, professional values, and the application of information and technology. The outcomes not met were liberal education, health care and organizational systems leadership, population health, policy in health care, interprofessional collaboration, and evidence-based practice.

For RNs prepared at the ADN and diploma levels, Sarver, Cichra, and Kline (2015) surveyed staff nurses for their opinions on barriers to advancing their nursing education and what motivates them to continue. RNs reported that increased job opportunities and expanded knowledge contributed to their wishes to continue their education, while motivators included tuition reimbursement and a reasonable time to complete the program. Barriers included the commitment of time and expenses such as books and supplies. They found that the average time to complete the RN to BSN program was 2.63 years.

Issues related to undergraduate education (ADN and BSN) such as the time and money spent on undergraduate education for entry into practice still raise issues related to technical versus professional practice. These issues ask nursing to consider whether it is time to move not only from the BSN but to graduate education for entry into practice. One needs only to interview nurses with baccalaureates who are older than 40 years of age to discover the excess number of credits in their degree work to realize the enormity of the problem and the injustices nurses suffered in gaining education beyond the diploma and associate degree with no academic recognition of their additional work. Going one step further, nurses in that age group or older who hold master's and/or doctorates suffer the same overabundance of credits, earning far more than their colleagues in medicine, pharmacology, education, engineering, religion, and law.

Master's Level

According to the American Association of Colleges of Nursing (AACN, 2017a), there were approximately 69 entry into practice at the master's-level programs in the United States. A program specifically designed by the AACN for college graduates with majors not in nursing is the CNL track (AACN, 2017b). Other entry-level master's programs offer specialties in advanced practice such as clinical specialists and nurse practitioners, roles in nursing management, clinical education, and community/public health nursing. It should be noted that many advanced practice programs are converting from the master's to the DNP. For details on graduate programs, master's programs are described in Chapter 8 and the DNP and PhD descriptions may be found in Chapter 9. Generally, except for the advanced generalist role specific to the CNL, the master's entry level of preparation prepares nurses for leadership, clinical educator, and practice roles in the community.

Doctoral Levels: DNP

Yet another level of graduate nursing education is the doctorate of nursing practice/ clinical doctorate (DNP). Few, if any, entry-level doctoral programs exist, although there were several in the past. At this time, BSN graduates can continue their education and articulate directly into the DNP; however, most sit for the licensure examination and licensure is usually required for admission into the program. It is possible that in the future, this requirement might be waived and licensure would occur after graduation from doctoral studies. However, that is very unlikely to occur anytime soon.

Martsolf, Auerbach, Spetz, Pearson, and Muchow (2015) surveyed and interviewed nursing school administrators about their decisions to offer DNP programs. They found that the majority of those surveyed recognized the need for advanced practice nurses at the doctoral level; however, there was reluctance to offer the degree immediately following the baccalaureate in nursing owing to the idea that students and potential employers' acceptance of the role was not clear. In addition, there were related accreditation and certification issues as well as resource constraints. As the authors point out, these factors constrain the transition of programs for moving the baccalaureate graduate directly into the DNP.

In the meantime, some confusion on the part of academics and practice professionals exists as to the role of the DNP-prepared nurse. Udlis and Mancuso (2015) surveyed 340 nurses of varying educational and practice backgrounds who raised questions about the role of the DNP in academia and the type of scholarship expected from those with practice doctorates. There was agreement from the participants on the functions of the DNP on leadership in the health care system, improvement in health care outcomes, interprofessional collaboration, and evidence-based practice. The DNP clinical residency is required by some DNP programs but not all and this issue is raised by Harper, McGuinness, and Johnson (2017). The authors argue that a requirement for a residency places nursing on a par with other professional doctorate programs including medicine, physical therapy, and psychology. Furthermore, residencies validate specialty competencies that are specified in the educational program and they provide partnerships with participating clinical agencies. Harper et al. argue for consistent policies on residencies by accreditation agencies and academe.

Doctoral Levels: PhD

Thus far, the discussion in this chapter reviewed the various levels of nursing education for entry into professional practice. It did not touch upon the need for nursing scientists and educators. There is debate in the discipline about this issue as well since the question arises at to what level should a nursing faculty member be prepared in both the sciences of nursing and education and what are the levels of education and research activities expected for nursing scientists? There is an old rule of thumb in academe that the faculty members who teach should be educated to at least one degree higher than that of the students they expect to prepare. For example, baccalaureate or master's prepared at the associate degree level and master's or doctorate prepared at the baccalaureate level. Obviously, doctorate programs would require the doctoral level of prepared faculty, which then raises the question, DNP or PhD or both?

The question of programs to offer direct entry from the baccalaureate into the PhD level of nursing education remains an issue. Other disciplines/sciences offer these programs and produce younger graduates for the advancement of their science and professions. An interesting study by Nehls, Barber, and Rice (2016) compared three cohorts of PhD nursing students ($N = 84$) enrolled in a PhD program. The three groups consisted of Group 1: students who were nursing undergraduates or who just completed the BSN; Group 2: students who completed the BSN and had at least 1 year of practice; and Group 3: master's degree graduates with 1 or more years of clinical experience. Findings were that the first group members were younger and more ethnically diverse and the length of time to complete their program was about the same as the other groups; however, when the length of time to complete a master's degree for Groups 2 and 3 were taken into account, the program was considerably longer. As expected, the younger group participants expressed concerns about their lack of clinical experience compared to the other groups. All of the students expected to take teaching positions and the younger group had a stronger commitment to continuing research in a research-intensive program. All three groups expressed their concerns about their future roles as faculty and their teaching abilities.

Smeltzer et al. (2015) conducted a survey of nursing faculty in the United States who taught in doctoral programs. As discussed previously, DNP programs have outpaced their growth over PhD programs in the past decade. However, both have seen an increase in numbers. Smeltzer et al. found that DNP faculty had less experience in teaching and less scholarship compared to those teaching in PhD programs. The authors make the point that nursing will continue to need nursing scientists to improve health care outcomes and quality and that advanced practice nurses are needed to translate research into practice. Olsen and Smania (2016) present their ideas on determining what constitutes research in nursing. They point out that at the federal level, quality assurance and quality improvement (QI), evidence-based QI, translational science, and practice inquiry are all classified as research. Collaboration among all levels of nursing scientists, practitioners, and educators is imperative to build the discipline's science and education, improve patient health care outcomes, and bring about positive health care system changes.

An important point from a review of the literature and reports from practice that relate to nursing education and the faculty role is the fact that education is also a science and consists of theories, concepts, models, and practice. Nursing academe must take this into account and ensure that nurses choosing to assume educator roles have the knowledge, expertise, and skills in both nursing and teaching. There are a few nursing programs that offer the EdD or the PhD with a major in nursing education, and there are master's degree programs that also have an education track. Nursing educators as well as their colleagues in practice must recognize the need to blend nursing and education knowledge in order to present up-to-date clinical knowledge and skills to students through effective curriculum planning and teaching and learning modalities.

PROPOSED UNIFIED NURSING CURRICULUM

Table 10.1 presents a proposed unified nursing education curriculum that addresses some of the issues raised regarding levels of nursing practice, from entry level to advanced practice and research roles, and the appropriate level of education necessary to meet the requirements of these roles. It compares a nonstop curriculum ending with a practice or research-focused doctorate to step-out options that are similar to today's various levels of nursing education in higher education from the ADN to the PhD. It reveals a rigorous academic program common to professional education, and yet there is an efficiency of time and quality of courses that provides the student with opportunity to build on courses sequentially and integrate nursing knowledge and skills into the supporting arts and sciences. Based on the curricula in Table 10.1, the argument for "entry into practice" ends with the idea that a candidate is eligible for licensure at various points of the educational track commencing with the completion of the associate degree (lower division) and a 3-month internship; or completion of the bachelor of science with a residency; or a master's degree either as an advanced generalist (CNL) or specific functional or advanced practice nurse with prescribed residencies prior to licensure; and finally, a doctorate that includes a clinical or research residency. Thus, students have a choice for entering practice through licensure at the associate, bachelor's, master's, or doctorate degree levels. At the same time, the curricula contain the same courses or content, thus allowing nurses to enter at the next step of their education to continue their career opportunities. If these generic curricula were adapted by schools of nursing, there would be no need for challenge examinations and repetition of courses containing the knowledge and skills already assimilated.

Schools of nursing bear the responsibility for evaluating the credentials of applicants with prior education or degrees not in nursing. There is a need for flexibility in granting credit for courses equivalent to those pre- and corequisites in nursing and nursing courses (for RNs with degrees not in nursing) to enter into the curriculum and to complete the next academic level. Examples are RNs with baccalaureates or master's in other disciplines and nonnurses with baccalaureates or higher degrees who matriculate directly into master's programs rather than repeating the baccalaureate. Of course, RNs need upper-division–level nursing courses or their equivalent and nonnurses need nursing courses equivalent to the baccalaureate but offered at the graduate level prior to entering master's or doctorate-level nursing courses.

The advantages to the entry-level doctorate program are numerous. It would facilitate high school graduates' entry into a nursing program with graduation 8 years away, thus producing expert clinicians, researchers, and educators who are relatively young in age. The 8-year total curriculum plan provides the time for in-depth education and the production of quality graduates prepared for practice, teaching, and research roles. If the profession embraces this transformation of nursing education, then it must come to grips with the reality that there are roles for personnel such as the licensed practical/vocational nurses. It is logical that these programs fall into the community college genre, thus raising the specter of the "Civil War" in nursing yet again. This author leaves that debate to the nursing educators reading this text and the profession over the next few decades.

TABLE 10.1 Proposed Unified Nursing Curriculum

| Career Ladder Program (With Step-Out Options) | | | | Nonstop Entry-Level Doctoral Program (DNP or PhD) | |
| Prerequisites | | Nursing Courses | | Prerequisites | |
Courses	Credits	Courses	Credits	Courses	Credits
Year 1					
Verbal and Written Communications	6	Introduction to Nursing and Health Care	3	Verbal and Written Communications	6
Anatomy and Physiology	6	Basic Health Assessment and Skills	3	Anatomy and Physiology	8
Microbiology	4	Nursing Process and Skills	4	Chemistry	4
Language or General Education	3	Care of the Older Adult	3	Psychology	3
Total Credits	19	Total Credits	13	Sociology/Anthropology	6
				Language or General Education	3
				Total Credits	30
Year 2					
Sociology/Anthropology	3	Parent Child Nursing	6	Human Development	3
Human Development	3	Psychiatric/Mental Health Nursing	4	Microbiology	4
General Education	3	Adult Acute Care Nursing	6	Statistics	3
Introduction to Health Care Informatics	3	12-Week Paid Internship Prior to Licensure	Work Study/no credit	Chemistry	4
Nutrition	3			U.S. Health Care System and Health Professions	3
Introduction to Pharmacology	2			Nutrition	3

Cognates		Nursing Courses	
Courses	Credits	Courses	Credits
		Introduction to Health Care Informatics	3
		Language or General Education	3
		Genetics	3
		Introduction to Nursing and Health Care	3
Total Credits	17		16
		Total Credits	32

Step out for ADN: Total credits: 65

Year 3

Cognates		Nursing Courses		Cognates		Nursing Courses	
Courses	Credits	Courses	Credits	Courses	Credits	Courses	Credits
Genetics	3	The Nursing Profession	3	Economics	3	Basic Health Assessment and Skills	3
Pharmacology	3	Critical Care Nursing	4	Pharmacology	3	Nursing Process with Skills	4
Chemistry	4	Transcultural Nursing	4			Care of the Older Adult	3
Statistics	3	Research in Nursing	3			Parent Child Nursing	6
General Education	3					Psychiatric/Mental Health Nursing	4
						The Nursing Profession	3
						Research in Nursing	3
Total Credits	16		14		6		26

(continued)

TABLE 10.1 Proposed Unified Nursing Curriculum (*continued*)

Year 4

Cognates	Credits	Nursing Courses	Credits	Courses	Credits	Nursing Courses	Credits
General Education Electives	6	Community Health Nursing	6	Bioethics	6	Adult Acute Care Nursing	6
Bioethics	3	Nursing Leadership and Interprofessional Collaboration	3	General Education	3	Transcultural Nursing	4
Economics	3	Health Care Delivery System	3			Community Health Nursing	6
		Nursing Informatics	3			Nursing Leadership and Interprofessional Collaboration	3
		Capstone Practicum	3			Nursing Informatics	3
		12-Week Paid Residency Prior to Licensure	Work Study/no credit			Critical Care Nursing	4
Total credits	12		18		6		26

Step out for BSN: Total credits: 65 (lower division) + 60 (upper division) = 125

Year 5

Nursing Cognates	Credits	Nursing Courses	Credits	Nursing Cognates	Credits	Nursing Courses	Credits
Nursing Theory	3	Functional Role Theory I, for example, Advanced Practice, Clinical Nurse Leader, Clinical Specialty, Education, Management	2	Nursing Theory	3	Capstone Practicum (Upper Division)	3

Cognates	Credits	Nursing Courses	Credits	Cognates	Credits	Nursing Courses	Credits
Analysis of Health Care Organizations	3	Functional Role Practicum I	4	Analysis of Health Care Organizations	3	Functional Role Theory I, e.g., Advanced Practice, Clinical Nurse Leader, Clinical Specialty, Education, Management	2
Nursing Research Evidence-Based Practice	3			Nursing Research Evidence-Based Practice	3	Functional Role Practicum I	4
Advanced Nursing Informatics	3			Advanced Nursing Informatics	3		
Advanced Pathophysiology[a]	3			Advanced Pathophysiology[a]	3		
Total Credits	15/12		6	Total Credits	15		9

[a]This course is not required for nonadvanced practice MSN roles.

Year 6

Cognates	Credits	Nursing Courses	Credits	Nursing Cognates	Credits	Nursing Courses	Credits
Advanced Health Assessment[a]	2	Functional Role Theory II, e.g., Advanced Practice, Clinical Nurse Leader, Clinical Specialty, Education, Management, etc.	3	Advanced Health Assessment[a]	3	Functional Role Theory II, e.g., Advanced Practice, Clinical Nurse Leader, Clinical Specialty, Education, Management, etc.	2
Advanced Pharmacology[a]	4	Functional Role Practicum II	3	Advanced Pharmacology[a]	3	Functional Role Practicum II	4
Population Health	3-6	Master's Project or Thesis[b]	3	Population Health	3	Nursing History and Philosophy	3

(continued)

TABLE 10.1 Proposed Unified Nursing Curriculum (*continued*)

Year 6

Courses	Credits	Courses	Credits	Courses	Credits	Credits
		For entry-level master's: 12 Week Paid Residency Prior to Licensure	Work Study/ no credit	Health Care Economics	3	9
Total Credits^a	9/3		6/9-12^b	Total Credits	12	

^aThese three courses are not required for nonadvanced practice roles.
^bRequired of nonadvanced practice master's degree candidates.

Step out for master's degree with 30–42 credits

Year 7

DNP				Research-Focused Degree (PhD or DNS)			
Cognates	Credits	Nursing Courses	Credits	Cognates	Credits	Nursing Courses	Credits
Health Care Economics	3	Translational Science	3	Quantitative Research	3	Nursing Science, Analysis of Theories	3
		Foundations for the DNP in Practice and Leadership	3	Qualitative Research	3	Seminar: Dissertation I	3
		Advanced Communications and Interprofessional Health Care	3	Mixed Methods	3	Advanced Communications and Interprofessional Health Care	3
		Advanced Nursing Informatics	3			Quality Nursing Care and Outcomes Management	3
		DNP Project I, II	6				

		Quality Nursing Care and Outcomes Management	3				12
Total			21		9		

**Year 8
DNP and PhD/DNS**

DNP				Research-Focused PhD or DNS			
Nursing Courses	Credits	Cognates	Credits	Cognates	Credits	Nursing Courses	Credits
Role-Specific Evidence-Based Practice Residency	6	Electives (Education courses for faculty roles or cognates to support research)	6	Electives (Education courses for faculty roles or cognates to support research)	6	Nursing Science Theory Development	3
DNP Project III	3		6			Advanced Practice and Leadership Role Development	3
Advanced Practice and Leadership Role Development	3					Seminar Dissertation II	3
For entry-level DNP: 12 Week Paid Residency Prior to Licensure	Work Study/ no credit			For entry-level PhD: 12 Week Paid Residency Prior to Licensure	Work Study/ no credit		
Total	12		6		6		9

Postmaster's DNP: Total 36 credits

Nonstop DNP: Total 195 credits

Nonstop PhD: Total 207

SUMMARY

This chapter summarized the current state of nursing education with its many points of entry into professional practice and the educational programs that produce the nursing workforce. While the world order, the national society, and the health care system change rapidly, it is difficult to predict the future. There are prevailing trends that should have an impact on the development and evaluation of nursing curricula over the next decade. If nursing chooses not to respond to these changes, the profession will continue to be splintered with less opportunity for it to help in shaping public policy toward optimal health care for the populace. Nursing educators have a responsibility to work with their colleagues in practice and research to develop curricula that prepare nurses for the future, who are competent and caring, excellent clinicians and practitioners, leaders and change agents, and scholars and researchers. A nursing education system for the future will have the following characteristics:

1. Clearly defined levels of education and differentiated practice in the health care system based on education and experience
2. Entry into practice for staff nurse positions following a 3-month residency in a selected arena of practice
3. Quality institutions of higher education that specialize in the preparation of staff nurses for entry into evidence-based practice in a timely fashion
4. Quality higher education institutions that focus on the faculty role of excellence in teaching, community service, research, and the translation and application of knowledge from nursing science and related disciplines
5. Quality institutions of higher education that specialize in the preparation of nurses to provide evidence-based advanced practice nursing and interprofessional services for individuals, families, communities, and aggregates
6. Students, graduates, and faculty who are active participants and generators of new knowledge in nursing and related disciplines' research
7. Quality institutions of higher education that specialize in the preparation of nurse leaders who will influence health care policy and change the health care system for the benefit of the populations they serve
8. Academic and health science centers that specialize in nursing research and the advancement of nursing science through translational science and evidence-based practice; testing of theories; the development of new theories, concepts, and models; and educational innovations on the national and international levels

DISCUSSION QUESTIONS

- Given the rapid changes in the health care and educational systems and the ongoing shortage of nurses, what changes in nursing education do you envision within the next 5 to 10 years?
- What strategies for changing nursing education worked in the past and how can they apply to needed changes in nursing education today? What are the lessons from the past that prohibited nursing from moving its educational agenda forward? How can today's nursing educators use these lessons to bring about change?

LEARNING ACTIVITIES

Student-Learning Activities

Synthesize the information in this text into a "Dream School of Nursing." Develop a curriculum that prepares nurses for practice 10 years hence, keeping in mind that practice and the setting in which it is delivered will be different. Let your imagination run wild!

Faculty Development Activities

Hold a faculty meeting focused on brainstorming and let creative thoughts flow freely. List the characteristics of the ideal nurse prepared to practice 5 to 10 years hence. Examine these characteristics and decide how a curriculum can be developed that provides the kind of education necessary to prepare this kind of nurse. Focus on creativity and newer theories of learning. Compare these ideas to your existing curriculum. How can it be transformed into the one you envision and still meet accreditation and professional standards and criteria?

References

Accreditation Commission for Education in Nursing. (2017). Accredited programs. Retrieved from http://www.acenursing.us/accreditedprograms/programsearch.asp

American Association of Colleges of Nursing. (2017a). *Schools offering entry-level or 2nd degree master's programs.* Retrieved from http://www.aacn.nche.edu/leading-initiatives/research-data/GENMAS.pdf

American Association of Colleges of Nursing. (2017b). CNL programs. Retrieved from http://www.aacn.nche.edu/cnl/about/cnl-programs

Commission on Collegiate Nursing Education. (2017). CCNE-accredited master's nursing degree programs. Retrieved from http://directory.ccnecommunity.org/reports/rptAccreditedPrograms_New.asp?sort=state&sProgramType=2

Giddens, J., Keller, T., & Liesveld, J. (2015). Answering the call for a bachelors prepared nursing workforce: An innovative model for academic progression. *Journal of Professional Nursing, 31*(6), 445–451.

Harper, D. C., McGuinness, T., & Johnson, J. (2017). Clinical residency training: Is it essential to the doctor of nursing practice for nurse practitioner training? *Nursing Outlook, 65*(1), 50–57.

Institute of Medicine. (2011). *The future of nursing: Leading change, advancing health.* Washington, DC: National Academies Press.

Kumm, S. Godfrey, N., Tucci, M., Muenks, M., & Spaeth, T. (2014). Baccalaureate outcomes met by associate degree program. *Nurse Educator, 39*(5), 216–220.

Martsolf, G., Auerbach, D., Spetz, J., Pearson, M., & Muchow, A. (2015). Doctor of nursing practice by 2015. An examination of nursing schools' decisions to offer a doctor of nursing practice degree. *Nursing Outlook, 63*(2), 219–225.

Masters, K. (2015). Implementation of a generic baccalaureate concurrent enrollment program: Increasing the percentage of nurses prepared at the baccalaureate level. *Nursing Education Perspectives, 36*(3), 192–193.

Nehls, N., Barber, G., & Rice, E. (2016). Pathways to the PhD in nursing: An analysis of similarities and differences. *Journal of Professional Nursing, 32*(3), 163–172.

Olsen, D., & Smania, M. (2016). Determining when an activity is or is not research. *The American Journal of Nursing, 116*(10), 55–60.

Sarver, W., Cichra, N., & Kline, M. (2015). Perceived benefits, motivators, and barriers to advancing nurse education: Removing barriers to improve success. *Nursing Education Perspectives, 36*(3), 153–156.

Smeltzer, S., Sharts-Hopko, N., Cantrell, M., Heverly, M., Nthenge, S., & Jenkinson, A. (2015). A profile of U.S. nursing faculty in research- and practice-focused doctoral education. *Journal of Nursing Scholarship, 47*(2), 178–185.

Udlis, K., & Mancuso, J. (2015). Perceptions of the role of doctor of nursing practice-prepared nurse: Clarity or confusion. *Journal of Professional Nursing, 31*(4), 274–283.

CHAPTER 11

Distance Education, Online Learning, Informatics, and Technology

Stephanie S. DeBoor

CHAPTER OBJECTIVES

Upon completion of Chapter 11, the reader will be able to:

- Review the various types of distance education programs that are utilized in the delivery of nursing education programs
- Analyze the application of technology and informatics and their effectiveness on the implementation of the nursing curriculum
- Review the literature related to the efficacy of distance education programs
- Examine the issues facing nursing educators that relate to the application of informatics and technology in nursing education

OVERVIEW

This chapter discusses the effects of informatics and technology on curriculum development and evaluation. Distance education formats are reviewed including land-based satellite campuses of home institutions, hybrid, web-based with immersion, and online platforms. Other technological advances such as smart classrooms, patient simulations, electronic medical record systems, and information systems applied to education and health care are analyzed. A brief review of the research findings on the efficacy of these programs and student satisfaction is presented and issues related to distance education and technology are introduced.

DISTANCE EDUCATION PROGRAMS

Distance education is defined as any learning experience that takes place a distance away from the parent educational institution's home campus. It can be as close as a few blocks away in an urban center to as far away as another nation. It implements the curriculum through a planned strategy for the delivery of courses or classes that can include off-site satellite classes managed by the home faculty or credentialed off-site faculty, broadcast of classes through videoconferencing and teleconferencing to off-campus sites, web-conferencing, web-based instruction, and faculty-supervised clinical experiences including preceptorships and internships. Distance education offers continuing education programs, degree programs, single academic courses, or a mixture of on-campus and off-campus course offerings. Distance education's roots can be traced to the early 1700s through correspondence study (Bower & Hardy, 2004). The instructor would mail the students their lessons and once completed, the students would in turn return the assignments via mail. While a good way to include those who did not otherwise have access to a home campus, lost mail and time delays proved to be limitations of the postal system. Technology continued to advance with satellite communication in the 1960s, advancing to fiberoptic systems of the 1980s. Today, the Internet and a few key strokes from any computer allow for students to connect to faculty from all over the world. Online education has been a growing trend as universities across the United States search for strategies to increase enrollment in prelicensure, RN-to-BSN, and graduate nursing programs.

The following discussion reviews planning considerations for distance education. Also discussed are types of distance education that include satellite campus programs, web-, video- and teleconferencing, and online, web-based programs.

Needs Assessment and Compatibility With the Components of the Curriculum

When planning for any type of educational program that will be delivered off the main campus, nursing educators must have supporting data from an assessment of the external and internal frame factors that document the need for a program. It should include the projected success of the program based on a business case, cost analysis, assured applicant pool, and a business plan. Once the needs assessment is completed and a time frame is in place, planners review all of the components of the curriculum to ensure congruence with the originating educational program. For details on conducting a needs assessment, budgeting, and the components of the curriculum, see Section II and Chapter 5. In addition, an evaluation plan should be developed to ensure the quality of the program and to meet accreditation standards.

External Frame Factors

Whether considering distance education for individual students from multiple locations, or a group of students within one geographical location, utilizing the components of assessment from the internal and external frame factors, a needs assessment reveals the feasibility for developing a distance education program. If the program plans an off-campus but on-land satellite, the external frame factors include an assessment of the community where the program is to take place with such factors as community location and receptivity to distance education, the population's characteristics and its sophistication in technology, the delivery of education far from the home campus, and the ability to create an academic setting away from the home campus. The most up-to-date technology and system support teams are a necessity if the program is to be delivered completely online. Additional external frame factors include an assessment of support and area competition from vendors of distance education programs and other nursing education programs that serve the region. The health care system and health needs of the populace have an influence on the program as to how graduates of the program can serve them. Assessments of collaborative relationships that will supply the program with available practicum locations in the off-site health care agencies are critical to the success of the program within that community area.

A demonstrated need for a distance education program includes support from members of the nursing profession in the region that is to be served; national, regional, and state regulations; and accreditation agencies' approvals. Usually, the sponsoring program must notify all accrediting and approval agencies of its plans to offer the distance education program with each of these agencies requiring specific descriptions of the program including the potential student body, faculty, curriculum plan, academic and capital infrastructure support systems, timelines, plans for evaluation, and most importantly, financial feasibility with a business plan.

Internal Frame Factors

Much like the external frame factors, a review of the internal frame factors provides additional information in the planning for a distance education program. Of prime concern is the support of the parent academic institution and its experience with distance education programs. If it has a history of managing these types of programs, it is more likely to be supportive of the nursing program. A check with the mission and purpose, philosophy, and goals of the parent institution and the nursing program is in order to ensure the distance education program's congruence with those of the parent. The internal economic situation and its influence on distance education programs are critical to the financial feasibility of the program. An assessment of faculty familiarity and comfort with the use of current technology along with support of instructional designers and programmers will be required to support an effective distance education program.

Cost Issues

If the recommendations from the needs assessment demonstrate that the distance education program is viable, the school of nursing administration prepares a project proposal, or business case to present to the parent institution. The purpose for a business case is to persuade key administrators and stakeholders that establishing a distance education program meets the mission of the institution, has a substantial potential student body, and adapts the existing accredited program to an online or satellite format without compromising its quality. The business case describes the program in detail and demonstrates that it is economically feasible. If prior distance education programs demonstrated success in bringing revenues to the program or are, at the least, self-sufficient, it is more likely that new programs will be supported. After presentation to and approval by the administration, the business case is developed into a detailed business plan.

The first and foremost cost issue to address in the business plan is the economic feasibility of the distance education program based on an analysis of expected start-up costs, administrative costs, required number of faculty and staff, capital expenses (on-site facilities and technology support systems), and academic support (recruitment, admission, records, library access, and student support systems). Many times, the needs assessment becomes a write-off at the expense of the nursing program and is financed through contingency funds or program development funds generated from grant overhead costs. The plan should include possible initial grant support for start-up funds and plans for eventual self-sufficiency. The resources that are required from the parent institution are listed and include clinical-experience facilities; technological support systems for videoconferencing, teleconferencing, and/or web-based instruction; administrative, faculty, and staff expenses; and academic support systems such as library, academic, and student services. Included in the assessment is a list of potential administrators, staff, faculty, and the proposed program's student body characteristics.

The administration's role and costs include supervisory or management functions to implement the program such as budget and personnel management, liaison activities with regional stakeholders, public relations, coordination, marketing plans, and preparation of reports to seek approval and accreditation of the distance education program from relevant agencies. Some of the staff and/or faculty cost considerations are the required full-time and part-time equivalents, benefits, travel and other expenses, supplies, and equipment.

Curriculum and Evaluation Plans

In addition to the economic feasibility for the program, an analysis of the curriculum is in order to ensure that the proposed distant program is congruent with the mission, goals, organizational framework, and student learning outcomes of the parent program. Although the format and delivery of the curriculum may differ from the original, it must meet the same goals and objectives of the program. Administrators and faculty must make decisions regarding the format and have a rationale for why certain formats are chosen. Faculty pedagogy must be considered when developing an online format. This transformation may be difficult for some faculty members who always taught as the "sage on the stage."

The new program should be integrated into the master plan of evaluation of the parent program to ensure its quality. Additionally, it should have its own evaluation plan for monitoring the program as it is implemented for corrections along the way (formative evaluation) and to have summative evaluation plans in place that measure the success of the program in terms of student learning outcomes and success, satisfaction of the stakeholders, and its continued congruence with the components of the parent program's curriculum. See Table 11.1 for guidelines for the development of distance education programs.

TYPES OF DISTANCE EDUCATION PROGRAMS

The following is a description of the major types of distance education programs and those that fall under the formats of synchronous (live, real-time, simultaneous) or asynchronous (occurring at various times) delivery. Universities utilize learning management systems (LMSs) to deliver web-based, online educational courses. Some of the pros and cons for each type of distance education options are listed.

Satellite Campuses

For the purposes of this discussion, *satellite campuses* are defined as those programs that offer the curriculum in whole or in part on off-campus sites from the parent institution. While they can incorporate technology methods such as videoconferencing and web-based instruction, the majority of the teaching and learning takes place in classrooms and involves in-person (synchronous) interactions between the faculty and students. For nursing, clinical experiences may occur in health care facilities in the community in which the satellite campus is located. Faculty members who teach in the parent institution serve as on-site faculty or act as consultants to off-site faculty who teach the same curriculum. For those faculty members on the home campus who actually teach on the satellite campus, travel costs and the related time it takes for travel are included in the costs for implementing the program. These costs are weighed against the cost of the salary and benefits for hiring on-site faculty. With the emergence of the Internet, satellite campuses are becoming less utilized for nursing education.

Online/Web-Based Programs

Online and web-based instruction had its beginnings through faculty and student use of communication tools such as LISTSERVs, email, and access to resources and references on the World Wide Web. In the 1990s and early 21st century, the use of web-based instruction through LMSs became more prevalent. They proved so popular with students that some courses were mounted as a combination of web-based and on-campus instruction classes for home-campus students as well as off-campus students. Online/web-based instruction is usually delivered through the use of LMSs with which the institution has a contract, although some institutions develop their own. In a 2016 report,

TABLE 11.1 Guidelines for the Development of a Distance Education Program

Guideline Topic	Questions for Data Collection and Analysis	Desired Outcome
Needs Assessment: External Frame Factors	To what extent are the distant sites supportive of the program and sophisticated in the use of technology? To what extent has the health care system demonstrated support for the program and the nursing profession? To what extent is the health care system open to student clinical experiences and what resources do they have available for the experiences? To what extent is the program competitive with other educational program(s)?	The distant site(s) is receptive to distance education programs, sophisticated or open to the technology of distance education, and has a health care system supportive of the program, the nursing profession, and student clinical experiences, if indicated. The program is competitive with other programs.
External Frame Factors	Have program approval and accreditation bodies been notified of the program and do they approve or is there an indication that they will approve the program in the future?	Relevant program approval and accrediting agencies have been notified and approve the program or there are indications for approval in the future.
Needs Assessment: Internal Frame Factors	To what extent does the distance education program's mission, philosophy, organizing framework, goals, and objectives reflect those of the parent institution? To what extent does the parent institution have experience in the selected modality(ies) of distance education and/or have the resources to support it? Are there plans in place that indicate adequate resources for the program including infrastructure, human resources, and academic program support?	The mission, purpose, philosophy, organizing framework, goals, and objectives of the distance education program are congruent with the parent institution. The parent institution has experience with and/or the resources to support the program. Plans are in place and resources are adequate for academic infrastructure, human resources, and academic program support.
Economic Feasibility	To what extent will the parent institution support a needs assessment for the distance education program? If there are no funds from the institution, are there other possible resources? Are there start-up funds available from the institution or are there other sources such as funds from partner health care or educational institutions?	There is support from the parent institution or other sources for a needs assessment. There are start-up funds from the parent institution or other sources.

(continued)

TABLE 11.1 Guidelines for the Development of a Distance Education Program (*continued*)

Guideline Topic	Questions for Data Collection and Analysis	Desired Outcome
	Does the business case justify the need for the program including its congruence with the mission of the institution, a demonstrated need for the program in the community, an adequate potential student body, and assurance of the maintenance of its quality? Has the business plan accounted for personnel costs (staff, technicians, and faculty); administrative costs; facilities (if indicated); academic support systems, e.g., library, enrollment services, financial aid; and the required technology system(s)? To what extent are there plans for self-sufficiency? Are there projections for the size of the student body and other resources necessary to maintain the program?	The business case is persuasive and includes justification for the development of the program, i.e., meets mission, meets a need, has an adequate potential student body, and maintains quality. The business plan includes funds for the required personnel, administrative costs, facilities (if indicated), academic support systems, and the required technology system. There are financial plans in place for self-sufficiency and maintenance of the program.
Congruence With the Components of the Curriculum	To what extent does the curriculum plan for the distance education program reflect that of the parent institution, e.g., course descriptions, credits, objectives, and content?	The distance education program's curriculum plan is congruent with that of the parent institution.
Delivery Model Options	Have all modalities been considered including off-site, on-land satellite campuses, videoconferencing and/or teleconferencing, and online or web-based methods?	All modalities for the delivery method are reviewed to lead to a rationale for the selected model or combination of several.

Delivery Model Options: Selection and Its Rationale	To what extent does the selected model fit the learning needs of the students? To what extent are there faculty members who can utilize the model(s)? If not, are there faculty development plans and technical support in place? To what extent is the selected model "user-friendly" for students and faculty?	The selected model fits the learning needs of the students. The selected model is within the scope of the faculty's expertise or there are faculty development plans in place. The selected model is "user-friendly" for students and faculty.
Delivery Model: Implementation Plan	To what extent is the selected model(s) congruent with the curriculum plan? Does the selected model fit the implementation plan of the curriculum, i.e., is it possible to deliver theory, lab, and clinical experiences?	The selected model is congruent with the curriculum plan. The curriculum plan can be implemented through utilization of the selected model(s).
Delivery Model: Evaluation	Is there an evaluation plan in place and to what extent is it congruent with the master plan of the parent institution? Does the evaluation plan include both formative and summative evaluation measures? To what extent does the evaluation plan include strategies and personnel for follow-up and revisions if necessary based on the data analyses and recommendations from the evaluation plan? Is the selected delivery model(s) relevant to current education practices? To what extent is the selected model adaptable to future changes in the profession and education and health care systems?	There is an evaluation plan in place and it is congruent with the master plan of evaluation for the parent institution. The evaluation plan includes both formative and summative measures. The evaluation plan has mechanisms in place to revise the program according to data analyses and recommendations from evaluation activities. The selected delivery model is relevant to current education practices and adaptable to future changes in the education, profession, and health care systems.

Online Report Card Tracking Online Education in the United States, Allen and Seaman identified a 7% growth in distance education enrollments between Fall 2012 and Fall 2014. Babson Survey Research Group (2015) reported in the state of online learning in institutions of higher education that overall enrollments are being outpaced by the growth of online enrollments. This report identified a total of 5.8 million students enrolled in distance education during the Fall 2014. Online courses are those in "which at least 80 percent of the course content is delivered online. Face-to-face instruction includes courses in which zero to 29 percent of the content is delivered online; this category includes both traditional and web facilitated courses. Blended, (sometimes called hybrid) instruction has between 30% and 80% of the course content delivered online" (Allen & Seaman, 2016, p. 7). This type of distance education allows for more flexibility for those who do not have easy access to a home campus. Students can log in at any time to lessons from any place in the world as long as they have Internet access.

Web-Based With Immersion

This form of distance education has students complete the majority of studies entirely online through asynchronous discussion boards and written assignments. Students are required to come to the home campus once or twice per semester for immersion days. During on-campus meetings, students participate in skill labs, clinical assessments with standardized patients (SPs), and lectures from clinical experts to enhance their learning. Immersion days allow students to interact and collaborate with faculty and other peers of the cohort. Faculty has an opportunity to assess students' knowledge, skills, and expertise within their specialty of study and provide remediation. Students enjoy speaking with faculty and getting immediate feedback as opposed to the delayed response of online communication. The downside to this format is that students must incur the expense of traveling to the home campus in addition to the standard university tuition and fees they pay each semester.

Hybrid Distance Education

Hybrid courses utilize blended synchronous and asynchronous formats for educational delivery. Students have both online and required times to meet face to face either on campus or within an online "virtual" classroom. The "virtual" classroom is a web-conferencing platform where faculty and students can meet live. Big Blue Button (2017), Blackboard Collaborate (2017), and Zoom (2017) are examples of this technology. The pros and cons of this format are echoed in those that were expressed previously in the web-based with immersion format.

Development of Online Programs

Web-based teaching and learning require an LMS, computer access to the web by faculty and students, technological support through the use of instructional support staff, and training sessions for faculty and students who are not familiar with the system. Some institutions of higher learning use experienced instructional technology staff and faculty who mount and manage courses for teachers whose only responsibility is for the actual teaching of the course. This method provides technical support for teaching faculty; however, it may remove some of the academic freedom from the teacher of record. For example, the teacher does not have the ability to change course assignments or formats without going through the support staff to make the changes. It can also prove to be expensive since the institution is paying for several staff members when only one may be required.

The American Distance Education Consortium (ADEC, 2016) provides best practices for developing online courses. It is a brief overview of what should be considered and part of providing quality in distance education and online programs. This includes suggestions on homepage development, course structure and educational strategies, interaction and collaboration with faculty/peers, incorporation of pedagogical technology, and security measures for testing, assessments, and assignments.

One must consider that there are differences in traditional classroom and online education, thus faculty need to adopt a pedagogical shift in teaching strategies. Fiedler, Giddens, and North (2014) identified that faculty support is essential in successful adaptation to technological innovation in nursing education. The initial time spent in converting a traditional course or a new course to a web-based course is great and, as with all courses, requires updating and revisions each subsequent time that it is taught. Multiple learning activities are available through the Internet such as synchronous real-time chat rooms and live classrooms where students and faculty meet at a prearranged time and discuss topics or review questions about course assignments. Asynchronous entries (occurring at various times and also labeled as "threaded discussions") about selected topics provide the students and faculty with opportunities to discuss topics and present their ideas and views on them. The assignments related to these usually require reading assignments and/or a review of the literature so that the discussions are scholarly treatises on the subject at hand. Faculty can post a lecture through an essay or PPT presentation that includes notes, illustrations, references to uniform resource locators (URLs), videotapes, movies, and other audiovisual media and pose thought questions for discussions related to the "lecture." Group work assignments are possible through the use of chat rooms, live classrooms, threaded discussions, and email communications.

Many LMSs have programs that allow faculty to develop surveys and examinations that are secure and provide statistical analyses of the results. A few examples of web-based educational and live-time platforms are Blackboard (2017), Canvas (2017), Moodle (2016), Pearson Education Inc. (2017), and Wimba (2017). There are online exam proctoring services available to further protect the integrity of the program. Examity (2017), Kryterion Online Proctoring (2017), and ProctorU (2017) are some examples of these proctoring services.

Learning Theories for Online Formats

Most distance education programs employ *andragogy* (adult learning) strategies for the delivery of courses and classes through off-campus satellite sites, videoconferencing, telecommunications, online, and web-based technology. The majority of teaching and learning strategies offered in these formats is learner centered and facilitates active student participation in the process rather than the traditional pedagogical methods for presenting information to the student. See Chapter 6 for learning theories that apply to online educational formats and for ideas for research on the use of learning theories for online instruction.

Uzuner Smith, Hayes, and Shea (2017) identify that social constructivism theories of learning are often identified in online and blended approaches of higher education. Constructivism theory applies well to electronic learning since the theory centers on the ability of the learner to build on previous knowledge, assimilate new knowledge, and interpret the knowledge gained to the surrounding environment. It requires active learner participation, reflection, and social interaction with faculty and peers (Kala, Isaramalai, & Pohthong, 2010).

Research Findings on the Efficacy of Online Formats

As online teaching and learning continues to become the norm of delivery, it is important to examine the effectiveness of this educational modality. Du et al. (2013) conducted a systematic review to examine the efficacy of web-based distance learning for nursing education. Of the nine randomized controlled trials that met inclusion criteria, results indicated that there were equal or better results in knowledge acquisition for those who participated in web-based distance learning. The U.S. Department of Education (2010) found that blended online or hybrid delivery was superior to fully online instruction. In addition, the blending of the online format is rated as superior to traditional face-to-face instruction.

Hampton, Pearce, and Moser (2017) identify the effectiveness of online learning on student learning outcomes. Their study examined student teaching and learning preferences in online courses. Results recognized the differences in teaching/learning strategies across generations and identified preferred strategies that enhance student engagement. The two methods preferred by students as most engaging and most effective to learning were narrated PowerPoint (PPT) presentations/videos and case studies. The methods found to be least enjoyed were group projects and wikis (collaborative editing by the users).

Advantages and Disadvantages of Web-Based Education

Advantages of web-based education include flexible times for students and faculty, multiple learning and teaching strategies, active participation on the part of all students, personal/individual communications between students and faculty, moderate maintenance times for managing and updating the course once it is mounted, and relative assurance of curriculum integrity. For the home institution, the advantage of web-based education includes the ability to enroll more students without creating a need for on-campus space.

Some of the disadvantages of online systems are the need for technological support; initial and on-going costs related to contracts for LMSs and computers; the lack of face-to-face encounters between faculty and students; the large amount of faculty time consumed in mounting the course; the need for faculty and student development in the use of technology; the possible loss of nursing values such as visible and tactile communications; and a minimal sense of belonging to the home campus.

Student engagement is often difficult to maintain with distance education. Looyestyn et al. (2017) conducted a systematic review of the use of gamification in increasing student engagement in online programs. This concept first emerged in the context of computer gaming. This strategy uses software that incorporates game elements, such as levels, challenges, quests, and rewards based on the success of the "player" learner. It is suggested that self and/or peer competition promotes engagement and there is an increase in learning outcomes when gamification is utilized. This bodes well for millennial learners as noted in the study of Montenery et al. (2013). They identified this generation of learners as very comfortable and reliant on the use of technology in their everyday lives. Millennials desire immediate feedback and positive reinforcement, which gamification rewards provide.

Finally, students sometimes feel isolated while taking a predominately online course. Fox (2017) examined the use of VoiceThread, a cloud-based technology, to promote collaboration in an online course. This technology allows students to share their knowledge through voice recording instead of a written discussion post. Findings indicated both pros and cons to this technology. Challenges included setting up the microphone, getting the right volume, minimizing extraneous noise, understanding language and accents, and feeling nervous the first time using the recording technology. On a positive note, participants identified this technology made them feel a similar connection to their peers and faculty, as if they were communicating in a face-to-face classroom. The overall response to VoiceThread was affirmative and students expressed preference with this technology over text discussion boards.

CLINICAL COURSES AND DISTANCE EDUCATION

It is possible to provide quality clinical experiences for students through distance education modalities. For example, the off-site satellite campus with on-site faculty usually provides clinical experiences in the "traditional" mode. Faculty develops the clinical courses, including skills laboratory courses, according to the implementation plan of the curriculum. Students are assigned to clinical laboratories for the acquisition of assessment and clinical skills, as well as to health care agencies for supervised clinical experiences. The latter are under the supervision of faculty who either directly supervise a group of students in the clinical setting or coordinate student preceptorships with students assigned to qualified staff nurse preceptors.

With careful planning, it is possible to provide clinical experiences for students enrolled in online courses through videoconferencing or teleconferencing and web-based instruction. Keeping in mind that course objectives must remain the same to ensure the integrity of the curriculum, faculty responsible for clinical courses can design the course so that the didactic and discussion components of the course are delivered through the selected distance education technology. Assignments, logs, or journals describing the clinical experiences, examinations, and pre- and postconferences can also take place through technology and can be *asynchronous* (occurring at various times) or *synchronous* (simultaneous). The actual clinical experiences occur through faculty-coordinated preceptorships, local faculty hired by the institution for clinical supervision of students, or by faculty traveling to the clinical site to supervise a group of students.

If faculty members serve as coordinators for clinical experiences with off-site preceptors and students, they must secure agreements between the educational program and the health care agency and preceptor; set standards for the qualifications of the preceptors; orient the preceptors to the curriculum, the course, and the role of preceptors; provide guidance throughout the experience to the preceptors and students; develop a communications network for all participants; supervise preceptors and students; assign the grades with input from the preceptors; and evaluate and revise the program based on feedback.

Simulated clinical experiences in a laboratory setting can take place with the use of high- and low-fidelity mannequins accompanied by case scenarios to prepare for hands-on clinical experiences in the reality setting. Rodriguez, Nelson, Gilmartin, Goldsamt, and Richardson (2017) explored the perceptions of undergraduate nursing students in relation to the use of best practices in simulation teaching, and the importance assigned to each teaching practice to support learning. These researchers used the Educational Practices Questionnaire, a 16-item validated instrument that measures aspects of simulation-based learning. Students were surveyed twice (midpoint and end) during their four-semester baccalaureate nursing program. Results indicated a significant increase in learning between mid- and endpoint surveys, which supports high-fidelity simulation as an innovative clinical teaching model for clinical practice hours.

THE GROWTH OF INFORMATICS AND TECHNOLOGY

Technology in the Classroom

The utilization of technology in the classroom and through distance education guides the implementation of the curriculum by determining the format for delivery of its courses. Technology applied to the classroom and distance education programs has grown exponentially over the past few decades. It moved from teacher-centered lectures accompanied by movies and slide shows in the classroom to the use of online PPT presentations with voice-over features, YouTube videos, MP3, and flash drives containing course materials for faculty and students' personal computers. Additional student-centered devices include electronic clickers for classroom participation and electronic note-taking software that links to course syllabi, materials, and lectures. Online technology is available through eLearning software that provides the educator with the ability to broadcast lectures or brief discussions complemented by movies, slides, website access, and so on. Examples of these software packages are Camtasia, Filmora, and Lectora. The development of these multimedia teaching/learning aids promotes active student participation in the learning process and facilitates the change from teacher-focused strategies to student-centered learning processes.

Classroom response systems such as handheld "clickers" are quickly being replaced with open-source, cloud-based, or commercial audience response systems (ARSs) applications. These systems allow students to respond to questions using a range of personal computing devices such as cell phones, smartphones, and laptops. Distributions of students' answers are immediately displayed. Montenery et al. (2013) report that this technology helps those who would not normally answer verbally in the classroom setting build confidence. In addition, ARS encourages engagement, participation, and provides instant feedback, which millennial learners' desire.

Njie-Carr et al. (2017) conducted an integrated review of the literature in regard to the "flipped classroom technique" as it applies to pedagogy for nursing education. This technique involves students preparing for class in advance by completing reading assignments and listening to short lectures instead of the traditional in class faculty lecture style. A total of 95 articles were obtained and 13 were used for analysis. Reviewed studies pertained to student success and satisfaction, student and faculty preparation, and discrepancies between faculty conceptualization of the flipped classroom technique. The authors concluded flipped classroom techniques promote active learning and critical thinking. One must consider teaching assignments and the technological support resources required for this teaching method. Suggestions are offered for additional research that is specific to flipped classroom models for nursing education, along with studies that examine long-term effects related to clinical performance. Finally, these authors found that disciplines outside of nursing can provide application and implementation strategies for this educational method.

Electronic library resources provide faculty, researchers, and students with Internet access to journals, electronic versions of textbooks, and reference databases. The most frequently used databases in nursing are Cumulative Index to Nursing and Allied Health Literature (CINAHL), Cochrane Database of Systematic Reviews, Health Sciences, Medline, Nursing and Allied Health, Ovid Nursing Journals Full Text, and PubMed. Social sciences and the sciences databases such as Behavioral Sciences and ScienceDirect are frequently used, as well as Educational Resources Information Center (ERIC) for references on education.

The "Cloud" Internet databases store files and other data in remote computer servers in order to synchronize and download them onto other electronic devices. They provide a virtual place for faculty, researchers, and students to store and exchange files, databases, and to submit and grade written assignments such as papers, journals, and logs. These services can be free or, if there is a large amount of data to store, a fee may be charged. Examples of some of these virtual files Internet services are Apple's iCloud, DropBox, Google Drive, and SugarSync.

Teachers writing on the chalkboard, students frantically trying to write down everything faculty says, all things of the past. *USA Today* (Alderton, 2016) reported spending on computer hardware increased last school year in nearly half (46%) of all U.S. school districts, indicating K through 12 is also moving to digital platforms in tandem with higher education. Smart Classrooms are technology-enhanced classrooms that provide opportunities for teaching and learning through the integration of technology, such as computers, specialized software, audience response technology, networking, and audio/visual capabilities. Video Capture software such as Camtasia, SnagIt, Adobe Presenter, and Movavi Screen Capture allow faculty members to record their lecture videos, and broadcast on the web or save to a video file. Students can be present for the live classroom lecture, view on a website in real time outside of the classroom, or watch at a later time. The recorded feature allows students to review the information for clarity or study purposes at their convenience.

While not a new phenomenon, the growth of massive open online courses (MOOCs) has implications for the future for granting credits toward degrees. MOOCs first appeared in 1988 but are growing in numbers available with free course offerings open to anyone. Several well-known institutions such as Harvard, Massachusetts Institute of Technology (MIT), Stanford, and the U.K. Open University offer the courses. In 2015, 11.3% of institutions reported having a MOOC and 2.3% are planning for one (Allen & Seaman, 2016). These percentages remain relatively stable and may in fact be plateauing. Courses vary by discipline and topic and they usually offer a certificate of completion if the student opts to finish the course. Some universities grant academic credit for completed courses based on competency-based models. Jordan (2014) reported that no more than 10% of the students finish courses and there is a high midway dropout rate. The impact of MOOCs on enrollment in higher education remains to be identified.

APPLICATION OF TECHNOLOGY TO EDUCATION

Simulated Clinical Experiences

The National Council of State Boards of Nursing (NCSBN) identified that up to 50% of high-quality simulation may be substituted for prelicensure nursing clinical hours (Alexander & Durham, 2015). The application of technology to the implementation of the curriculum occurs both on-campus and through distance education delivery systems. An example is the use of realistic interactive patient simulations in the laboratory setting for students to practice skills in a safe environment prior to providing nursing care in the clinical setting. Patient simulators come with ready-made case scenarios or faculty members can develop their own scenarios that can be programmed into the simulators. Many schools of nursing located on multidisciplinary health sciences campuses pool resources with other disciplines that result in shared state-of-the-art facilities to practice skills and foster interprofessional educational opportunities.

Other simulated experiences include human patient simulation/SP experiences with real people who have been programmed to present with health problems. Students interview and examine the patients for diagnosing health problems and, although real patients cannot simulate actual symptoms, they can provide realistic opportunities for history taking and communication skills. SPs are briefed ahead of time on what role they will be playing. During the simulation, the SP provides the student with additional information to assist in student learning. At the end of the simulation, SPs can provide feedback related to communication, interactions, and overall performance of the student. In some institutions, nursing is partnering with drama schools to fill the role of SPs. This is a cost-saving venture and students from both departments benefit from this partnership. MacLean, Kelly, and Geddes (2017) conducted an integrated review to examine the development of communication skills through the use of SPs. Nineteen articles were identified for review. The authors concluded that students' communication skills can be enhanced through educator and SP partnerships. In this study, SPs were used to both educate and evaluate student communications.

Newer models of mannequins available for nursing skills labs consist of low-fidelity or high-fidelity models. Examples of low-fidelity models are partial models such as an arm for practicing insertion of an intravenous line or a pelvis for physical examination. Whole body mannequins can be low fidelity for practicing such skills as bathing, turning, and positioning. High-fidelity mannequins are programmed to exhibit symptoms of bleeding, irregular pulses and respirations, emotions such as cries of pain and tears, and so forth. They are programmed according to preset scenarios and can be controlled by faculty in a booth adjacent to the simulated patient room. Rojas, Parker, Schams, and McNeill, (2017) describe the importance of simulation pedagogy and debriefing. In this study, faculty received education related to development of simulation and were evaluated using the Debriefing Assessment for Simulation in Health Care tool. The authors concluded a need for standardizing simulation scenarios and the importance of the debriefing phase. Assessment of both student and faculty performance is needed for quality improvement.

Virtual patient simulations are an emerging technology to support students who have limited access to clinical experiences. Foronda et al. (2017) recently published information on six newer technologies in the categories of augmented reality and virtual simulation that enhance student learning outcomes. Augmented reality is a cross of virtual and physical reality blended. Students physically take part in a virtual world where they have the opportunity to practice skills without the need of real patients or equipment. Products such as *Body Explorer, Flight Simulator* and *Microsoft HoloLens* represent this blended technology. Virtual simulation such as *CliniSpace, vSim for Nursing,* and *Shadow Health Digital Clinical Experience* are three-dimensional worlds of a health care that are entered through the users' laptops or personal computers as an "avatar." Students interact with their patients and receive feedback on their interactions and interventions with the virtual patient. These situations allow students to make clinical decisions in a situation that does not place the patient at risk. Foronda et al. see these technologies transforming education and improving learning outcomes.

Research Findings on the Efficacy of Case Scenario Simulations

There is much published on the efficacy of simulation. Bragard et al. (2016) measured technical and nontechnical skills of emergency and pediatric medical residents and pediatric nurses when interacting with a simulated pediatric patient experiencing a life-threatening cardiac arrhythmia. Participants were surveyed using questionnaires assessing self-reported changes in self-efficacy, stress, and satisfaction about skills. Results found that simulation-based training with debriefing had positive effects on reducing stress and increasing skill satisfaction.

Similar results were reported by McRae, Chan, Hulett, Lee, and Coleman (2017). They studied the effect of simulation on the self-confidence of nurses to perform cardiac surgical resuscitation and their satisfaction with the simulation experience. The Satisfaction With Simulation Experience scale was administered before and after two simulation scenarios. Findings indicated simulation increased self-confidence in performing resuscitation procedures for cardiac surgical patients and there was high satisfaction with the simulation experience.

Electronic Medical Records and Information Systems

As electronic patient records and information systems become more prevalent in the health care system, it becomes necessary for schools of nursing to provide the theoretical and technical knowledge related to these systems for nursing students. Booth, Sinclair, Brennan, and Strudwick (2017) provide an overview of the development and integration of simulated electronic medication administration record (eMAR) technology into undergraduate nursing curricula. Along with pharmacology didactic, students need to be exposed to experiences that mimic administration of medication to real patients. This includes the knowledge and skills related to computerized provider order entry (CPOE). These authors suggest the use of the sociotechnical systems theory for development of the simulated eMAR. This theory examines the relation "between humans and material objects (i.e., technology) in the generation of action" (p. 132). Provided are ideas, resources, and considerations for faculty in the development and implementation of the eMAR system. Booth et al. stress the importance of educational preparation and students' exposure to this technology before entering the clinical setting.

TRENDS, ISSUES, AND CHALLENGES FOR THE FUTURE

To remain competitive and current in the higher education market, nursing programs need to determine how they will expand their programs to meet the needs of students who may live and work some distance away from the home campus. Distance learning through technology offers the best opportunity for working nurses to continue their education and, as described earlier in the chapter, has been successful. Through consortia of varying levels of education, regional collaboratives, and the health care industry, these programs can be cost-effective and reach many more nurses than ever imagined.

The increasing market for LMSs provides cost-effective, quality educational delivery programs through web-based technology and in many ways, is proving to be an effective modality for engaging students in transformative learning experiences. These types of programs are far less expensive than videoconferencing and telecommunications; however, they require the technology, staffing, and faculty development programs to realize their full potential.

No matter the modality, the program must be within the context of the program's mission, philosophy, organizational framework, and goals and objectives. As with all curriculum development projects, faculty must examine the purpose of the distance education program in light of these components. In some cases, the program may not be compatible with the mission and therefore is not an option. For those programs that are compatible, the usual formative evaluation strategies must take place to ensure that the planning and implementation phases of the program are congruent with the overall curriculum plan. An evaluation plan to measure outcomes must be in place to maintain quality, meet program approval and accreditation standards, and ensure a quality program for its stakeholders such as students, consumers, and faculty.

The majority of distance education programs have copyright and intellectual property policies in place that are congruent with the parent institution. For new programs, along with faculty development and implementation support, it is advised that these policies be developed early in the process. The ideal policy is one that gives the individual faculty member the rights to the course syllabus and learning activities; however, the course description and objectives remain the property of the institution.

Privacy issues are addressed through the maintenance of the same policies of the parent institution. For web-based courses, owing to identification theft and computer hackers, many institutions issue identification numbers for students, staff, and faculty rather than social security numbers. Most LMSs have built-in privacy safety and security mechanisms allowing only students and faculty access to courses through personal identification numbers and passwords, and to protect debit and credit card information when paying tuition and fees.

Often, videoconferencing for satellite programs is delivered through closed-circuit television or public broadcasting system and thus is open to public access. However, only students officially enrolled in the courses can receive academic credit and have access to the supplemental material necessary for the course such as library services, course resources, email, LISTSERVs, and chat rooms.

An issue infrequently addressed in the literature is the matter of faculty to student ratios in distance education programs and their effect on quality education, faculty workload, and method of instruction. Online courses do not take up physical seats in an institution, but the number of students to faculty may affect the quality of the course. Online courses lead other technologies in reaching the greatest numbers of students. Except for MOOCs, institutions often limit course size per faculty.

As distance education programs increase in the future, new issues and challenges face faculty and institutions of higher learning. Less attention will be needed on the actual technology of the delivery systems and more attention will be necessary on the quality of the programs as they match the mission and purposes of the educational programs. Outcomes from distance education programs will be measured by increased opportunities for nurses to continue their education and the continued partnerships between education and service that result in a nursing workforce ready to meet the challenges of an ever-changing health care system and the health promotion and disease prevention needs of the populace.

SUMMARY

This chapter reviewed the various types of distance education programs and their relationship to curriculum development and evaluation. The influence of informatics and technology on nursing education was discussed. Some of the issues facing these types of programs were reviewed including cost-effectiveness, faculty workload, the application of teaching and learning principles, and student learning outcomes.

DISCUSSION QUESTIONS

- To what extent do you believe that technology-supported distance education programs changed nursing education for the 21st century?
- Of the multiple technology-supported distance education programs, which do you believe:
  - Is most cost-effective?
  - Meets desired outcomes?
  - Reaches the highest number of students?
  - Fosters faculty development?

  Explain your rationale
- Discuss the pros and cons for the delivery of clinical courses through distance education strategies.

LEARNING ACTIVITIES

Student-Learning Activities

1. Search the current literature (past 5 years) for at least three research articles on distance education programs, web-based education, or the application of informatics and technology on nursing education.
   a. Analyze them for a description of the outcomes for specific distance education modalities.
   b. Compare the modalities according to the outcomes that relate to teaching and learning effectiveness and student and faculty satisfaction.

Faculty Development Activities

1. Select one course that you teach and adapt it to either videoconferencing or web-based technology. Explain your rationale for selecting one or the other as it applies to the course.
2. If you teach a course(s) online, evaluate it for its student-learning outcomes and other measures of its effectiveness. Compare it to the program mission and program goals/objectives. Develop a plan for revising the course based on your evaluation.

References

Alderton, M. (2016). Smart classrooms give tech boost to learning. *USA Today*. Retrieved from https://www.usatoday.com/story/news/2016/07/30/smart-classrooms-give-tech-boost -learning/87699888

Alexander, M., & Durhan, C. F. (2015). NCSBN simulation guidelines for prelicensure nursing programs. *Journal of Nursing Regulation, 6*(3), 39–42.

Allen, I. E., & Seaman, J. (2016). *Online report card: Ten years of tracking online education in the United States.* Retrieved from http://onlinelearningsurvey.com/reports/onlinereportcard.pdf

American Distance Education Consortium. (2016). *Five best practices for developing online courses.* Retrieved from http://adec.edu/wp-content/uploads/Best_practices_developing_online_cour ses_6-20-16.pdf

Babson Survey Research Group. (2015). 2015 online report card-Tracking online education in the United States. Retrieved from https://onlinelearningconsortium.org/survey_report/2015-online-report-card-tracking-online-education-united-states

Big Blue Button. (2017). Engage your online students. Retrieved from http://bigbluebutton.org

Blackboard. (2017). Higher education technology & solutions. Retrieved from http://www .blackboard.com/Solutions-by-Market/Higher-Education.aspx

Blackboard Collaborate. (2017). Web conferencing software for education and business. Retrieved from http://www.blackboard.com/online-collaborative-learning/web-conferencing.aspx

Booth, R. G., Sinclair, B., Brennan, L., & Strudwick, G. (2017). Developing and implementing a simulated electronic medication administration record for undergraduate nursing education: Using sociotechnical systems theory to inform practice and curricula. *CIN: Computers, Informatics, Nursing, 35*(3), 131–139.

Bower, B. L., & Hardy, K. P. (2004). From correspondence to cyberspace: Changes and challenges in distance education. *New Directions for Community Colleges, 128,* 5–12.

Bragard, I., Farhat, N., Seghaye, M-C., Karam, O., Neuschwander, A., Shayan, Y., & Schumacher, K. (2016). Effectiveness of a high-fidelity simulation-based training program in managing cardiac arrhythmias in children: A randomized pilot study. *Pediatric Emergency Care*. doi: 10.1097/PEC.0000000000000931 (ePub ahead of print)

Canvas. (2017). How to choose an LMS. Retrieved from https://www.canvaslms.com/higher -education

Du, S., Liu, Z., Liu, S., Yin, H., Xu, G., Zhang, H., & Wang, A. (2013). Web-based distance learning for nurse education: A systematic review. *International Nursing Review, 60,* 167–177.

Examity. (2017). Better test integrity. Retrieved from http://examity.com

Fiedler, R., Giddens, J., & North, S. (2014). Faculty experience of a technological innovation in nursing education. *Nursing Education Perspectives, 35*(6), 387–391.

Foronda, C. L., Alfes, C. M., Dev, P., Kleinheksel, A. J., Nelson, D. A., O'Donnell, J. M., & Samosky, J. T. (2017). Virtually nursing. Emerging technologies in nursing education. *Nurse Educator, 42*(1), 14–17.

Fox, O. H. (2017). Using VoiceThread to promote collaborative learning in on-line clinical nurse leader courses. *Professional Nurse, 33,* 20–26.

Hampton, D., Pearce, P. F., & Moser, D. K., (2017). Preferred methods of learning for nursing students in an on-line degree program. *Journal of Professional Nursing, 33*(1), 27–37.

Jordan, K. (2014). Initial trends in enrolment and completion of massive open online courses. *International Review of Research in Open & Distance Learning, 15*(15), 133–160.

Kala, S., Isaramalai, S., & Pohthong, A. (2010). Electronic learning and constructivism: A model for nursing education. *Nurse Education Today, 30,* 61–66.

Kryterion Online Proctoring. (2017). Retrieved from https://www.onlineproctoring.com

Looyestyn, J., Kernot, J., Boshoff, K., Ryan, J., Edney, S., & Maher, C. (2017). Does gamification increase engagement with online programs? A systematic review. *Public Library of Science One, 12*(13), 1–19.

MacLean, S., Kelly, M., & Geddes. (2017) Use of simulated patients to develop communication skills in nursing education: An integrative review. *Nurse Education Today, 48,* 90–98.

McRae, M. E., Chan, A., Hulett, R., Lee, A. J., & Coleman, B. (2017). The effectiveness of and satisfaction with high-fidelity simulation to teach cardiac surgical resuscitation skills to nurses. *Intensive and Critical Care Nursing, 40,* 64–69.

Montenery, S., Walker, M., Sorensen, E., Thompson, R., Kirklin, D., White, R., & Ross, C. (2013). Millennial generation student nurses' perceptions of the impact of multiple technologies on learning. *Nursing Education Perspectives, 34*(6), 405–409.

Moodle. (2016). About Moodle. Retrieved from http://moodle.org/about

Njie-Carr, V. P. S., Ludeman, E., Lee, M. C., Dordunoo, D., Trocky, M. M., & Jenkines, L. S. (2017). An integrative review of flipped classroom teaching models in nursing education. *Journal of Professional Nursing, 33*(2), 133–144.

Pearson Education Inc. (2017). Products & services for institutions. Retrieved from http://www.ecollege.com/index.php

ProctorU. (2017). The global go-to for secure online testing. Retrieved from https://www.proctoru.com

Rodriguez, K. G., Nelson, N., Gilmartin, M., Goldsamt, L., & Richardson, H. (2017). Simulation is more than working with a manneqin: Students' perceptions of their learning experience in a clinical simulation environment. *Journal of Nursing Education and Practice, 7*(7), 30–36.

Rojas, D. E., Parker, C. G., Schams, K. A., & McNeill, J. A. (2017). Implementation of best practices in simulation debriefing. *Nursing Education Perspectives, 38*(3), 154–156.

Shadow Health. (2015). Digital clinical experiences™. Retrieved from https://shadowhealth.com/index.html

U.S. Department of Education, Office of Planning, Evaluation, and Policy Development, & Policy and Program Studies Service. (2010). *Evaluation of evidence-based practices in online learning: A Meta-analysis and review of online learning studies.* Retrieved from https://www2.ed.gov/rschstat/eval/tech/evidence-based-practices/finalreport.pdf

Uzuner Smith, S., Hayes, S., & Shea, P. (2017). A critical review of the use of Wegner's Community of Practice (CoP) theoretical framework in online and blended learning research, 2000–2014. *Online Learning, 21*(1), 209–237.

Wimba. (2017). Wimba classroom for higher education. Retrieved from http://www.wimba.com/solutions/higher-education/wimba_classroom_for_higher_education

Zoom. (2017). Video conferencing and web conferencing service. Retrieved from https://www.zoom.us

SECTION IV

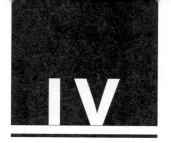

Program Evaluation and Accreditation

Sarah B. Keating

OVERVIEW

This section analyzes theories, concepts, and models used to evaluate and approve nursing education programs. Although evaluation appears as the last step, it occurs throughout the processes of curriculum development and its implementation. Evaluation activities are part of the program approval and accreditation processes that schools experience as part of their credibility for consumers of the programs and for documentation of the institution's ability to meet professional and educational standards. Information from evaluation activities provides the impetus for major and minor changes that must take place to maintain an up-to-date and high-quality curriculum.

Current economic and educational systems in the United States place an emphasis on outcomes and *total quality management (TQM)* or *continuous quality improvement (CQI)*: continually assessing the program and correcting errors as they occur to improve the quality of the program. In addition to measuring outcomes, it is necessary to assess the processes that bring about the final product, that is, instructional strategies that enable learners to become actively involved and self-directing to acquire new knowledge, behaviors, attitudes, and skills. Assessment of the conduits used to present the program such as web-based platforms, smart classrooms, simulated clinical situations, and so forth are part of the evaluation. Additional information that measures the outcomes in terms of graduates' performance and the quality of the program as compared to professional standards and the program's competitors provide a summative evaluation on how well the program meets its mission and goals.

To ensure quality, the parent institution should hold regional accreditation that demonstrates that it meets the standards for higher education, which is important to the nursing program's quality as well. There are many levels of program approval and accreditation that nursing programs undergo. For example, the parent institution approves and periodically evaluates the nursing program and the state board of nursing, a regulating agency, must approve the program initially and at periodic intervals. While the state board looks at quality, its primary charge is to view the program's performance in light of consumer protection. It also determines the program's eligibility for graduates to sit for RN licensure and in many states, approves nursing programs for advanced practice.

Accreditation is voluntary but at the same time, it gives credibility to a nursing program on the regional, national, and professional levels. Its purpose is to ensure quality as measured by higher education and nursing accrediting agencies' standards and criteria set by professional peers. An accredited program provides advantages including its reputation for quality, eligibility for grants and other external funding, and for its graduates' eligibility for licensure, certification, admission into higher degree programs, and scholarships.

THE ROLE OF FACULTY, STUDENTS, CONSUMERS, AND ADMINISTRATORS IN EVALUATION

As is true for curriculum development, the faculty is key to the assessment of program processes and outcomes and to the collection and analysis of the data. Students are an important part of the evaluation process as measured by their performance on tests and clinical skills, satisfaction with the program, and their assessment of teaching effectiveness and the quality of the courses in which they participate. Evaluation of the program must also come from the major consumers of the program, which include alumni, employers of the graduates, and the recipients of the graduates' nursing care. The program's success is further assessed by the graduates' performance on licensure and certification exams, job skills, professional achievements, and promotion of the program to others. Employers of the graduates and the population receiving their services provide invaluable information and serve as a barometer of the program's match to the health care needs of the population and the system's demand for its graduates.

The role of administrators in evaluation is to provide the leadership and financial resources necessary for the process and if indicated, consultation services (internal or external expertise). Administrators must see to it that there is an adequate support staff for the ongoing collection and analyses of data and they have responsibility for ensuring that the findings are disseminated in a timely fashion to the program's stakeholders and for follow-up on the recommendations from the findings.

THE MASTER PLAN OF EVALUATION AND PROGRAM REVIEW

Chapter 12 focuses on major evaluation theories, concepts, and models related to program review and assessment. It describes the system of program approval and periodic review within the parent institution. Peer and administrative review bodies and individuals grant approval to initiate programs in academe. Traditionally, reviews of established programs occur every 5 years within the institution to ensure quality and in some instances, justify the continuation of the program when enrollments decline or economic times require downsizing of academic programs.

With an emphasis on outcomes, evaluation is essential for measuring success, establishing benchmarks, and continually improving the quality of the program. Because programs need to meet academic and accreditation standards, professional discipline expectations, and consumer demand, most institutions have a master plan of evaluation. The master plan may be organized around an evaluation model or theory or by criteria set by accrediting bodies, or it may choose to use both. The master plan provides the guidelines for collecting information to prepare required reports such as program approval or review, accreditation, and to demonstrate the worth of the program to the parent institution and the community. Institutions use the results of evaluation to continue and to improve the program, demonstrate excellence, and market their programs to the public.

PREPARING FOR AN ACCREDITATION VISIT

Chapter 13 follows through on the concepts from Chapter 12 by providing a case study of the process for preparing for accreditation in nursing education. It provides educators with guidelines for preparing for accreditation including timelines, preparing the report, roles, and responsibilities of faculty, submission of the report, and preparation for the visit.

CHAPTER 12

Program Evaluation and Accreditation

Sarah B. Keating

CHAPTER OBJECTIVES

Upon completion of Chapter 12, the reader will be able to:

- Analyze common definitions, concepts, and theories of quality assurance and program evaluation
- Analyze several models of evaluation for their utility in nursing education
- Analyze the various forms of accreditation and typical accreditation processes that are used to indicate a program meets specific standards and criteria
- Compare research to program evaluation processes
- Justify the rationale for strategic planning and developing a master plan of evaluation for educational programs
- Compare the roles of administrators and faculty in program evaluation and accreditation

OVERVIEW

This chapter reviews definitions, concepts, and theories related to evaluation, quality assurance, and accreditation as they apply to nursing education. Conceptual models of evaluation; utilization of standards, criteria, and benchmarks for evaluation and accreditation; comparison of evaluation research to program evaluation; and types of program evaluation and their purposes are included. The chapter continues with a discussion of strategic planning, the development of master plans of evaluation, and the roles of nursing faculty and administrators in these activities. As discussed in the section overview, educational evaluation occurs while assessing the program for its quality, currency, relevance, compliance with regulatory agency requirements and accreditation standards, projections into the future, and the need for possible revisions in light of these factors. While the administration usually assumes the leadership for strategic planning, faculty becomes part of the process, especially as it relates to responding to the information provided by the evaluation of the curriculum and the future plans for the institution. A master plan of evaluation provides the information necessary for curriculum evaluation and revision if indicated, and for program or institutional strategic planning.

COMMON DEFINITIONS, CONCEPTS, AND THEORIES RELATED TO EVALUATION, QUALITY ASSURANCE, AND ACCREDITATION

While many of the terms, concepts, and theories of educational evaluation originated from business models, they have been adapted to education, especially in light of the emphasis on outcomes. The following definitions are commonly used terms in evaluation as they apply to nursing education. To initiate the discussion, the first term to consider is a comparison of evaluation to assessment. *Evaluation* is a process by which information about an entity is gathered to determine its worth. It differs from assessment in that the end product of evaluation is a judgment of its worth, while *assessment* is a process that gathers information that results in a conclusion such as a nursing diagnosis or problem identification. It does not end with a judgment but rather a conclusion.

Quality is a term that takes on many meanings depending on the context in which it is used. For the purposes of this chapter and in the interest of simplicity, quality as conceptualized by Schindler, Puls-Elvidge, Welzant, and Crawford, (2015) is measured as "purposeful, transformative, exceptional, and accountable" (p. 8). *Quality assurance* for the purposes of nursing education is the process of collecting data on how well the institution or program meets its defined standards, criteria, goals, or mission. Total quality management/improvement (TQM/TQI) and continuous quality improvement (CQI) are processes or systems that involve all of the stakeholders in the program in the assessment of the quality and effectiveness of the program according to criteria or standards. These processes identify gaps or errors and correct problems to ensure that the program maintains its purpose and quality. Stakeholders continuously ask the questions: How are we doing? Are we meeting our goals? What barriers or challenges are we encountering? What are the processes or systems that inhibit or enhance our progress? What can we do to improve?

Formative and summative evaluation terms are used frequently when evaluating educational programs. The classic and still used definitions for the terms were developed by Scriven (1996). He describes *formative evaluation* as "intended–by the evaluator–as a basis for improvement" (p. 4). For example, in nursing, the faculty compares students' progress in meeting course objectives and what processes took place to achieve or not achieve them and based on the findings what corrective measures should take place to meet the objectives (or possibly, change the objectives). Scriven describes *summative evaluation* as a holistic approach to the assessment of a program and it uses results from the formative evaluation. Continuing with the examples from nursing, faculty evaluates the development of critical thinking and clinical decision-making skills in its graduates as an outcome of the educational program. In this instance, these skills would need to be measured both before and after the program to determine an increase and proficiency in the skills. Both formative and summative types of evaluation "involve efforts to determine merit or worth, etc." (Scriven, 1996, p. 6). Scriven points out that summative evaluation can serve as formative evaluation. For example, if a nursing program finds that graduates' clinical decision-making skills are inadequate (summative evaluation), it can use that information to analyze the program for the strategies (formative evaluation) that were utilized to promote these skills and make improvements as necessary.

Additional definitions commonly used in evaluation are *goal-based evaluation* and *goal-free evaluation*. Scriven (1974) described goal-based program evaluation as that which focuses only on the examination of program goals and intended outcomes, while an alternative method could be used to examine the actual effects of the program. These effects (goal-free evaluation) include not only the intended effects, but also unintended effects, side effects, or secondary effects. An unintended effect in nursing might be an increase in the applicant pool owing to the community's interactions with students in a program-sponsored, nurse-managed clinic. While this was not a stated goal of the program, it was a positive, unintended outcome.

CONCEPTUAL MODELS OF EVALUATION

Conceptual Models

For years, nursing education programs used many of the models of evaluation developed in health care and education. Examples were Donabedian's (1996) Structure, Process, and Outcome model for health care evaluation and Stufflebeam et al.'s (1971) Context, Input, Process, and Product (CIPP) educational model. Some of these models continue to serve nursing well but as nursing develops the uniqueness of the discipline, it is using its own models for evaluation. Chinta, Kebritchi, and Elias (2016) describe the application of the CIPP model in higher education in a large U.S. university. For nursing programs using the CIPP model it is useful to know that Chinta et al. identified two missing components in the CIPP model. They point out the need to include internal and external metrics and to add benchmarks to the model for a more complete evaluation. Their description provides a practical application and guide for using the CIPP model for the evaluation of higher education programs.

Horne and Sandmann (2012) conducted an integrative review of the literature to ascertain if graduate nursing programs evaluate their effectiveness based on reaching the outcomes/goals of the program, cost-effectiveness, student and faculty satisfaction, decisions that are based on the evaluation outcomes, and measuring the quality of the program. Prior to their report on the findings, they define evaluation and its various processes, as well as describe some of the models of evaluation reported in their review of the literature. They found a paucity of articles related to program evaluation but found a few helpful ideas for programs to measure program quality and effectiveness in nursing.

A model for evaluating the quality of nursing doctoral programs developed by Kim, C. Park, S. Park, Khan, and Ketefian (2014) surveyed faculty and students in doctoral programs across the United States. The questionnaire for the survey consisted of four domains of measurement: the program, faculty, resources, and evaluation. Using these four domains and information from the programs' administrators on the institutions' numbers of students and graduates, the authors found their research instrument to be both valid and reliable. Results from the survey revealed that the overall quality of the schools assessed was good, but there was room for improvement. It is a model of evaluation that could be applied to other nursing programs at the graduate level.

Benchmarking

Programs can set benchmarks to measure their own success and standards of excellence, or compare themselves to similar institutions. Benchmarks can be used in competition with other programs for recruiting students or seeking financial support or they can be used to motivate the members of the institution to strive toward excellence. Yet another function of benchmarking is the ability to collaborate with other institutions to share strengths with each other and to continually improve programs. Benchmarks include the financial health of the institution; applicant pool; admission, retention and graduation rates; commitment to diversity; student, faculty, staff, and administrators satisfaction rates; National Council Licensure Examination (NCLEX®) and certification pass rates; and so forth.

An example of a benchmarking project when developing or revising DNP programs is presented by Udlis and Manusco (2012) from their website survey of DNP programs across the United States. The authors present a summary of the history of the development of the degree and then present their findings from the 2011 website survey of 137 programs. Findings are organized according to type of program, program length and number of credits, location by region of the United States, cost, platform for offering the program, electives availability, number of credits, and the practice course name. Their study provides benchmarks and trends in DNP education programs as programs continue to evolve and increase across the United States. Asif (2015) presents a detailed description of the utilization of benchmarking as a model of program evaluation and points out that it begins with the need to identify areas in the program that need improvement. From that assessment, the stakeholders become involved in determining what the priorities for improvement are and what benchmarks will contribute to that improvement.

An Evaluation Processes Model

The Centers for Disease Control and Prevention (CDC, 2017) developed a framework for program evaluation that is useful to educators. While it focuses on the processes of evaluation, it includes a framework for assigning value or worth to the findings from the process. The major steps in the process are: (a) engage the stakeholders, (b) describe the program, (c) focus the evaluation plan, (d) gather credible evidence, (e) justify conclusions and recommendations, (f) use and share lessons learned and, finally, the cycle begins again with the first step: "engage the stakeholders." The steps of the model incorporate standards against which the program is evaluated and include utility, feasibility, propriety, and accuracy. For nursing programs, there are many and include accreditation standards or criteria and professional/educational essentials or standards.

Formative Evaluation for Nursing Education

Formative and/or process evaluation strategies include course evaluations; student achievement measures; teaching effectiveness surveys; staff, student, administration, and faculty satisfaction measures; impressions of student and faculty performance by clinical agencies' personnel; assessment of student services and other support systems; students' critical thinking development and other standardized tests such as gains in knowledge and skills; NCLEX readiness; satisfaction surveys of families of students; retention/attrition rates; and cost-effectiveness of the program. Antecedent or input evaluation items include the entering grade point averages (GPAs), American College Testing (ACT; www.act.org/products/k-12-act-test), Scholastic Achievement Test (SAT; pro fessionals.collegeboard.com/higher-ed), and Graduate Record Examination (GRE; www .ets.org/gre) scores for applicants and accepted students; retention and/or attrition rates; scholarship, fellowship, and loan availability; and endowments and grants for program development and support.

Nursing education's need to improve evaluation measures in formative education is pointed out by Mansutti, Salani, Grassetti, and Palese (2017) in their review of the literature for measures of the quality of clinical learning experiences. Their purpose was to identify the psychometric properties and methodological quality of these measures. They found 26 studies that utilized eight clinical learning environmental instruments; however, different methods were used to measure results for the eight identified instruments. Overall, Mansutti et al. found poor content and construct validity of the instruments and they point out that students did not participate in the evaluation of the instruments that were used. The statistical analyses of the findings from the instruments varied among the studies. The authors identify the need for the development of instruments that evaluate students' performance that are consistent, reliable, and valid.

An example of a competency-based nurse practitioner program across the various levels of nursing education from the BSN to the DNP is presented by Schumacher and

Risco (2017) that illustrates how competencies can be leveled leading from formative (competencies and objectives) to summative evaluation (program outcomes). The model includes definitions and differentiation among competencies, outcomes, major competencies, program outcomes, minor or level competencies, course objectives, and course-related student outcomes. Another example for developing formative evaluation measures and leveling evidence-based practice outcomes across the curriculum from the BSN to DNP level is described by Hande, Williams, Robbins, Kennedy, and Christenbery (2017). Both of these models are exemplars for formative or process evaluation methodologies in nursing education that should ultimately lead to summative or product evaluation.

SUMMATIVE EVALUATION USING STANDARDS, ESSENTIALS, AND CRITERIA

Summative evaluation differs from formative evaluation with its purpose to assess and judge the final outcomes of the educational program, while formative evaluation assesses the processes used to achieve the final outcome. The "product" of the educational program can be measured according to the overall goal and objectives of the program/curriculum and other standards and criteria of regulating bodies such as boards of nursing, professional standards such as nursing organizations' code of ethics and practice standards, essentials or competencies defined by professional and educational organizations, and last but not least, accreditation standards and criteria.

Measures to determine final outcomes of the program include follow-up surveys of the success rates of the graduates including their pass rates on licensure and certification exams, employers' and graduates' satisfaction with the program, graduates' performance, and alumni's accomplishments in leadership roles, as change agents, professional commitment, and continuing education rates. Additional outcome measures include graduation rates, accreditation and program approval status, stakeholders' perceptions of the graduates, ratings of the program by external evaluators or agencies, faculty and student research productivity, community service, and public opinion surveys. Many of these outcome measures can be used to serve as benchmarks for setting achievement levels, for example, 99% pass rates on NCLEX or for comparing the institution to other admired or similar institutions as a measure of quality.

Lewallen (2015) offers practical suggestions on ways in which nursing educators can conduct a program evaluation by organizing faculty and staff groups to collect and manage data, analyze the findings, and use the results to make decisions. Lewallen cites the importance of program evaluation and its function to ensure the quality of the program and to meet the requirements of regulatory and accreditation agencies. The concept of meta-evaluation is discussed in detail by Ardisson, Smallheer, Moore, and Christenery (2015) who trace the history of the concept and its application to higher education and eventually to its role in nursing education evaluation. The idea of meta-evaluation is that the process of program evaluation needs to be assessed to ensure its integrity, that data are of the highest quality, and that decisions made are data driven. They offer a conceptual model from their nursing program evaluation activities for other schools of nursing and argue that meta-evaluation leads to CQI.

TYPES OF PROGRAM EVALUATION

Program Approval by Regulatory Agencies

Each state, according to its constitution, regulates higher education and approves programs usually requiring that the institutions meet regional accreditation standards and for professional programs, professional accreditation standards. For information on individual states, the U.S. Department of Education (USDOE) lists the various state, territory, and commonwealth departments of education and their higher education agencies at: www2.ed.gov/about/contacts/state/index.html. For nursing, at the present time, there is no national licensure to practice as a nurse or as an advanced practice nurse. Thus, licensure to practice as a nurse falls onto the state in which the nurse practices. Each state has a nursing practice act that defines the role of the nurse through defined regulations. The state board of nursing acts to enforce the regulations in the interest of patient safety and public protection. The membership of the National Council of State Boards of Nursing (2017) consists of all 50 state boards as well as those in Washington, DC, and the four U.S. territories. In some states, in addition to the definition of nursing practice, advanced practice is defined using the consensus standards as a model. In spring 2017, there were 38 boards that had definitions of advanced practice and of those, 21 allowed independent practice and prescription authority. For an updated list of the states utilizing major components of the Consensus Model go to www.ncsbn.org/2017Marchmapwithpoints.pdf.

Program Approval by Accreditation

A major factor that affects curriculum development and evaluation in nursing education is the imperative that a nursing program meet state board of nursing regulations and accreditation standards set by a national accreditation agency. In addition, in the case of certain specialties, specialty accreditation organizations such as those for nurse midwives and nurse anesthetists accredit programs with those specialties. While not necessarily part of accreditation agencies' standards, some standards and criteria are set by professional organizations such as the American Association of Colleges of Nursing (AACN), the National League for Nursing (NLN), and the Consensus Model for Advanced Practice Registered Nurses (APRNs): Licensure Accreditation, Certification, and Education (LACE) that can in turn be part of accreditation expectations. While accreditation in the United States is voluntary, failure to be approved or accredited can lead to closure of the institution by the state regulatory agency, ineligibility for program development funds, or disqualification of the program's students for Title IV financial aid support, traineeships, and scholarships. If students attempt to transfer credits or have degrees from nonaccredited schools, it is likely that the credits and degrees will not be recognized when applying to other institutions of higher education that are accredited.

Accreditation agencies set the standards or criteria by which to judge the quality of educational programs. The Council for Higher Education Accreditation is an organization of institutions in higher education whose purpose and mission is to ensure academic quality through accreditation. An overview of its membership and role in advocacy for quality higher education in the United States may be found on its home page at www.chea.org/userfiles/uploads/chea-at-a-glance_2015.pdf. In addition to its role in quality assurance in the United States, CHEA has an international quality group to address quality issues in higher education in other nations. Information about this group may be found at www.chea.org/4DCGI/indexint.html?menukey=home. CHEA recognizes accrediting agencies and serves as a representative for higher education concerned with national accreditation issues as well as in the world community. A list of its recognized accrediting bodies may be found on its website at www.chea.org/userfiles/Recognition/CHEA_USDE_AllAccred.pdf.

An example of the issues in which CHEA becomes involved is its advocacy role in the question of student financial aid for for-profit higher education institutions. In the United States there has been an increase in these programs, especially for those offering distance education formats. A positive effect from them is that they are recruiting a more diverse student body and people from lower income groups. However, these for-profit institutions receive 25% of all of the funds distributed by the Department of Education owing to their higher costs. Thirteen percent of all students in higher education are enrolled in for-profit schools but they account for approximately 31% of the student loans, and they are responsible for about half of all defaults on the loans (Lindgrensavage, 2016).

The USDOE is the official governmental agency that recognizes accrediting agencies in the United States. On the institutional level, colleges and universities are usually accredited by a regional accrediting agency including the Middle States Commission on Higher Education; the New England Association of Schools and Colleges, Commission on Institutions of Higher Education; the North Central Association of Colleges and Schools, The Higher Learning Commission; The Northwest Commission on Colleges and Universities; the Southern Association of Colleges and Schools, Commission on Colleges; the Western Association of Schools and Colleges, Accrediting Commission for Community and Junior Colleges; and the Western Association of Schools and Colleges, Senior Colleges and University Commission. A list of these agencies and details about them can be found on the USDOE website at www2.ed.gov/admins/finaid/accred/accreditation_pg6.html. These regional agencies have the infrastructure and paid staff to support their missions, which is to ensure the quality of higher education institutions. The agencies are staffed by experts in the field including not only those in education, but also staff experts in distance learning systems, educational technology, and informatics. Volunteer directors or commissioners who are experts in higher education such as presidents, provosts, administrators, deans, and faculty set the standards and policies of the accreditation agencies Additional volunteers are selected and trained according to their expertise in higher education to act as visitors to institutions undergoing accreditation. The USDOE recognizes accrediting agencies to ensure educational quality including the regional agencies as well as specialized accreditors.

The majority of nursing programs are housed in multipurpose colleges or universities that are regionally accredited. Since PhD and DNS programs are not accredited by a specialized accrediting agency for nursing, it is important that they are regionally accredited to ensure they meet the standards of quality in higher education doctoral programs. (As an aside, the AACN [2017] developed outcomes and doctoral elements for the research-focused degree in nursing, which may be found at www.aacn.nche.edu/education-resources/phdposition.pdf.) In order to determine if an institution meets regional accreditation standards, it prepares a self-study report that responds to each of the accreditation standards and involves the stakeholders in its preparation including administrators, faculty, staff, and students. After receiving the report, a team of volunteer peer evaluators from the accrediting agency visits the institution to verify and clarify the information found in the self-study. The team prepares a report on its findings that is presented to the board or commission of the accrediting agency that reviews the findings and determines if the institution meets the standards and should receive either first-time accreditation, continuing accreditation, or submit a progress report if indicated.

Program accreditation, like institutional accreditation, is voluntary. In 2017, there were three nationwide accrediting agencies for nursing recognized by the USDOE. They were the Accreditation Commission for Education in Nursing, the Commission on Collegiate Nursing Education, and the NLN Commission for Nursing Education Accreditation.

Accreditation by these agencies is voluntary but for students and graduates in nursing programs, coming from an accredited program is essential for scholarships, traineeships, financial aid support, career opportunities, and future continuing education plans that involve a higher degree. Each of these agencies are similar to the regional accreditors as they have an infrastructure and staff but depend on volunteer experts from the profession to set standards, make site visits, and participate in recommendations and policy making.

As mentioned earlier, there are specialized accreditors for nursing programs with specialty tracks in their graduate programs. Nursing specialty accrediting agencies recognized by the USDOE include the American Association of Nurse Anesthetists and the American College of Nursing Midwives (USDOE, 2017). The Consensus Model for APRNs: LACE was developed in 2008 by representatives from professional nursing organizations, nursing educators, certification agencies, and state boards of nursing. The model identified four areas of advanced practice: nurse anesthetists, clinical specialists, nurse midwives, and nurse practitioners. It also recognizes certified nurse practitioners who practice in both acute care and primary care settings and are educated and certified for both roles. Advanced practice nurses must be licensed by the state board of nursing where they practice, certified by a certification program recognized by the National Council of State Boards of Nursing, and educated in an accredited institution recognized by the USDOE and according to the standards delineated in the Consensus Model. A detailed description of the Consensus Model: LACE may be found at the American Nurses Association APRN Consensus Model website (www.nln.org/docs/default-source/accreditation-services/accreditation_agencies_joint_statement_on_ap_final-1015.pdf?sfvrsn=2).

Program Approval in Academe

Basically, there are two types of program evaluation in academe that differ from regulatory and accreditation processes: *program approval* and *program review*. Before a new program is initiated, its parent institution must approve it. As reiterated throughout this text, it is the faculty who develop the curriculum for a new program and it should be based on a needs assessment that provides the rationale for why it is needed, how it meets the mission of the institution, and who the key stakeholders are. In addition to the curriculum plan, a budget should accompany it and it is expected that it projects the costs and income for at least the next 5 to 10 years to justify its start-up and maintenance.

In academe, the usual rounds of approval are as follows. The first round is for the faculty within the originating department/school to approve the proposal; its next round depends on the hierarchal structure of the institution. The following levels of approval are based on a moderate- to large-scale institution and it is understood that smaller institutions may not have as many approval rungs. After faculty approval within the originating program, the proposal may go to a curriculum- or program-approval committee within its college or division. Preliminary approval may have to be granted by administrators before it enters other formal approval levels in order to determine its economic feasibility and its fit to the mission and/or strategic plan. After approval at the program's local level by committees and faculty as a whole, it proceeds to the next level, which is usually a program or curriculum committee at the division or college level. With its approval, it goes to the overall university or college graduate or undergraduate committee for its review and approval. Next, it goes to a subcommittee of the senate that reviews program proposals. On its approval, the senate reviews it for its role in the university and quality and if approved, sends it to the chief executive for academic affairs such as a vice president or provost. Upon that person's approval, the president of the institution approves the program. The governing board such as a board of trustees or regents is the final rung of approval and it may have a subcommittee that reviews it with recommendations prior to its going to the full board. These levels of approval are for academic approval only. For professional programs, such as nursing, accreditation processes, and state board of nursing, approvals should be initiated along the way to reensure the academic entities that the program is qualified for professional approval and accreditation.

Program Review

Program review in academe occurs on average every 5 years within the parent institution. The purpose for program review is to ensure the quality and sustainability of the program and to demonstrate to the institution's constituency its place in the academic community. Faculty prepares an overview of the program especially related to its mission, student learning outcomes, enrollments, the quality of the faculty, and enrollment and graduation projections. When economic times are tough, these reviews help demonstrate the relationship of the program to the mission of the institution, its contributions to the community, and the quality of the program. Nursing often finds itself having to justify its program owing to the relatively small faculty to student ratios required when clinical supervision is factored in. Nursing programs provide data as evidence to support the program, its cost-effectiveness, its place in meeting the mission of the institution (serving the public), and its contributions of student enrollments to the core general education, prerequisite requirements, program development funds, and research and scholarship production.

Turner (2016) conducted an assessment of an online program in educational leadership and administration and stated that the process of program review can lead to strategic planning, CQI, and also parallel functions with accreditation processes. Turner especially focused on the need for the evaluators to "close the loop" on findings that indicate a need for follow-up. Another point is that the student learning outcomes must be measurable, attainable, and in concordance with the institution's goals and strategic plan.

The requirements and processes for program approval and review use the same data sets as many of the other assessment and evaluation activities related to professional accreditation and standards of excellence. Thus, it is not unusual for a parent institution to request copies of the most recent self-studies and accreditation reports that either substitute for program review criteria or supplement the requirements. Program approval and review should be integrated into the school's strategic plan so that data sets gathered from the master plan can serve all assessment and evaluation activities.

Research and Program Evaluation

Sometimes there is confusion between evaluation research and the process of evaluation. The evaluation process starts with an identification of the program or entity that is to be evaluated, the purpose of the evaluation, and who the stakeholders are within the program. It requires many of the same steps of research including a review of the literature, identification of a theory or model of evaluation to guide the process, collection and analysis of credible data related to the program, synthesizing the analysis to come to a conclusion, and a judgment with recommendations for further assessment and strategies for improvement. It differs from program evaluation research as it focuses on one program and its purpose is to evaluate or judge the program in terms of the program's quality and ability to meet its purpose and goals.

Research in evaluation, on the other hand, differs from the evaluation process. It begins with a description of a problem and a research question related to program evaluation theories, concepts, and processes for the purpose of comparing them, testing them, and perhaps developing a new theory, concept, or model of evaluation. As is common in most research, the purpose for investigation and a research question/inquiry is stated. There is a literature review and, based on the review, a theoretical/conceptual framework is postulated followed by descriptions of the methodology, data collection and analysis, findings, and recommendations. Research in evaluation is usually viewed as applied research and differs from basic research as it is searching for practical solutions to problems. It has a broader focus than program evaluation and looks to contributing to the discipline of educational theory and conceptual bases.

Strategic Planning

Strategic planning for an institution provides the guidelines for carrying out the mission of the institution and at the same time, is used to evaluate how well the institution is meeting its mission and goals. A strategic plan incorporates the institution's vision statement and core values that look to the future and where it plans to be 3 to 5 years hence. From that vision, goals are set that guide the processes necessary to reach the vision. Strategic planning usually begins with the top executive and management team providing the leadership for its development. In academe, the parent institution's top administrators (president, vice presidents, provosts, deans, et al.) initiate the plan, which is, in turn, implemented throughout the institution by the various academic divisions. Key stakeholders in the institution are brought into the planning process to ensure that the plan and its action plans are relevant and realistic in terms of meeting the goals within the time frame specified. Each year, progress is measured toward reaching the goals and realizing the vision with corrections to the plan as necessary and redevelopment of a strategic plan occurring at the end of the specified time period or sooner, if unexpected events cause the need for a new strategic plan.

Each program within the institution may choose to develop its own strategic plan; however, it should be congruent with that of its parent but unique to the program's mission and goals. The chief nursing officer of the nursing program and administrative team act as the initiators of a strategic plan and involve faculty, staff, and students in the planning process. It is useful to consult with graduates and consumers of the program as well for their perspectives on how well the program meets its mission and goals and what they foresee for the future. In addition, consultation with other disciplines assists the planners to identify the role of nursing in the higher education and health care systems.

A positive, comprehensive, and inclusionary approach to strategic planning is described by Harmon, Fontaine, Plews-Ogan, and Williams (2012) in a summary of the University of Virginia's School of Nursing strategic planning process. They adapted the Appreciative Inquiry (AI) model used in business for planning and promoting a positive milieu. The authors describe the process they underwent for planning, holding, and summarizing the outcomes from a summit that developed strategic plans for the School of Nursing's future. It is a very useful model for other institutions undergoing the strategic planning process. Skiba (2015) presents some trends in emerging technologies and their effects on higher education that have implications for nursing when developing strategic plans. These trends are defined as short term (the effects of pedagogical changes, e.g., flipped classrooms, online learning), midterm, (measurements of learning, the growth of open resources for students, meta-data analysis, etc.), and long term (interinstitutional/international cooperation and new discoveries).

It is wise for nursing programs to have goals set for the future with action plans to carry them out. These goals and action plans are reviewed at least annually to assess progress toward the goals and to adjust or develop new goals as the program and its needs and constituencies change. To avoid the pitfall of exquisite planning processes that fail to implement the plan, the use of a master plan of evaluation provides the structure, details, and timelines for assessing and evaluating the progress that the program is making toward reaching its vision and short-term and long-term goals.

MASTER PLAN OF EVALUATION

Rationale for a Master Plan of Evaluation

When developing a master plan of evaluation, one of the major tasks to integrate into the plan is to meet accreditation or program approval standards. These standards or criteria are the baseline requirements of the profession to ensure that programs are of sufficient quality to meet the expectations of the discipline. They also demonstrate to the public that a program is recognized by external reviewing bodies and thus the quality of its graduates meets educational and professional standards. Graduation from an accredited program is usually one of the admission standards for continued degree or educational work. Many funding agencies for programs require accreditation as it indicates that the program is of high enough quality to assume the responsibility for the administration of grants and completion of projects. Most accrediting agencies require that a program have a master plan of evaluation or evidence of institutional policies with their regular review and reports on compliance or revisions if indicated (ACEN, 2017; CCNE, 2017). A master plan helps identify the components of the program that need to be evaluated, who will do the data collection and when, what methods of analysis of the data will be employed, and the plans for responding to the findings for quality improvement. Having a master plan of evaluation in place greatly facilitates these processes when submitting accreditation self-study reports, program approval reports, or proposals for funding.

With an emphasis on outcomes, the evaluation process is essential for measuring success, establishing benchmarks, and continually improving the quality of the program. A master plan of evaluation is used to provide data for faculty's decision making as part of an internal review and for meeting external review standards. It is important to have a master plan that continually monitors the program so that adjustments can be made as the program is implemented as it is part of the total quality improvement process. It is equally important to measure outcomes in terms of meeting the vision, strategic plans, goals, and objectives of the program, with certain benchmarks that help pinpoint the quality of the program.

Components of a Master Plan of Evaluation

The master plan must specify what is being evaluated and an organizing framework is useful so that as nearly as possible, no crucial variable is omitted for review. Additionally, it is important to identify the persons who will:

1. Collect the data
2. Analyze the findings
3. Prepare reports
4. Disseminate the reports to key people
5. Set the timelines for collection, analysis, and reporting of the data

Finally, there must be a feedback loop in place for recommendations and decision making. Reports from the evaluation should include the following:

1. Identification of existing and potential problems
2. Previously unidentified or new needs

3. Successes and why
4. Recommendations for improvement, discontinuance of a program, or proposals for new programs
5. Action plans for changes that include the people responsible and timelines
6. A summary of the evaluation and judgment on the program's success or progress toward meeting its goals

Table 12.1 provides guidelines for developing a master plan of evaluation and the major components to be assessed for evaluation. In addition to including the curriculum and its components, it incorporates external and internal frame factors (Johnson, 1977), the infrastructure, the core curriculum, students, alumni, and human resources. As indicated in the table, these are only the major components. It is possible that as educational evaluation evolves, other components will emerge. The elements within each component are not listed. Each institution must determine which elements fall under the major components.

ROLES OF ADMINISTRATORS AND FACULTY IN PROGRAM EVALUATION AND ACCREDITATION

Administrators in academe provide the vision and leadership for the educational program. However, it is imperative that the administration and the major stakeholders of the institution be in agreement about its mission, vision, purpose, and goals. Stakeholders include the governing board, the chief executive officer, the administrators of the infrastructure and the academic programs, the faculty, students, alumni, and consumers served by the institution. These stakeholders make up the "personality" and body of the institution that marks it as unique in its contributions to society and they too must be in agreement with the vision and purpose of the institution to maintain a strong educational program. Administration periodically reviews the mission and vision of the institution to match them to current needs and provides the leadership for revising them according to need. Additionally, administration monitors assessment and evaluation activities to ensure program quality and provides adequate resources in a timely manner for accreditation and program evaluation activities.

All faculty members participate in the evaluation of the curriculum and the program through their input into specific areas and needs for assessment, the collection of data, data analyses, and the formulation of recommendations for decision making regarding the program. In many schools of nursing there are evaluation committees that lead the process or, in other cases, curriculum committees may be charged with the evaluation of the curriculum and program. As part of the parent institution, nursing representatives provide input into university/college-wide evaluation activities. As a professional program, nursing faculty has valuable input into evaluation processes owing to the necessity for meeting professional accreditation and organizations' standards and criteria.

SUMMARY

This chapter reviewed classic definitions, concepts, and models of evaluation with definitions of commonly used terms. The rationale for strategic planning and a master plan of evaluation was presented. Types of tools and instruments for data collection for evaluation of educational programs and the roles of administrators and faculty were reviewed.

TABLE 12.1 Major Components and Guidelines for Developing a Master Plan of Evaluation

| Component | Action Plans | | | | | | | Follow-Up Plans |
	Responsible Party	When and How Often	Instruments and Tools for Data Collection	Data Findings and Analysis	Criteria, Outcomes, or Benchmarks	Reports and Recommendations	Maintain and Monitor or Improve	By Whom, How, and When
Program Mission/Vision/Goals/ Organizational Framework								
Program								
Strategic Plan								
External Frame Factors								
Internal Frame Factors								
Infrastructure Systems: Buildings								
Facilities								
Support Systems								
Student Services								
Financial								
Administration								
Technology/Informatics								
Library								

(continued)

TABLE 12.1 Major Components and Guidelines for Developing a Master Plan of Evaluation (continued)

| Component | Action Plans | | | | | | Follow-Up Plans |
	Responsible Party	When and How Often	Instruments and Tools for Data Collection	Data Findings and Analysis	Criteria, Outcomes, or Benchmarks	Reports and Recommendations	Maintain and Monitor or Improve	By Whom, How, and When
Baccalaureate[a] Curriculum: Congruency with Mission/Vision/ Philosophy/Organizational Framework								
Overall Purpose/Goal								
End-of-Program (Student Learning Outcomes) and Level Objectives								
Prerequisites								
General Education								
Electives								
Baccalaureate Nursing Major Courses								
Course Objectives and Content								
Learning Activities								

Teaching Effectiveness						
Graduate Curriculum[a]: Congruency with Mission/Vision/Philosophy/Organizational Framework						
Overall Purpose/Goal						
End-of-Program (Student Learning Outcomes) and Level Objectives						
Prerequisites						
Cognates						
Electives						
Core Nursing Courses						
Course Objectives and Content						
Specialty/Functional Courses						
Course Objectives and Content						
Learning Activities						
Teaching Effectiveness						

[a]The same components for the baccalaureate and graduate curricula apply to associate degree, master's, and doctorate programs.

DISCUSSION QUESTIONS

- Explain the differences between conceptual models of evaluation and the use of benchmarks. Give examples of their application to the evaluation of an educational program.
- To what extent do you believe faculty should be involved in a strategic planning process? Explain why.
- Describe how a master plan of evaluation contributes to the external review of a nursing program.

LEARNING ACTIVITIES

Student-Learning Activity

Using Table 12.1, develop a master plan of evaluation for the case study of a fictional school of nursing outreach program found in the Appendix.

Nurse Educator/Faculty Development Activity

Using Table 12.1, find your school of nursing's evaluation plan and assess it for any missing components or action plans.

References

Accreditation Commission for Education in Nursing. (2017). Accreditation manual. Retrieved from http://www.acenursing.org

American Association of Colleges of Nursing. (2017). *The research-focused doctoral program in nursing: Pathways to excellence*. Retrieved from http://www.aacnnursing.org/Portals/42/Publications/PhDPosition.pdf

Ardisson, M., Smallheer, B., Moore, G., & Christenbery, T. (2015). Meta-evaluation: experiences in an accredited graduate nurse education program. *Journal of Professional Nursing, 31*(6), 508–515.

Asif, M. (2015). Determining improvement needs in higher education benchmarking. *Benchmarking, 22*(1), 56–74.

Centers for Disease Control and Prevention. (2017). A framework for program evaluation. Retrieved from https://www.cdc.gov/eval/framework/index.htm

Chinta, R., Kebritchi, M., & Ellias, J. (2016). A conceptual framework for evaluating higher education institutions. *International Journal of Educational Management, 30*(6), 989–1002.

Commission on Collegiate Nursing Education. (2017). Mission, values, & history. Retrieved from http://www.aacn.nche.edu/accreditation/AboutCCNE.htm

Donabedian, A. (1996). Quality management in nursing and health care. In J. A. Schemele (Ed.), *Models of Quality Assurance* (pp. 88–103). Albany, NY: Delmar.

Hande, K., Williams, C., Robbins, H., Kennedy, B., & Christenbery, T. (2017). Leveling evidence-based practice across the nursing curriculum. *Journal for Nurse Practitioners, 13*(1), e17–e22.

Harmon, R. B., Fontaine, D., Plews-Ogan, M., & Williams, A. (2012). Achieving transformational change: Using appreciative inquiry for strategic planning in a school of nursing. *Professional Nursing, 28*, 119–124.

Horne, E. M., & Sandmann, L. R. (2012). Current trends in systematic program evaluation of online graduate nursing education: An integrative literature review. *Journal of Nursing Education, 51*(10), 570–576.

Johnson, M. (1977). *Intentionality in education: A conceptual model of curricular and instructional planning and evaluation*. Albany, NY: Center for Curriculum Research and Services.

Kim, M., Park, C., Park, S., & Ketefian, S. (2014). Quality of nursing doctoral education and scholarly performance in U.S. schools of nursing: Strategic areas for improvement. *Journal of Professional Nursing, 30*(1), 10–18.

Lewallen, L. (2015). Practical strategies for nursing education program evaluation. *Journal of Professional Nursing, 31*(2), 133–140.

Lindgrensavage, C. (2016). Regulatory oversight of student financial aid through accreditation of institutions of higher education. *Journal of Law and Education, 45*(3), 327–361.

Mansutti, I., Saiani, L., Grassetti, L., & Palese, A. (2017). Instruments evaluating the quality of the clinical learning environment in nursing education: A systematic review of psychometric properties. *International Journal of Nursing Studies, 68*, 60–72.

National Council of State Boards of Nursing. (2017). About NCSBN. Retrieved from https://www.ncsbn.org/about.htm

Schindler, L., Puls-Elvidge, S., Welzant, H., & Crawford, L. (2015). Definitions of quality in higher education: A synthesis of the literature. *Higher Learning Research Communications, 5*(3), 3–13.

Schumacher, G., & Risco, K. (2017). Nurse practitioner program curriculum development: A competency-based approach. *Journal of Nurse Practitioners, 13*(2), e75–e81.

Scriven, M. (1974). Evaluation perspectives and procedures. In W. J. Popham (Ed.), *Evaluation in education: Current applications*. Berkeley, CA: McCutchan.

Scriven, M. (1996). Types of evaluation and types of evaluator. *Evaluation Practice, 17*(2), 151–161.

Skiba, D. (2015). On the horizon: Implications for nursing education. *Nursing Education Perspectives, 36*(4), 263–266.

Stufflebeam, D. L., Foley, W., Gephart, W., Guba, E., Hammond, R., Merriman, H., & Provus, M. (1971). *Educational evaluation and decision making*. Itasca, IL: Peacock.

Turner, L. N. (2016). *Quality assurance in online graduate education: Program review processes and assessment techniques used in higher education* (Order No. 10014419). Available from ProQuest Dissertations & Theses Global: The Humanities and Social Sciences Collection (1767049660). Retrieved from https://search.proquest.com/docview/1767049660?accountid=13802

Udlis, K. A., & Manusco, J. M. (2012). Doctor of nursing practice programs across the United States: A benchmark of information. Part I: Program characteristics. *Journal of Professional Nursing, 28*(5), 265–273.

U.S. Department of Education. (2017). Accreditation. Retrieved from https://findit.ed.gov/search?utf8=✓&affiliate=ed.gov&query=Accreditation

CHAPTER 13

Planning for an Accreditation Visit

Felicia Lowenstein-Moffett

CHAPTER OBJECTIVES

Upon completion of Chapter 13, the reader will be able to

- Prepare a plan for accreditation that includes the development of a timeline
- Apply strategic processes for the preparation of faculty, students, and stakeholders for the self-study and site visit
- Apply principles of continuous quality improvement (CQI) to all accreditation activities

OVERVIEW

The purpose of accreditation for educational programs is to receive recognition for meeting specific quality standards or criteria that are outlined and supported by national, regional, and even state organizations. Programs obtain accreditation to demonstrate their excellence to consumers and the general public and further, to illustrate that the programs meet professional standards and offer quality education. Nursing education programs have a direct impact on public health and safety and thus, must demonstrate rigorous standards of quality set by the profession.

This chapter explores the preparation for accreditation by presenting a case study that is typical for a nursing program preparing to host a site visit. The process is not intended to be prescriptive but rather a general guide, which can be adapted to the programmatic needs of an institution. The purpose for the accreditation site visit is to provide an opportunity for external, peer reviewers to objectively verify information provided by the program in a self-study report. Accrediting agencies look at each program to ensure that the mission, vision, program outcome goals, and learning objectives are sufficient to meet the quality standards of the profession and to prepare graduates for professional nursing roles (Accreditation Commission for Education in Nursing [ACEN], 2017; American Association of Colleges of Nursing [AACN], 2017). Accreditation site visits and self-study reports reduce "curriculum drift" that occurs when an accredited nursing curriculum becomes different from the actual curriculum plan, causing a gap in educational standards over time. Accreditation site visits provide a time for the program to share additional information with the site visitors that further demonstrates how the accreditation standards and programmatic outcomes are met.

NATIONAL ACCREDITING BODIES

As previously discussed in Chapter 12, accreditation in universities and colleges of higher education within the United States is a nongovernmental, voluntary process to ensure that acceptable measures of quality are achieved (U.S. Department of Education [USDOE], 2017). Schools request that their programs be evaluated by an independent agency in order to achieve accreditation standing from that specific agency. Each accrediting agency's specific standards and core measures are anchored in educational and professional tenets, values, and the science of the disciplines undergoing evaluation such as nursing. Having accreditation provides quality assurance and is one of the key elements in the Higher Education Act's federal student aid program that allow students to receive federal funding and student loans (U.S. Department of Education, 2006). The Council for Higher Education Accreditation (CHEA) is a private, nonprofit, national organization designed to coordinate accreditation activities in the United States. The CHEA provides formal recognition of regional, national, and specialized higher accreditation bodies and focuses on academic quality (Eaton, 2015).

Role of the U.S. Department of Education

There are two types of accrediting agencies in the United States: recognized or unrecognized by the U.S. Department of Education. A recognized institution of higher education is considered to be the best measure for determining quality education. The U.S. Department of Education does not accredit institutions; however, the DOE determines which regional and national institutional accrediting agencies receive recognition (U.S. Department of Education, 2017).

Nursing Program Accrediting Agencies

Accreditation agencies for nursing programs in the United States are the ACEN, the Commission on Collegiate Nursing Education (CCNE), and the National League for Nursing Commission for Nursing Education Accreditation (NLN CNEA). ACEN and CCNE are recognized by CHEA and the DOE, while CNEA, a new agency, is seeking recognition from both agencies. All three agencies have established standards and criteria that must be met to obtain accreditation. ACEN accredits nursing education programs and schools at both the postsecondary and higher degree levels that offer a certificate, diploma, or professional degree (ACEN, 2017). CCNE is a national, autonomous accreditation agency that supports and encourages CQI processes in nursing programs at the baccalaureate and graduate nursing levels (AACN, 2017). The CNEA accredits all nursing programs from the practical/vocational nurse (PN/VN) to the clinical doctorate (NLN CNEA, 2017). Accrediting agencies share responsibility with nursing faculty and clinicians to develop and maintain program outcomes and accreditation standards that ensure quality education and public safety (ACEN, 2017; CCNE, 2013; NLN CNEA, 2017).

In addition to these three agencies, there are several national agencies that accredit clinical specialties such as those for nurse midwives and nurse anesthetists (see Chapter 12). Although the purpose is different, state boards of nursing evaluate nursing programs to ensure that they meet the minimum criteria set by state legislation and interpreted into state regulations governing nursing education and practice. New nursing programs must prepare self-study reports and are visited by site evaluators to verify that state regulations are met. Depending on the state, periodic reports and visits are scheduled to ensure continuous compliance with the regulations. Although the standards, criteria, and regulations may differ somewhat for each accrediting or regulatory agency, much of the data and reports for each of the agencies can be replicated.

The role of the accrediting body is to serve the public by providing an unbiased opinion regarding the assessment of professional educational programs. Schools of nursing that are seeking accreditation are required to submit an application, usually in the form of a self-study. The self-study defines how the program meets the standards of the accrediting body. There is an onsite evaluation/visit to verify, amplify, and clarify the material in the self-study report. The reviewers examine samples of student work, courses, and clinical sites. They meet with faculty, students, and administrators to ask questions and compare answers for consistency regarding the program. In addition, a request for public opinion is displayed on the school's website for the team to review prior to their arrival. The review team provides feedback prior to concluding the visit and makes recommendations to an agency advisory committee that makes the final decision regarding accreditation. Depending on the number of programs being reviewed, determination of accreditation is usually made 2 to 3 months following the site visit.

ACCREDITATION CASE STUDY—PREPARING FOR THE SITE VISIT

Previous chapters discussed the value of accreditation and its impact on schools of nursing. The following case study reviews the process for preparing to host an accreditation site visit. It is not specific to one type of agency so that the information can apply to total program accreditation, specialty accreditation, or state board visits.

Getting Started

Well-prepared faculty from an accredited organization should welcome the accreditation site visit as an opportunity to showcase its program and validate the current CQI processes in place. Approximately 12 months prior to a scheduled on-site visit, the accrediting agency notifies the nursing program that an upcoming site visit is pending. At that time, the program schedules and confirms the dates for the self-study report and the site visit according to the specific guidelines from the accrediting agency.

- *A midsized nursing program is scheduled for reaccreditation in a year. The nursing school graduates approximately 200 prelicensure students each year. The program received notification of the upcoming accreditation. The due dates for the self-study report and site visit were included and the process for writing the report and hosting the site visit were initiated.*

The first step in the accreditation process is to determine which faculty members will be responsible for writing the self-study and what processes will be used to gather the supporting programmatic data. Accreditation dates should be anticipated from the previous accreditation expiration dates and should never come as a surprise to well-prepared programs focused on quality improvement. Faculty members are typically appointed to work on an accreditation committee by the dean or director of the nursing program. The committee's task is to embark on the preparation of the self-study report, set timelines, and prepare for the visit. Previous experience in the accreditation process by a senior faculty member who serves as the primary author of the report and leads the committee in preparation for the visit is beneficial. However, the total faculty in the program undergoing evaluation has a role in the process and the preparation of the self-study report. It is generally recommended that one or more faculty members attend training sessions offered by the accrediting body, which provides instructions on how to prepare the report.

- *The dean of the nursing program appointed three faculty members to the accreditation committee with a senior professor as chairman who will take the lead role in preparing the self-study and arrangements for the accreditation site visit.*

Evaluation Plan

The second critical step in the process of accreditation is the development of an evaluation plan. Begin this process early! It is usually the best approach as part of the CQI process. The appointed committee is crucial in attending to the logistics of the site visit in addition to writing the self-study report. The process should begin with a careful review of all standards, objectives, and guidelines of the accrediting agency followed by a thorough comparison and analysis of the program's compliance with the standards. Next, the committee determines what data are currently collected and what additional information and supporting documents are needed for the self-study report and the site visit. Accredited institutions design and implement their own programmatic and student outcome measures based upon their curriculum plan. These data are used as the baseline for the assessment. The program and student outcomes are further evaluated and expanded upon in the accreditation self-study report. Knowledge of the standards of the accrediting agency and/or the specialty certification standards of the profession guide the faculty committee in determining the specific documentation crucial to demonstrating how the program under evaluation achieves program outcomes.

- *The committee begins to evaluate the data that are currently collected by the program undergoing the accreditation process. This is the time to review the total programmatic outcomes. As a group, they decide to review each of the accreditation standards of the accrediting agency and take a close look at how the program meets each standard. It is decided to divide up the workload and have committee meetings regularly.*

Timeline

Develop a timeline for the preparation process. The timeline is essential to keep the momentum and timeliness of a large project moving forward. It is helpful to develop a "backward calendar" by looking at the date that the report is to be submitted to the accrediting agency. Work backward from that date, allowing enough time for edits of the self-study and necessary revisions. Create a master calendar with specific due dates, team assignments, and expected completion dates.

- *The team members meet to develop a master calendar/timeline and set goals and objectives with designated members who have responsibility for each. They set the deadlines for meeting the goals and objectives to allow time for editing the self-study document and gathering additional data as necessary. The senior faculty member plans to have the report completed 3 weeks prior to the due date set by the accreditation agency to ensure sufficient time to review, complete, and edit the report. The accreditation team is working within a 1-year timeframe. It was decided that the team would meet monthly for 6 months, every 2 weeks for 5 months, and weekly for the duration of the accreditation process.*

Accreditation Committee

Early in the forming process, the committee determines how program information will be gathered, shared, and stored for the accreditation committee and the site visitors. Single faculty members may be involved with writing sections of the self-study report, as well as preparing for the site visitation. Self-study reports focus on topics specific to the standards such as the mission and vision of the organization, admission standards, enrollment data, student retention, gainful employment of graduates postgraduation, curriculum plan, pedagogy, faculty preparation, faculty and preceptor preparation and competence, institutional functions that impact the school of nursing, program resources, administrative support, faculty resources, strategic planning processes, stakeholder needs, and analysis of all program learning outcomes. When writing a self-study report, it is critical that the lead author reviews the document in its entirety to ensure that the document reads as one programmatic voice, even if it has been written by several faculty members. Nonfaculty staff members have a vital role in the accreditation process and should be identified by the committee early in the planning phase. The team should also identify key members within the institution who will be pivotal to the accreditation process such as the academic provost/vice president, relevant senate and committee members, librarian, informatics and data processing administrators, and distance learning staff.

- *The accreditation committee determined how often it will meet as a group when the timeline was developed. Committee members review their specific roles and contributions to the team to ensure an understanding of their assignments. The committee chair plans to read each section as it is completed to check for accurateness and the overall writing style, and will make final edits to the self-study report. The dean of the school of nursing plans to receive periodic updates on the committee's progress and will read the self-study report prior to submission to the accrediting agency to check for completeness. The team in collaboration with the dean identifies and works with several nonfaculty support staff members who have critical roles in preparing the data for the self-study report and the logistics of the site visit.*

Role of the Faculty, Administrators, Students, and Stakeholders

Prepare staff in advance! Meet with the staff members to reinforce how vital their roles are in the accreditation process and how confident the program is about having a successful evaluation. Be certain that faculty members know that they will be interviewed by the site visitors about the program, their courses, and the students. All faculty members, full time and part time, should be familiar with the standards of the accreditation agency, the curriculum, and their role in the delivery and evaluation of the program. Students should be aware of the accreditation process and familiar with their program and its goals, and that they will have an opportunity to meet with the visitors. Some programs conduct a mock site visit to create increased comfort and familiarity with the process before the site evaluators arrive. The dean/director of the program should ensure that all faculty members, including part-time clinical instructors, are present on campus or at nearby clinical sites during the site visit. Distance education faculty should be on standby to demonstrate strategies for the delivery of the program.

Visitors may need to verify a process or request a document that has not been provided to them, thus files should be available and updated and other persons who are connected to the program should be aware of the upcoming visit. The visitors may ask to speak to stakeholders and other members of the institution outside of the nursing department. In advance of the visit, the dean/director of the program or the chair of the accreditation committee should ask the visitors' leader for his/her list of people with whom the team would like to meet. A tentative schedule of the key people with whom the visitors need to meet should be set, shared with the visitors' team leader, and approved. This should be done well in advance of the visit since the evaluators usually like to meet with the top administrators such as the president, vice presidents, deans, librarians, and other key administrators who have tight schedules. Be sure to prepare all areas of the institution, clinical sites, and other stakeholders about the dates of the accreditation visit and what program(s) is/are being accredited. Taking a "standby" approach can avoid unnecessary scrambling for unplanned evaluator questions.

- *The nursing accreditation committee was added to the agenda for all nursing faculty meetings to provide updates and/or education as necessary. The committee planned a staff development day, 1 month prior to the on-site visit to prepare faculty by reviewing the accreditation standards, discussing how the program meets those standards, and reviewing the self-study document. Review of the faculty handbook is also planned to ensure that all faculty are knowledgeable about current departmental policies and processes. The dean sent an email to faculty and support staff notifying them in advance of the dates of the accreditation visit with the expectation that they will be on campus or in a nearby clinical agency, or online for distance education faculty during the entire visit process.*

Preparing to Host a Site Visit

Arrangements should be made early in the preparation phase to ensure an ample, private, and secure space for the accreditors who perform the on-site assessment. The accreditation agencies provide specific requests for the visitors' space requirements and notify the program of how many evaluators will be on site. Depending on the agency, it may be the responsibility of the program to arrange for the accreditors' accommodations that include conference space associated with the team leader's room for the accrediting team to meet for planning the visit and reviewing their findings. On campus, a room must be provided that is sufficient in size to accommodate the visitors. It should be a comfortable work room located preferably within the department in close proximity to faculty and administrators. Refreshments for breaks and lunch arrangements should be included. For the most part, the visitors use breaks and lunches to review their work thus far, although they may ask to use those times to meet with select faculty, students, staff, or administrators.

The visitors' room should be prepared with computers to access electronic data, documents, learning management systems, and other evidence that support the written self-study report. If files are used for evidence of quality processes or support of the standards, they should be indexed and cross-referenced according to the standards for the evaluators to find necessary information with ease. Examples of files include a directory/list of key administrators, faculty, and staff; program brochures; the program curriculum, course syllabi, samples of student work; an organizational chart, committee meeting minutes; the faculty manual including policies and procedures; the student handbook; and so forth. If the program offers a distance-learning format, a demonstration of long distance communications with students should be scheduled during the visit. Be certain that faculty members are well versed in the electronic resources that they use to communicate to students.

- *The nursing school prepares for the on-site evaluators' arrival and a secure conference room and resource room for the visitors are ready. Materials in the room include referenced and indexed documents and files as well as electronic data to corroborate the submitted written self-study report. The resource room contains examples of student coursework and capstone projects, faculty contributions to committees and scholarship of teaching, the program evaluation plan and quality improvement processes, and other information to demonstrate excellence in nursing education. The information technology department at the university set up individual computers for each visitor with secure temporary passwords and a computer for communicating with students and faculty at a distance is available. Telephone services are also available for both internal and external calls as needed. The committee ensured that all supporting documentation is categorized according to accreditation standards and easily accessible (electronically and/or in well-organized indexed files) for the evaluators. The dean assigned a nonfaculty support staff to assist the evaluation team for the entire time of the site visit to coordinate the schedule and to assist the visitors as needed. A list of key administrators and faculty phone numbers and departments is in the resource room by each computer. The committee posted the agenda for the on-site visit where it is easily visible in the resource room and in the faculty areas to ensure a timely evaluation process. Reminder announcements were sent to stakeholders, preceptors, and institutional leaders that an accreditation site visit is scheduled. This allows for ample opportunity for the accreditors to meet with any of them during the site visit.*

SUMMARY

Accreditation is a process for ensuring a quality nursing education program. It provides an endorsement from the accrediting agency that connotes excellence in meeting academic and professional standards. Programs voluntarily submit to rigorous appraisal processes to determine the extent to which the program(s) meet the standards set by the profession and demonstrate their quality to consumers, stakeholders, and the public. The process for preparing for an onsite visit from the accreditors does not need to be laborious, although it is time consuming. In the spirit of CQI, the accreditation process, self–study report, and site visit provide a chance to recognize opportunities for improvement and to celebrate successes.

DISCUSSION QUESTION

Many educational systems in other nations in the world are under the direct supervision and regulations of the government. In the United States, accreditation is voluntary, although there are factors that curtail the institution's activities if it is not accredited. Debate the pros and cons of voluntary versus regulated accreditation to ensure quality education. Do you believe the U.S. system of accreditation for higher education works? Explain the rationale for your answer.

LEARNING ACTIVITIES

Student-Learning Activities

1. Go to the websites of the ACEN, the CCNE, and the NLN CNEA and compare the standards for accreditation for each agency according to the levels of education they accredit (e.g., PN/VN, associate's degree, baccalaureate, master's, and doctorate). What are the differences, if any, among the agencies?
2. Interview several faculty members for their perspectives on accreditation and its role in ensuring quality in nursing education. Based on the interviews, do you think it is important for all faculty members to be aware of accreditation processes? Why or why not?

Faculty Development Activities

1. Review the last self-study accreditation report for your nursing program. Identify changes in the program that took place after the visit. Were the changes as a result of the accreditation process or were there other factors that brought about the changes? Based on your review, what recommendations do you have for the next accreditation visit?
2. Identify the accreditation agency for your nursing program. Review its standards/criteria for accreditation. What strategies in your program are in place to gather data that relate to the standards? Are current data in place and ready for analysis, evaluation, and follow-up on findings to ensure that the program meets the standards? What role in these strategies do you believe faculty has?

References

Accreditation Commission for Education in Nursing. (2017). Philosophy of accreditation. Retrieved from http://www.acenursing.org/philosophy-of-accreditation

American Association of Colleges of Nursing. (2017). CCNE accreditation. Retrieved from http://www.aacnnursing.org/CCNE

Commission on Collegiate Nursing Education. (2013). *Standards for accreditation of baccalaureate and graduate nursing programs*. Retrieved from http://www.aacn.nche.edu/ccne-accreditation/Standards-Amended-2013.pdf

Eaton, J. (2015). *An overview of U.S. accreditation*. Retrieved from http://www.chea.org/userfiles/uploads/Overview%20of%20US%20Accreditation%202015.pdf

National League for Nursing Commission for Nursing Education Accreditation. (2017). Overview. Retrieved from http://www.nln.org/accreditation-services/overview

U.S. Department of Education. (2006). 1998 Amendments to the Higher Education Act of 1965. Retrieved from https://www2.ed.gov/policy/highered/leg/hea98/index.html

U.S. Department of Education. (2017). Accreditation in the United States. Retrieved from https://www2.ed.gov/admins/finaid/accred/accreditation.html#Overview

SECTION

Research, Issues, and Trends in Nursing Education

Stephanie S. DeBoor

Sarah B. Keating

OVERVIEW

This section reviews research, current issues, and trends in nursing education for their effect on curricula and the priorities derived from them that influence curriculum development and evaluation activities now and in the future. Chapter 14 reviews the current state of research in nursing education, specifically as it applies to curriculum development and evaluation. The need for research that provides the basis for evidence-based educational practice is reviewed. Possible research questions are posed based on a summary of the scholarly/research-based articles found in the nursing and educational literature and presented throughout this text. While qualitative research generates useful information, the numerous qualitative studies relating to nursing education should serve as a foundation for further quantitative, qualitative, and mixed methodology studies that are geographically diverse and reflect various types of programs. Such studies can lead to evidence-based educational practice for the development of relevant nursing programs that center on the learner and program outcomes and meet the needs of the profession and health care system.

Chapter 15 summarizes the chapters and reexamines some of the issues raised in the text to offer possible solutions that could affect the future of nursing education. A look at nursing education in hindsight leads to a forecast of the future including several scenarios for education and their impact on the profession. Members of the nursing profession are asked to discard old prohibitive ways of thinking about nursing education and its mandate to provide knowledgeable, competent, and caring professionals and move into the future with innovative and creative nursing programs that continue to educate nurses ready for the challenges of the health care system. Nursing must continue to move its trajectory for higher education or find itself out-of-sync with other professionals and the health care system. This section begins the discussion for nursing educators and their role in conducting meaningful research, scholarship, translational science, and evidence-based practice in nursing education to meet the challenges and plan for the future.

CHAPTER 14

Research and Evidence-Based Practice in Nursing Education

Michael T. Weaver

CHAPTER OBJECTIVES

Upon completion of Chapter 14, the reader will be able to:

- Deliberate on the faculty role in scholarship, translational science, and research in nursing education and its influence on curriculum development and evaluation, evidence-based practice in nursing, health care policy, and delivery of care
- Analyze current research in nursing education that applies to curriculum development and evaluation
- Identify topics needing investigation and research in curriculum development and evaluation based on the National League for Nursing's (NLN) recommendations for research in nursing education

OVERVIEW

Nursing faculty members have three major roles in academe: teaching, scholarship/research, and service. This chapter examines the roles of teacher, scholar, and provider of service as they apply to nursing faculty. The American Association of Colleges of Nursing's (AACN, 1999) Task Force on Defining Standards for the Scholarship of Nursing presents four areas that are seen as encompassing academic scholarship within the nursing profession, namely discovery of new knowledge, teaching to pass on and enhance others' understanding, application of new knowledge to improve individual and population health, and integration of knowledge both from and into other disciplines. Scholarship is therefore seen to encompass the full range of the tripartite academic role: research, pedagogy, and service.

A scholar reviews the current state of knowledge in the discipline and applies that knowledge to practice, while at the same time observing phenomena in practice (nursing and education) to identify those needing further investigation. Scholars share those observations with others through reflection, discussion, debate, and writing scholarly papers/articles based on evidence surrounding the topic. Their scholarly works should lead to inquiry that generates knowledge, builds the sciences of the profession and education, and ultimately addresses nursing's social mandate to improve health-related outcomes.

In the area of research, scholars observe the environment, raise questions about phenomena and, by exploring the factors surrounding them, ask questions that merit further investigation. The research questions generate inquiries and/or hypotheses that result in proposals for investigation. They require in-depth literature reviews to identify concepts and theories that relate to the topic and help shape the nature of the proposed research from a pilot study to in-depth studies that include qualitative, quantitative, and mixed-methodology approaches. Tenure-track faculty members in research-focused programs, such as Carnegie classifications R1–R3, are usually expected to engage in research as a component of their academic scholarship. Nontenure-track faculty or those in multipurpose institutions typically do not have expectations of research as part of their scholarship, but rather are expected to contribute to the profession through scholarship related to pedagogy and practice. Scholarly productivity and metrics are of particular importance for faculty in terms of meeting institutional requirements for tenure and promotion. Nursing faculty seeking academic positions need to investigate the institution's policies on scholarship prior to accepting a position in order to be aware of institutional expectations.

An increasingly important area of scholarship is translational science, which utilizes research findings to develop evidence-based practice recommendations. It crosses all disciplines, providing opportunities for interdisciplinary collaboration and interprofessional education of students in preparation for the collaborative relationships necessary to provide comprehensive, evidence-based care within clinical and community settings. Translational science plays an increasingly important role in its provision of a mechanism for connecting academic nursing with clinical agencies. The doctor of nursing practice (DNP), as the nursing professional doctorate, is especially well-positioned to provide a bridge between research-focused faculty in academic nursing settings and the clinical priorities of nursing practice. Such partnerships are of particular importance and relevance in connecting academic nursing with academic health centers, as discussed in the AACN Manatt report (Enders, Morin, & Pawlak, 2016). This chapter examines the role of nursing faculty in nursing education research and scholarly activities, reviews the literature related to nursing education and indications for further study, and lists possible topics for investigation that relate to curriculum development and evaluation.

FACULTY ROLE IN NURSING EDUCATION RESEARCH

Faculty Qualifications

Although the National Council for State Boards of Nursing (NCSBN, 2009) recommends that nursing faculty members have at least a master's degree to teach in nursing programs and preparation in pedagogy as well as the science of nursing, the faculty shortage in some states resulted in the necessity to hire clinically experienced baccalaureate-prepared nurses. To ameliorate this situation, administrators, faculty peers, and the individual faculty member have a responsibility to support faculty to complete advanced degrees including the master's and/or doctorate. At the same time, doctorally prepared faculty members are encouraged to further their postgraduate scholarly work by becoming certified as nurse educators, and conducting research related to nursing education, that is, curriculum development, evaluation, and instructional design and strategies.

The NLN (2016) identified the need to build the science of nursing education as its first research priority in nursing education. Pedagogical theoretical frameworks and their attendant constructs, as well as commonly employed research methods and statistical techniques, often differ from those typically used in clinically focused research. As a result, doctorally prepared faculty members who have specific expertise in educational theories and research methods are needed in order to produce evidence-based recommendations for curriculum design and incorporation of effective teaching and evaluation methods in nursing programs. In its 2013 vision for doctoral preparation for nurse educators, the NLN identifies the need for increasing the number of doctorally prepared nursing faculty members who are skilled not only in the areas of pedagogical knowledge generation and translation of that knowledge to nursing curricula, but also knowledgeable in methods to evaluate associations between innovative teaching methodologies and patient care outcomes.

Educational research presents a number of challenges for nursing faculty. An overarching challenge is the relatively limited (compared to clinical research) number of opportunities for funding of educational research and the low to nonexistent indirect cost recovery rates typically attached to educational research grant mechanisms. Those conditions often present difficult cost–benefit decisions for school administrators when weighing the academic release time required for faculty to implement and manage the study, if funded. Another challenge derives from complexities required for study design and analytic methods, which result from having to implement the study within an existing curriculum. It is the exception, rather than the rule, to be able to implement a gold standard randomized controlled trial. Rather, the study must typically contend with students nested within instructors and clinical agency, student self-selection of course section, need to respect academic freedom in how an instructor delivers his or her course, and a dearth of valid and reliable hard measures for learning outcomes, resulting in the use of student self-rating of things like self-efficacy and clinical competence. The specialized, advanced research design and statistical analysis knowledge required to design studies with reasonable internal and external validity under those circumstances is typically not part of the curriculum that nursing faculty experience during their doctoral programs. As with clinical research endeavors, faculty members need to convene an interdisciplinary team that covers the requisite expertise required to appropriately address the research aims.

Importance to Personal Professional Development

Depending on faculty members' educational preparation and experience, it is expected that they engage in scholarship that relates to their expert knowledge, contributes to the mission of the school and university, and serves as content expertise for sharing with students in the teaching/learning process. In addition to content expertise, educators should have knowledge and skills in the art of teaching and learning, student assessment, and program development and evaluation. Each individual should conduct a personal assessment of these knowledge foundations and skills and identify those that need updating, strengthening, or assimilating.

Notwithstanding personal motivation, need, and responsibility for scholarship and research activities, support for these activities is also a responsibility of the academic administration and the institution. Release time, costs for attendance at professional meetings and conferences, and in some cases, tuition for advanced degree or specialty certifications are included as employment benefits. Many research-focused institutions expect faculty to generate studies that will fund not only research activities, but also support a portion of the individual faculty member's position, which is bought out by replacing the faculty member's teaching assignments with adjunct faculty for the duration of the funding. As Roberts and Glod (2013) point out, nursing faculty in research-focused institutions face the dilemma of meeting teaching responsibilities but at the same time, those in tenure-track positions are expected to produce scholarship and research to either retain or gain tenure. Their research activities take away from assigned clinical and theory teaching responsibilities, leaving those activities to nontenure-track and/or adjunct faculty. This can result in a dilemma for those nontenure-track faculty members who have both the institutional expectation and the requisite clinical expertise and knowledge to produce scholarly works, but are not necessarily provided the time for scholarship. That dissonance can result in a two-tier faculty system that can affect the curriculum, student-learning and program outcomes, and faculty morale.

Faculty members in schools of nursing based in non-research-focused institutions have a responsibility for scholarship related to evidence-based practice, implementation science, and research (generating new knowledge, in terms of clinical practice and pedagogy). For those without the terminal degree required for the discipline or faculty position qualifications, enrolling in and completing the required degree is an expectation. It is hoped that the employer will support this activity through release or flexible time and, in some cases, tuition support. In addition, to maintain the curriculum's currency and relevance, faculty must engage in scholarly activities that keep them updated and enriched in their content and pedagogical knowledge base and skills. Attending workshops and conferences in education and the clinical specialty should be an expectation, and the school should include support for faculty development to update educational skills. Research activities are not precluded in these institutions, and provide an important role for educators to advance their knowledge in nursing practice and education, and to contribute to the science of the discipline. Since financial support and release time might not be as available as in research-focused institutions, collaborative research among faculty members, other disciplines, practice colleagues, other schools of nursing, and health care systems (such as hospitals) offer scholarly opportunities for faculty.

Martin and Hodge (2011) describe their experience in developing a research model for faculty to meet the scholarship and research expectations in a non-research-focused institution. The authors list the expectations for faculty in their school and describe how a model for mentoring faculty research was implemented. Major components of the model included, among others, administrative support and a culture of support for scholarship and research, assigned time for research, goal setting and clear expectations, the mentorship and collaboration of other faculty, and external resources. Klemm (2012) described a research project that took place in an undergraduate research course. Throughout the semester, a faculty member acted as a mentor for the students to study women's adjustment to breast cancer. The qualitative research experience was successful with students learning about the research process as well as participating in a faculty member's research through the collection and analysis of data.

Freeland, Pathak, Garrett, Anderson, and Daniels (2016) compared the use of medical simulation mannequins along with didactic instruction to traditional didactic methods for training nurses to screen patients admitted with stroke symptoms for aspiration risk. Dividing a group of 32 nurses into two groups, one experiencing traditional didactic training, and the other using medical simulation mannequins along with didactic instruction, the authors found that the didactic plus mannequin group performed better on both screen administration and interpretation at the posttraining evaluation. Skill levels for administration and interpretation persisted over the 6-week follow-up period. The authors also used standard patients to evaluate administration and interpretation at the 6-week follow-up testing session to evaluate translation of skills to live patients. Performance and interpretation in those live individuals were found to be similar to performance at the 2- and 4-week assessments, providing evidence supporting transferability to actual clinical practice and adding to the body of evidence supporting the use of simulation as an effective teaching method.

An issue in nursing research when students conduct independent research, usually for thesis or dissertation purposes or when they assist faculty with the faculty's research, is the authorship of scholarly works resulting from the research. Welfare and Sackett (2011) surveyed faculty and students at research-intensive institutions to study their beliefs about authorship of research findings when students assisted faculty or conducted independent research. Welfare and Sackett developed case scenarios that described student research activities from collecting data and analysis to collaborative or independent research. They found differences between students' and faculty's perceptions about authorship and the order of the list of authors. While the instrument they developed was checked for content validity, the authors point out that similar studies using the tool should be conducted for validity and reliability of the tool. However, their findings brought forth many recommendations including an understanding or contract between faculty and student prior to initiating the research. They refer to student and faculty responsibilities and eventual authorship as listed by several professional organizations, which have guidelines and principles of ethical conduct (American Psychological Association [APA], 2014; Association for the Study of Higher Education [ASHE], 2014). With the growth of doctoral programs and research in nursing, this becomes a pressing issue to address for the profession, educators, and students.

The Scholarship of Teaching and Application to Nursing

Conducting research or earning an advanced degree or certification in one's own clinical or functional area of nursing lends credence to the faculty member's knowledge and skills in that specialty and contributes to the curriculum's currency in nursing science and practice. At the same time, adding to the knowledge base of learning theories, pedagogy, student assessment, and program development and evaluation is equally as important. Boyer's (1990) theory of scholarship in teaching comes to mind with its four components that promote faculty's application of teaching activities to research and scholarship. The four components are the scholarship of *discovery, integration, application,* and *teaching* and are succinctly described by Boyer in his *Scholarship Reconsidered* document. The model provides a framework for faculty as they carry out their activities in teaching and search for scholarship and research opportunities. Such activities contribute to the disciplines of nursing and education, and research findings when disseminated and translated can lead to evidence-based practice in the art of curriculum development, evaluation, and teaching and learning.

Briefly, Boyer (1990) describes the scholarship of *discovery* as those activities that result in the generation of new knowledge from experiences and phenomena observed while developing and evaluating programs and during the interactions and delivery of teaching and learning between the educator and the student. The scholar studies the new knowledge discovered and tests it for its usefulness and application to practice. The scholarship of *integration* is the summation of activities and interactions that occur in the educational environment and cause the educator to observe and synthesize the information into new approaches and knowledge. It is closely related to discovery and Boyer makes the case for its application to interdisciplinary studies, an issue with which nursing has long been affiliated but not always successful in carrying out. The scholarship of *application* refers to the application of new knowledge to teaching activities to test it for validity and reliability. It is evidence-based practice and deserves to be tested, studied for its relevance, and perfected as it evolves. Translational science has a close relationship to this concept. *Teaching* as scholarship is a way of viewing the activity as a scholarly pursuit for sharing knowledge with the learner and discovering new knowledge and ways of applying it to the sciences of nursing and education.

Examples of the application of Boyer's model to nursing education can be found in the AACN's *Defining Scholarship for the Discipline of Nursing* paper (AACN, 1999). The definition of nursing scholarship that helps guide nursing educators' research and scholarship is as follows:

Scholarship in nursing can be defined as those activities that systematically advance the teaching, research, and practice of nursing through rigorous inquiry that 1) is significant to the profession, 2) is creative, 3) can be documented, 4) can be replicated or elaborated, and 5) can be peer-reviewed through various methods. (AACN, 1999)

An article by Simpson and Richards (2015) provides an example of pedagogical inquiry that, since it occurs within assigned teaching responsibilities, provides a scholarship opportunity for faculty irrespective of tenure-track status. The authors evaluated the effects of redesigning a population health course on selected student-learning–related outcomes such as students' evaluations of the course and faculty observations regarding student understanding of content relevance. Limitations related to study design and outcome measures utilized also provide insight into some of the challenges that confront educators in terms of advancing pedagogy within existing programs. Those real-life challenges also highlight the need for expert faculty who can effectively work within those constraints and mentor other faculty, a need expressed in the NLN's paper, *A Vision for Doctoral Preparation for Nurse Educators* (NLN, 2013).

Importance to the Profession

Nursing faculty scholarship, translational science, and research contributions to the profession are innumerable. Clinical specialty and functional areas (administration, quality assurance, risk management, epidemiology, etc.), translational science, and research lead to evidence-based practice in the health care setting. Collaborative research with nursing colleagues and other health disciplines in the health care setting fosters positive patient outcomes, quality/safe health care, and changes in health care policy. An example of interprofessional collaboration and research occurred at Columbia University. The social media interactions of PhD and DNP students and faculty during one semester were studied by Merrill, Yoon, Larson, Honig, and Reame (2013). Merrill et al. described the curriculum enhancements that were added during the study, which included required seminar meetings during the time of the study and the PhD and DNP students took two courses together (Ethics and Quantitative Statistics). The students' and faculty's utilization of social networks among themselves during the semester was collected. It was found that during the first week, most communications occurred among faculty but by the end of the study (10 weeks later), the number of interactions and their distribution among the groups increased. This was one of the first studies to use social networks as a source of information and also to analyze relationships between doctoral students and faculty.

Research in nursing education allows for the sharing of best practices in the delivery of nursing education and types of programs that produce graduates ready for practice in the health care system. Scholarship, translational science, and research findings contribute to the profession's advocacy for higher education for nursing to meet the health care needs of the populace and to assume leadership roles in the health care delivery system. Research helps identify the types of educational programs best suited to levels of responsibility in the health care system and the role of nursing.

CURRENT RESEARCH IN THE LITERATURE ON CURRICULUM DEVELOPMENT AND EVALUATION

Curriculum Development and Revision

Throughout the update of this textbook the author and contributors reviewed the literature for classic and current research and studies in curriculum development in nursing. Many of these studies focused on one program and can serve as pilots for further research to be generalized across types and levels of program and geographical areas. Table 14.1 lists some of the references reviewed in this text that relate to curriculum development. As one can see, additional research-based studies are needed that can inform faculty as they consider revising existing curricula or developing new programs. Especially critical is the need to validate results and findings. Issues related to

TABLE 14.1 Studies That Apply to Curriculum Development

Topic	Author(s)/Dates	Type of Program	Type of Study	Recommendations
All Types				
National Survey of Accredited Nursing Programs in the United States to Describe Evidence-Based Teaching Practices	Kalb, O'Conner-Von, Brockway, Rierson, & Sendelbach, 2015	All accredited nursing programs	National online survey of faculty in all accredited nursing programs in the United States	Revise by incorporating methods to achieve more representative sample, especially within different programs. Revise items to lessen potential social desirability and provide information about types of evidence used. While perhaps not feasible, incorporating indicators of student success (NCLEX pass rates; advanced practice certification rates) may provide useful information.
Prelicensure				
National Surveys of Undergraduate Programs to Determine What Physical Examination Skills are Taught	Giddens, Wright, & Gray, 2012	Prelicensure	National survey of prelicensure programs	Replicate for changes in curricula, program outcomes, effect on patient care. Replicate through concept analyses of other specific concepts, e.g., patient safety, cultural competence.
Survey of Faculty in 98 Nursing Schools in New York State, with Follow-up Focus Group. The Aim Was to Describe Integration of QSEN Competencies Within Prelicensure Programs.	Pollard et al., 2014	Prelicensure	Online survey of faculty and administrators in 98 member schools of the New York State Deans of Baccalaureate and Higher Degree programs and the Council for Associate Degree Nursing	Replicate incorporating methods to improve response rate and ability to evaluate generalizability. Expand sample to enable comparison of program types and expand generalizability.

(continued)

TABLE 14.1 Studies That Apply to Curriculum Development (*continued*)

Topic	Author(s)/Dates	Type of Program	Type of Study	Recommendations
		Undergraduate ADN, BSN, Second-Degree BSN, RN to BSN		
A Curriculum Development Model Using Learning as Central for all Stakeholders; Response to the NLN's Call for Curricular Transformation	Davis, 2011	ADN	Description of the curricular change process using a curriculum development model	Utilize the model and analyze its effectiveness in curricular revision for similar programs. Compare to other models and programs.
Changes in Curricula to Include Evidence-Based Practice, Quality, Improvement Approaches, Safety Standards, Competency Frameworks, Informatics, and Interdisciplinary Education	Andre & Barnes, 2010	BSN	Review of curricular needs	Analyze concepts in the curriculum. Compare programs for content and outcomes and efficacy of instructional strategies.
Shared Decision-Making Model for Curriculum Revision	D'Antonio, Brennan, & Curley, 2013	BSN	Description of the curricular change process using the model	Utilize the model and analyze the effectiveness in curricular revision for similar programs. Compare to other models and programs.
Process for Mapping an Undergraduate Program to the AACN *Essentials*	Dearman, Lawson, & Hall, 2011	BSN	Process and how the model tied into NCLEX success rates	Review the literature for similar models, apply the model to several programs and compare results according to student demographics, type of program, student-learning outcomes, curricular differences, etc.
Incorporating Workshops on Bullying to Reduce Impact on Minority BSN Students	Egues & Leinung, 2014	BSN	Quasi-experimental pre- posttest design using survey of students attending workshops on bullying at a designated Hispanic- and minority-serving college	Incorporate an experimental design allowing comparison with a control group. Incorporate controls on intervention fidelity necessary for replication and comparative effectiveness of different evidence-based teaching methods.

A Model for Integrating Technology into the Curriculum Based on a Review of the Literature	Flood, Gasiewicz, & Delpier, 2010	BSN	Review of the literature and model development	Replicate for generalizability.
Management of Curricular Content to Avoid Content Saturation; Encourages Concept Teaching	Giddens & Brady, 2007	BSN	Literature review	Compare geographically representative and varying types of curricula that are concept based and taught in other types of curricula and teaching strategies.
Model for Incorporating Academic–Clinical Partnerships with the Veterans Administration (VA Nursing Academy)	Needleman, Bowman, Wyte-Lake, & Dobalian, 2014	BSN	Survey of faculty at partnership sites	Replicate in other academic–clinical partnership systems (e.g., schools of nursing within academic health centers).
Description of a Model Residency Program and its Outcomes that Resulted in Increased Confidence, Competence, Leadership, Etc.	Goode, Lynn, & McElroy, 2013	BSN Residency	Evaluation of student-learning outcomes	Replicate for validity, reliability, and generalizability.
Cognitive Scaffolding Model for Curricular Revision (Task, Metacognitive, and Sociocommunicative)	Hagler, Morris, & White, 2011	BSN	Description of the curricular change process using the scaffolding model	Utilize the model and analyze the effectiveness in curricular revision in similar programs. Compare to other models and programs.
Faculty and Students Who Champion Curricular Change also Facilitate Implementation of the Change	Powell-Cope, Hughes, Sedlak, & Nelson, 2008	BSN	Survey of faculty perceptions	Compare geographically representative and varying types of curricula.
A Model for Arranging Clinical Experience Agreements Between Health Care Agencies and Schools of Nursing Including Cost Factors	De Geest et al., 2010	Predominantly BSN	Description of a model when complex factors must be taken into account; includes cost and personnel factors	Utilize the model to demonstrate its validity and reliability and to compare to other models and programs. Study its effectiveness for program planning.

(continued)

TABLE 14.1   Studies That Apply to Curriculum Development (*continued*)

Topic	Author(s)/Dates	Type of Program	Type of Study	Recommendations
		Undergraduate ADN, BSN, Second-Degree BSN, RN to BSN		
Incorporating Technology into the Curriculum from Low- to High-Fidelity Technology; Extent to How It will be Used, Resources, and Faculty Development	Skiba, 2012; Thompson & Skiba, 2008	Predominantly BSN	Recommendation for integrating technology into curriculum when undergoing change	Conduct studies to demonstrate student-learning outcomes using various technologies. Survey schools for levels of integration of technology in the curricula and effects on student-learning outcomes and patient care.
Comparison of Second-Degree and Traditional Graduates	Brewer et al., 2009	Second-degree and traditional BSN	Survey of employers of BSN, traditional and second degree	Replicate for validity, reliability, and generalizability and investigate for factors that lead to differences.
Managers' Perceptions of Second-Degree Graduates' Clinical Skills; Comparison of Managers' and Graduates' Perceptions of Performance	Rafferty & Lindell, 2011; Regan & Pietrobon, 2010; Ziehm, Uibel, Fontaine, & Scherzer, 2011	Second-degree BSN	Survey of nurse managers of graduates	Replicate for reliability and validity and investigate for factors influencing perceptions, and generalizability.
Managers' Perceptions of Second-Degree Graduates' Performance and Retention Rates	Weathers & Raleigh, 2013	Second-degree BSN	Survey of nurse managers of graduates	Replicate for reliability and validity and investigate for factors influencing perceptions, and generalizability.
Experiences of Second-Degree BSNs	Penprase & Koczara, 2009	Second-degree BSN	Survey of students	Replicate for generalizability.
A Model to Examine the Q (Quality), P (Potential), and C (Cost; QPC) of Programs to Compare Disciplines From a Cost-Benefit Perspective	Booker & Hilgenberg, 2010	RN to BSN	Description of a cost analysis model to compare disciplines	Utilize the model to demonstrate its validity and reliability and to compare to other models and disciplines/ programs; study its effectiveness for program planning.

Title	Citation	Program	Method	Recommendations
Rn to BSN and BSN Students' Perceptions of the Value of Liberal Arts to Nursing	DeBrew, 2010	RN to BSN and BSN	Comparison of survey results	Replicate for reliability and validity and investigate for factors influencing perceptions, and generalizability.
Interdisciplinary				
An Interdisciplinary Program for Health Sciences Students to Share Patient-Centered Care and Learn About Other Disciplines	Dacey, Murphy, Anderson, & McCloskey, 2010	Undergraduate Interdisciplinary	Description of the program and outcomes	Utilize the curriculum to compare for similarities. Compare to other programs, geographical locations, types of students and programs, and measure student outcomes.
An Interdisciplinary Curriculum for Palliative Care in Oncology	Head et. al., 2014	Undergraduate and graduate interdisciplinary	Description of the program and methods used for formative feedback during development	Compare relevant student outcomes between students who have and have not participated in the curriculum.
Measure Students' Interprofessional Attitudes Across Medicine, Nursing, and Pharmacy	Sheu et al., 2012	Interdisciplinary	Mixed qualitative and qualitative on student interprofessional attitudes	Replicate for reliability and validity and investigate for factors influencing attitudes, and generalizability.
Entry-Level Master's				
Special Needs And Socialization of Entry-Level Master of Science in Nursing (MSN) Students	Klich-Heartt, 2010	Entry-level MSN	Review of the literature	Update review of literature; survey students in the programs for validation with representative sample; investigate support programs and their success; replicate.
Entry-Level MSN Students' Lived Experiences	McNiesh, 2011	Entry-level MSN	Qualitative survey of students	Investigate factors that apply to larger sample size and varying geographical areas.

(continued)

TABLE 14.1   Studies That Apply to Curriculum Development *(continued)*

Topic	Author(s)/Dates	Type of Program	Type of Study	Recommendations
Master's				
A Master's Program that Presents Leadership Theories to Advanced Practice Nurses as well as Those in Leadership to Apply in the Health Care System	Aduddell & Dorman, 2010	MSN	Description of the program and its outcomes	Utilize the curriculum or compare for similarities; compare to other programs, geographical locations, types of students and programs, and measure student outcomes.
A Master's-Level Curriculum That Prepares Nurse Leaders to Deliver Culturally Diverse and Linguistic Services in the Health Care System	Comer, Whichello, & Neubrander, 2013	MSN	Description of the curriculum and report on outcomes	Integrate the model into comparable program curricula and measure outcomes and compare across programs, student demographics, and geographical locations.
Conceptual Model for Integrating Scholarly Writing Across the Curriculum	Regan & Pietrobon, 2010	Graduate	Model uses rhetoric, ethnographic, recognition, and practice principles	Apply the model and measure outcomes; compare across programs.
Doctoral Programs				
Curriculum Content for Research-Focused Degrees	Anderson, 2000	Doctoral	Analysis of the content of research-focused programs to include: body of nursing knowledge, research, and preparation for teaching role	Conduct a national survey and content analysis of research and practice doctoral programs and the use of frameworks to guide curricula; compare between the types.
A Description of the Intention of the Practice Doctorate for Postmaster's and BSN to DNP Programs	Grey, 2013	DNP	Description and need for studies that compare BSN to DNP and postmaster's DNPs to compare to original intent(s) of the DNP	Conduct comparative studies of curricula, program outcomes, and graduates' practice across geographical locations, types of programs, and types of students.

AACN, American Association of Colleges of Nursing; NCLEX, National Council Licensure Examination; NLN, National League for Nursing's; QSEN, Quality and Safety Education for Nurses.

replicability and reproducibility raised for clinical research (e.g., see Vetter, McGwin, & Pittet, 2016) are equally applicable to educational research, especially in light of the constraints and design compromises that must be incorporated in order to feasibly conduct studies within an active curriculum.

Curriculum and Program Evaluation

Table 14.2 summarizes studies that were found to be related to curriculum and program evaluation research and provides recommendation for further study. Few studies were found that applied directly to nursing education program evaluation, indicating the need for testing of evaluation models, especially in light of the emphasis on the measurement of program outcomes and student-learning outcomes. Of particular need are methods to evaluate associations between pedagogical methods, curriculum content, objective measures of student-learning and nurse-sensitive patient outcomes for clinical care provided by students. Nursing may need to borrow from other disciplines to find and adapt evaluation models appropriate to nursing education and to compare models, theories, concepts, and methods for evaluation as they apply to nursing.

Research Topics That Apply to Curriculum Development and Evaluation

The NLN provides nursing educators with a list of priorities for nursing education research for 2016 through 2019 (NLN, 2016). The three major priorities include (a) building the science of nursing education, (b) linking student learning to health indicators, and (c) examination of the science of learning within the context of health transitions. Of particular importance for addressing these priorities is the availability of faculty scholars with the requisite expertise to formulate, plan, conduct, and disseminate findings from studies producing needed empirical evidence, and the skills and knowledge to then translate those findings into real-world pedagogy.

For the purposes of this chapter, scholarship is presented as it applies to curriculum development and evaluation and is based on the NLN's list of priorities for the advancement of the science of nursing education. Please note that the NLN priorities are italicized and that the suggested lists of ideas are not meant to be inclusive.

Impact of educational preparation to increase capacity of nurse scientists whose focus is the scientific and theoretical basis for nursing education.

1. Conduct a national survey of nursing faculty to evaluate association between educational preparation and involvement in nursing education research.
2. Track and survey graduates of select doctoral programs to describe their professional trajectory and evaluate associations between program characteristics and involvement in nursing education research.
3. Interview focus groups composed of nationally recognized experts in nursing education to identify themes related to knowledge and skills needed for a successful career focused on the science of nursing education.

Development and testing of instruments for nursing education research to measure learning outcomes and linkages to patient care.

1. Integrative review of the literature to identify concepts that are important learning outcomes for nursing students at various levels.
2. Integrative review of the literature to identify existing reliable and valid instruments for measuring learning outcomes.
3. Design and implement studies to test associations between student scores on selected valid and reliable learning outcome measures and relevant nurse-sensitive patient outcomes in patients for whom they provide care.

TABLE 14.2 Studies That Apply to Program and Curriculum Evaluation

Topic	Author(s)/Dates	Type of Program	Type of Study	Recommendations
All Types				
A Model of Evaluation	DeSilets, 2010	All types of educational programs	Descriptive	Test model and compare
Model for Evaluating Clinical Simulation	Cummings, 2015	All types of schools of nursing	Descriptive	
Model for Strategic Planning	Harmon, Fontaine, Plews-Ogan, & Williams, 2012	All types of schools of nursing	Descriptive	Test model and compare
Measure for Evaluation of Classroom Teaching Practices	Herinckx, Munkvold, Winter, & Tanner, 2014	All types of schools of nursing	Descriptive/ instrument development	Validate and test measure using independent samples
Three Cs Model of Evaluation	Kalb, 2009	All types of schools of nursing	Descriptive	Test model and compare
Summative Evaluation of Technology Outcomes	Newhouse, 2011	All types of educational programs	Comparison of digital measures to written assessment tools applied to technology	Test model and compare
Survey of Student Attitudes and Opinions about Program During Curriculum Redesign	Ostrogorsky & Raber, 2014	All types of educational programs	Descriptive	Apply in other settings undergoing curriculum revision to guide improvement efforts; evaluate associations between ratings and student outcomes
Measurement of Program/ Student-Learning Outcomes	Praslova, 2010	All types of educational programs	Descriptive	Test model and compare
Combined Program Evaluation and Evaluation Research	Spillane et al., 2010	Secondary schools but applicable to all	Mixed methodologies (quantitative, qualitative, and triangulation)	Check reliability and validity of tools; replicate across different types of programs

(continued)

| TABLE 14.2 | Studies That Apply to Program and Curriculum Evaluation (*continued*) | | | |

Topic	Author(s)/Dates	Type of Program	Type of Study	Recommendations
Associate Degree/Community Colleges				
Models of Program Evaluation	Bers, 2011	Associate degree	Descriptive	Review for models to test, report of model, compare utilization of models across geographical areas and types and levels of educational programs
Graduate Programs				
Description of Models of Evaluation to Measure Outcomes in Schools of Nursing	Horne & Sandmann, 2012	Graduate nursing programs	Integrative review of the literature	Review for models to test, report of model, compare utilization of models across geographical areas and types and levels of educational programs
Benchmarks and Trends for DNP Programs	Udlis & Manusco, 2012	DNP programs	National survey of DNP programs	Replicate; investigate identified characteristics and benchmarks

Meta-analysis and meta-synthesis informing the state of the science.

1. Meta-analytic review of literature reports of studies testing theories of learning.
2. Meta-analytic review of literature reports comparing various pedagogical methods.

Examination and use of technology, simulation, informatics, and virtual experiences on student learning affecting clinical practice.

1. Studies comparing relevant student clinical practice outcomes between various technology-enhanced learning methods (e.g., simulation, virtual reality, mannequins, standard patients).
2. Follow-up studies of associations between graduates' and their employers' satisfaction with practice competencies and types of learning strategies employed within the graduate's program.

Identification of innovative approaches to learning that improve clinical reasoning and judgement applied to patient care affecting individuals, families, and communities at national and global levels.

1. Integrative review of the literature for reports and studies comparing clinical reasoning and judgment outcomes between different pedagogical methods.
2. Compare selected student clinical patient care outcomes related to individual, family, and population health outcomes between various teaching approaches.

Identification of innovative approaches to learning that improve clinical reasoning and judgment applied to patient care affecting individuals, families, and communities at national and global levels.

1. Integrative review of the literature to identify approaches to learning that have been applied to increase clinical reasoning and judgment.
2. Design and implementation of studies to compare the influence of different pedagogical methods on clinical reasoning and judgment applied to care of individuals, families, and communities.

Integration of differences based on genomics, sex, ethnicity, age, gender, and other aspects of diversity in educational approaches.

1. National survey of schools of nursing to describe how genetics competencies for nurses are integrated into the curriculum.
2. Design and implementation of studies to describe how students incorporate diversity-related information into clinical decision making and construction of care plans.

Links among learning, improved care delivery, and chronic care management with effective intra/interprofessional education and practice.

1. Integrative literature review to describe incorporation of interprofessional learning experiences into curricula.
2. Design and implementation of studies to elucidate how interprofessional teams interact and reach consensus about patient care.
3. Design and implementation of studies to compare effectiveness of different methods for interprofessional education (e.g., standard patients, case study) for clinical decision making, care planning, and care delivery.

Caregiving and caregivers in the provision of palliative care, pain management, care of the aged, disabled, mentally challenged.

1. Survey of agencies providing care to these vulnerable populations to identify clinical skills and knowledge required for provision of effective care.
2. Integrative review or meta-analysis of literature to describe pedagogical methods employed to develop clinical knowledge and skills to provide care to these vulnerable populations.

SUMMARY

This chapter reviewed the qualifications expected for nursing faculty and the types of research, translational science, and scholarship activities expected of faculty, with recognition of variability in expectation according to type of institution. Descriptions of scholarship, research, and translational science activities were discussed. Examples of research possibilities were presented using Boyer's (1990) scholarship of teaching model. Additional ideas for research, translation of research, and scholarship in nursing education were listed under the NLN's (2016) priorities for research in nursing education. Two tables reviewed articles from the literature found throughout this text that merit further investigation or replication.

- In your opinion, what is the major factor that interferes with the faculty's role in scholarship and research? What strategies do you suggest to resolve the issue?
- Differentiate between scholarship, translational science, and research as they apply to the faculty role. Give examples for each.

Student-Learning Activities

1. Divide your class into four groups based on Boyer's (1990) concepts on the scholarship of teaching (discovery, integration, application, and teaching) and provide at least two examples for each.
   a. Describe how you would carry out each project including project design, personnel, costs, and time commitment.
   b. Present your examples to the total group and critique them according to their rigor, practicality, and contribution to nursing education science.

Faculty Development Activities

Identify a researchable problem in your practice as a nursing educator. Share it with a colleague and discuss the problem, refine it into a research statement and, if appropriate, hypotheses. Discuss an appropriate review of the literature, a conceptual or theoretical framework for the study, and possible research and analytic methodologies. Discuss how it could be funded, potential collaborators to cover breadth and depth of expertise needed, and the time commitment required. Develop a plan to carry it out and describe potential limitations based on design compromises required.

References

Aduddell, K. A., & Dorman, G. E. (2010). The development of the next generation of nurse leaders. *Journal of Nursing Education, 49*(3), 168–171.

American Association of Colleges of Nursing. (1999). Defining scholarship for the discipline of nursing. Retrieved from http://www.aacnnursing.org/News-Information/Position-Statements-White-Papers/Defining-Scholarship

American Psychological Association. (2014). A graduate student's guide to determining authorship credit and authorship order. Retrieved from http://www.apa.org/science/leadership/students/authorship-paper.pdf

Anderson, C. A. (2000). Current strengths and limitations of doctoral education in nursing: Are we prepared for the future? *Journal of Professional Nursing, 16,* 191–200.

Andre, K., & Barnes, L. (2010). Creating a 21st century nursing workforce: Designing a bachelor of nursing program in response to the health reform agenda. *Nurse Education Today, 30*(3), 258–263.

Association for the Study of Higher Education. (2014). ASHE principles of ethical content. Retrieved from http://www.ashe.ws/?page=180

Bers, T. (2011). Program review and institutional effectiveness. *New Directions for Community Colleges, 152,* 63–73.

Booker, K., & Hilgenberg, C. (2010). Analysis of academic programs: Comparing nursing and other university majors in the application of a quality, potential, and cost model. *Professional Nursing, 26,* 201–206.

Boyer, E. L. (1990). *Scholarship reconsidered: Priorities of the professoriate*. Princeton, NJ: The Carnegie Foundation for the Advancement of Learning. Retrieved from http://depts.washington.edu/gs630/Spring/Boyer.pdf

Brewer, C. S., Kovner, C. T., Poornima, S., Fairchild, S., Kim, H., & Djukic, M. (2009). A comparison of second-degree baccalaureate and traditional-baccalaureate new graduate RNs: Implications for the workforce. *Journal of Professional Nursing, 25*(1), 5–14.

Comer, L., Whichcello, R., & Neubrander, J. (2013). An innovative master of science program for the development of culturally competent nursing leaders. *Journal of Cultural Diversity, 20*(2), 89–93.

Cummings, C. (2015). Evaluating clinical simulation. *Nursing Forum, 50*(2), 109–115.

Dacey, M., Murphy, J. I., Anderson, D. C., & McCloskey, W. W. (2010). An interprofessional service-learning course: Uniting students across educational levels and promoting patient-centered care. *Journal of Nursing Education, 49*(12), 696–699.

D'Antonio, P. O., Brennan, A. M. W., & Curley, M. A. Q. (2013). Judgment, inquiry, engagement, voice: Reenvisioning an undergraduate nursing curriculum using a shared decision-making model. *Journal of Professional Nursing, 29*(6), 407–413.

Davis, B. W. (2011). A conceptual model to support curriculum review, revision, and design in an associate degree nursing program. *Nursing Education Perspectives, 32*(6), 389–394.

Dearman, V., Lawson, R., & Hall, H. R. (2011). Concept mapping a baccalaureate nursing program: A method for success. *Journal of Nursing Education, 50*(11), 656–659.

DeBrew, J. K. (2010). Perceptions of liberal education of two types of nursing graduates: The essentials of baccalaureate education for professional nursing practice. *Journal of General Education, 59*, 42–58.

De Geest, S., Sullivan Marx, E. M., Rich, V., Spichiger, E., Schwendimann, R., & Spirig, R., & Van Malderen, G. (2010). Developing a financial framework for academic service partnerships: Models of the United States and Europe. *Journal of Professional Scholarship, 42*(3), 295–304.

DeSilets, L. (2010). Another look at evaluation models. *Journal of Continuing Education in Nursing, 41*(1), 12–13.

Egues, A., & Leinung, E. (2014). Antibullying workshops: Shaping minority nursing leaders through curriculum innovation. *Nursing Forum, 49*(4), 240–246.

Enders, T., Morin, A., & Pawlak, B. (2016). *Advancing healthcare transformation: A new era for academic nursing*. Retrieved from https://www.manatt.com/getattachment/d58fee3a-2eb1-4490-82d5-94b94d0d5331/attachment.aspx

Flood, L., Gasiewicz, N., & Delpier, T. (2010). Integrating information literacy across a BSN curriculum. *Journal of Nursing Education, 49*(2), 101–104.

Freeland, T., Pathak, S., Garrett, R., Anderson, J., & Daniels, S. (2016). Using medical mannequins to train nurses in stroke swallowing screening. *Dysphagia, 31*, 104–110.

Giddens, J. F., & Brady, D. P. (2007). Rescuing nursing education from content saturation: The case for a concept-based curriculum. *Journal of Nursing Education, 46*(2), 65–69.

Giddens, J. F., Wright, M., & Gray, I. (2012). Selecting concepts for a concept-based curriculum: Application of a benchmark approach. *Journal of Nursing Education, 51*(9), 511–515.

Goode, C. J., Lynn, M. R., & McElroy, D. (2013). Lessons learned from 10 years of research on a post-baccalaureate nurse residency program. *Journal of Nursing Administration, 43*(2), 73–79.

Grey, M. (2013). The doctor of nursing practice: Defining the next steps. *Journal of Nursing Education, 52*(8), 462–465.

Hagler, D., Morris, B., & White, B. (2011). Cognitive tools as a scaffold for faculty during curriculum redesign. *Journal of Nursing Education, 50*(7), 417–422.

Harmon, R. B., Fontaine, D., Plews-Ogan, M., & Williams, A. (2012). Achieving transformational change: Using appreciative inquiry for strategic planning in a school of nursing. *Professional Nursing, 28*, 119–124.

Head, B. A., Schapmire, T., Hermann, C., Earnshaw, L., Faul, A., Jones, C., . . . Pfeifer, M. (2014). The interdisciplinary curriculum for oncology palliative care education (iCOPE): Meeting the challenge of interprofessional education. *Journal of Palliative Medicine, 17*(10), 1107–1115.

Herinckx, H., Munkvold, J, Winter, E., & Tanner, C. (2014). A measure to evaluate classroom teaching practices in nursing. *Nursing Education Perspectives, 35*(1), 30–36.

Horne, E. M., & Sandmann, L. R. (2012). Current trends in systematic program evaluation of online graduate nursing education: An integrative literature review. *Journal of Nursing Education, 51*(10), 570–576.

Kalb, K. (2009). The three Cs model: The context, content, and conduct of nursing education. *Nursing Education Perspectives, 30*(3), 176–180.

Kalb, K., O'Conner-Von, S., Brockway, C., Rierson, C., & Sendelbach, S. (2015). Evidence-based teaching practice in nursing education: Faculty perspectives and practices. *Nursing Education Perspectives, 36*(4), 212–219.

Klemm, P. (2012). Conducting nursing research with undergraduate students: A collaborative, participatory approach. *Nurse Educator, 17*(1), 10–11.

Klich-Heartt, E. I. (2010). Special needs of entry-level master's-prepared nurses from accelerated programs. *Nurse Leader, 8*(5), 52–54.

Martin, C., & Hodge, M. (2011). A nursing department faculty-mentored research project. *Nurse Educator, 36*(1), 35–39.

McNiesh, S. G. (2011). The lived experience of students in an accelerated nursing program: Intersecting factors that influence experiential learning. *Journal of Nursing Education, 50*(4), 197–203.

Merrill, J. A., Yoon, S., Larson, E., Honig, J., & Reame, N. (2013). Using social network analysis to examine relationships among PhD and DNP student and faculty in a research-intensive university school of nursing. *Nursing Outlook, 61*, 109–116.

National Council of State Boards of Nursing. (2009). *Report of findings from the effect of high-fidelity simulation on nursing students' knowledge and performance: A pilot study.* NCSBN Research Brief, 40. Chicago, IL: Author.

National League for Nursing. (2013). *A vision for doctoral preparation for nurse educators.* Retrieved from http://www.nln.org/docs/default-source/about/nln-vision-series-%28position-statements%29/nlnvision_6.pdf

National League for Nursing. (2016). *NLN research priorities in nursing education 2016–2019.* Retrieved from http://www.nln.org/docs/default-source/professional-development-programs/nln-research-priorities-in-nursing-education-single-pages.pdf?sfvrsn=2

Needleman, J., Bowman, C., Wyte-Lake, T., & Dobalian, A. (2014). Faculty recruitment and engagement in academic-practice partnerships. *Nursing Education Perspectives, 35*(6), 372–379.

Newhouse, C. P. (2011). Using IT to assess IT: Towards greater authenticity in summative performance assessment. *Computers & Education, 56*, 388–402.

Ostrogorsky, T., & Raber, A. (2014). Experiences of first-year nursing students during an education redesign: Findings from the Oregon Consortium for Nursing Education. *Nursing Education Perspectives, 35*(2), 115–121.

Penprase, B., & Koczara, S. (2009). Understanding the experiences of accelerated second-degree nursing students and graduates: A review of the literature. *Journal of Continuing Education in Nursing, 40*(2), 74–78.

Pollard, M., Stapleton, M., Kennelly, L., Bagdan, L., Cannistraci, P., Millenbach, L., & Odondi, M. (2014). Assessment of quality and safety education in nursing: A New York state perspective. *Nursing Education Perspectives, 35*(4), 224–229.

Powell-Cope, G., Hughes, N. L., Sedlak, C., & Nelson, A. (2008). Faculty perceptions of implementing an evidence-based safe patient handling nursing curriculum module. *Online Journal of Issues in Nursing, 13*(3). Retrieved from http://www.nursingworld.org/MainMenuCategories/ANAMarketplace/ANAPeriodicals/OJIN/TableofContents/vol132008/No3Sept08/ArticlePreviousTopic/NurseFacultyandSafePatientHandling.html

Praslova, L. (2010). Adaptation of Kirkpatrick's four level models of training criteria to assessment of learning outcomes and program evaluation in higher education. *Educational Assessment and Evaluation, 22*, 215–225.

Rafferty, M., & Lindell, D. (2011). How nurse managers rate the clinical competencies of accelerated (second-degree) nursing graduates. *Journal of Nursing Education, 50*(6), 355–357.

Regan, M., & Pietrobon, R. (2010). A conceptual framework for scientific writing in nursing. *Journal of Nursing Education, 49*(8), 437–443.

Roberts, S. J., & Glod, C. (2013). Faculty roles: Dilemmas for the future of nursing education. *Nursing Forum, 48*(2), 99–105.

Sheu, L., Lai, C. J., Coelho, A. D., Lin, L. D., Zheng, P., Hom, P., . . . O'Sullivan, P. S. (2010). Impact of student-run clinics on preclinical sociocultural and interprofessional attitudes: A prospective cohort analysis. *Journal of Health Care for the Poor and Underserved, 23*(3), 1058–1072.

Simpson, V., & Richards, E. (2015). Flipping the classroom to teach population health: Increasing the relevance. *Nurse Education in Practice, 15*(3), 162–167.

Skiba, D. (2012). Technology and gerontology: Is this in your nursing curriculum? *Nursing Education Perspectives, 33*(3), 207–209.

Spillane, J. P., Pareja, S., Dorner, L., Barnes, C., May, H., Huff, J., & Camburn, E. (2010). Mixing methods in randomized controlled trials (RCTs): Validation, conceptualization, triangulation, and control. *Education, Assessment, Evaluation, Accountability, 22*, 5–28.

Thompson, B. W., & Skiba, D. J. (2008). Informatics in the nursing curriculum: A national survey of nursing informatics requirements in nursing curricula. *Nursing Education Perspectives, 29*(5), 312–317.

Udlis, K. A., & Manusco, J. M. (2012). Doctor of nursing practice programs across the United States: A benchmark of information. Part I: Program characteristics. *Journal of Professional Nursing, 28*(5), 265–273.

Vetter, T., McGwin, G., & Pittet, J. (2016). Replicability, reproducibility, and fragility of research findings: Ultimately, caveat emptor. *Anesthesia & Analgesia, 123*(1), 244–248.

Weathers, S. M., & Raleigh, E. D. (2013). 1-Year retention rates and performance ratings: Comparing associate degree, baccalaureate, and accelerated baccalaureate degree nurses. *Journal of Nursing Administration, 43*(9), 468–474.

Welfare, L. E., & Sackett, C. R. (2011). The authorship determination process in student–faculty collaborative research. *Journal of Counseling & Development, 89*, 479–487.

Ziehm, S. R., Uibel, I. C., Fontaine, D. K., & Scherzer, T. (2011). Success indicators for accelerated master's entry nursing program: Staff RN performance. *Journal of Nursing Education, 50*(7), 395–403.

CHAPTER 15

Issues and Challenges for Nursing Educators

Stephanie S. DeBoor

Sarah B. Keating

CHAPTER OBJECTIVES

Upon completion of Chapter 15, the reader will be able to:

- Analyze the trends, issues, and challenges raised throughout the text that apply to curriculum development and evaluation
- Consider some strategies for resolution of the issues raised and ways to meet the challenges with an eye to the future

OVERVIEW

This chapter summarizes the text to provide the reader with an overview of the processes related to curriculum development and evaluation in nursing education. It begins with the major milestones in the history of nursing education in the United States to gain perspectives on its move into higher education in order to meet the needs of the current and future health care systems. The chapters provide guidelines from expert, experienced nursing educators and the latest literature and research on theories, concepts, and models that apply to curriculum building, evaluation, accreditation, and the roles of faculty in the processes. Major issues and challenges raised throughout the text are reviewed with some ideas for strategies to bring them to resolution. The chapter ends with a description of the characteristics of a future ideal nursing education system.

CHAPTER 1: HISTORY OF NURSING EDUCATION IN THE UNITED STATES

Chapter 1 raises many of the issues related to nursing's role in academe from the time of Nightingale, to hospital-based, apprentice-type programs, and ultimately, to higher education institutions including the associate degree, baccalaureate, master's, and doctorate levels. The influence of major wars and resulting federal support of nursing education are reviewed. Nursing's efforts to improve and standardize curricula through several commissions' and committees' work leading to accreditation of programs are described. The Institute of Medicine's (IOM, 2010) recommendation from *The Future of Nursing: Focus on Education* calls for nurses to be prepared at higher levels of education to meet the health care needs of the 21st century. In response, programs and enrollments in RN-to-BSN and RN-to-MSN programs are expanding. The explosion of DNP programs for advanced practice, the recognition of the PhD as the discipline's research and theory-building degree, the effect of health care legislation, and the impact of technology on the profession will be the major forces that influence continued evolvement of nursing in the 21st century.

CHAPTER 2: CURRICULUM DEVELOPMENT AND APPROVAL PROCESSES IN CHANGING EDUCATIONAL ENVIRONMENTS

Chapter 2 reviews the processes that schools of nursing undergo to bring about curriculum revision or to develop new programs. It includes some of the facilitators and barriers to the processes. It discusses the roles and responsibilities of faculty for ensuring curriculum integrity and its currency with current and future practice in both nursing and education. The various levels of approval for curricular revision or proposals for new programs and the need for the resources to support the processes are considered. The involvement of stakeholders such as students, health care partners, and other disciplines is important to ultimate success. Ideas for faculty development are presented especially as they relate to new and part-time faculty members who may have minimal preparation for the role of educator in academe. The issue of content saturation must be confronted; else the temptation to crowd the curriculum beyond the point of reason will overwhelm students' learning capacity. Newer innovations to implement the curriculum are reviewed such as innovative conceptual learning approaches, technology, high-fidelity simulations, dedicated clinical educational units, and partnerships with health care systems and other community resources.

CHAPTER 3: NEEDS ASSESSMENT: THE EXTERNAL AND INTERNAL FRAME FACTORS

Chapter 3 introduces the Frame Factors Model, a conceptual model that describes the major external and internal factors that influence, facilitate, or impinge upon the curriculum. It reviews the major components of a needs assessment that include analyses of these factors. While the principal activities of faculty in curriculum development and evaluation are on the curriculum plan, improvement based on evaluation of its implementation, and the final program outcomes, the processes related to a needs assessment should become part of the repertoire of the faculty. Faculty members sophisticated in the assessment of frame factors are at an advantage to view the curriculum and its place in the scheme of financial security, position within the health care system and the profession, role in meeting the health care needs of the community and industry, and its significance to the parent institution.

It is recommended that nursing educators use the Frame Factors Model when evaluating their educational programs, considering revisions of existing programs, or initiating new programs. While administrators may take the leadership role in conducting needs assessments, faculty should participate in the decisions for what type and how much data to collect and what decisions are made that affect the curriculum based on the needs assessment. A case study illustrating the application of the Frame Factors Model is found in the Appendix. It proposes a collaborative, international program between two schools of nursing, one in the United States and one in Africa. With the expanding use of distance education through the Internet, it provides some ideas about the challenges and the excitement related to developing these types of curricula.

CHAPTER 4: FINANCIAL SUPPORT AND BUDGET MANAGEMENT FOR CURRICULUM DEVELOPMENT OR REVISION

Chapter 4 reviews the resources and costs related to the financial support and budget planning for curriculum development, evaluation, and accreditation activities. Specific costs include faculty release time, administrative and staff support, office equipment, technology support, and supplies. These are costs over and above the usual budget demands and must be planned for in advance. The challenge is to earmark funds for these activities to avoid unexpected shortfalls and an impact on other program expenditures. Knowledge of possible resources external to the program is useful for generating funds that help initiate and support new programs and several potential funding sources are reviewed. In addition to budget planning, the roles and responsibilities of administrators and faculty are described and the importance of faculty participation and contributions to budgetary planning is noted.

CHAPTER 5: THE CLASSIC COMPONENTS OF THE CURRICULUM: DEVELOPING A CURRICULUM PLAN

Chapter 5 organizes the components of the curriculum in the traditional way, that is, mission/vision, philosophy, goal, organizational framework, student-learning outcomes (objectives), and implementation plan. The components of the curriculum provide an organizing framework for initiating or revising an educational program. Major concepts related to the underlying philosophy and the beliefs faculty hold about nursing and education are examined in light of their contribution to the philosophy and their place in the curriculum. Examples include beliefs about teaching and learning processes, critical thinking and its application to nursing, liberal education and the sciences, the health care system, and so on. Most faculty members agree that these concepts are fundamental to nursing education.

While it may seem cumbersome at times, in the long run, examining the curriculum by its major components results in a logical order for planning and evaluation. When faculty members contemplate change in response to a needs assessment of the external and internal frame factors, each component of the curriculum is examined for its congruence with the proposed changes. This may lead to a radical revamping of the curriculum, for it may be discovered that the demands for graduates or from the health care system have so dramatically changed that the mission, philosophy, and goals of the program are outdated or irrelevant. Approaching the curriculum holistically by viewing all of its components leads to orderly revisions rather than the "Band-Aid" approach that attempts to mend one portion of the program without considering its effects on the other components and avoids overloaded and content safurated curricula.

CHAPTER 6: IMPLEMENTATION OF THE CURRICULUM

Chapter 6 continues the discussion of curriculum planning by reviewing the processes necessary to implement the curriculum once the mission, vision, philosophy, goals, and student-learning outcomes are in place. Crucial to the process is the faculty's knowledge and beliefs concerning learning theories and educational taxonomies. Chapter 6 provides synopses of common learning theories and taxonomies that specifically apply to nursing education. Critical thinking and its application to clinical reasoning and clinical judgment skills are differentiated and explained as they apply to the nurse's ability to provide care in today's complex health care system.

Moving from learning theories, taxonomies, and critical thinking, the chapter discusses their application to student-focused instructional strategies. The strategies include the flipped classroom, team-based activities, problem-based learning, and simulation. The diversity of student learners and the effect of distance education are touched upon. The role of student evaluation and its methods in light of measuring course objectives conclude the chapter.

CHAPTERS 7 THROUGH 9: CURRICULUM PLANNING FOR UNDERGRADAUTE AND GRADUATE PROGRAMS

Chapter 7 Undergraduate Programs

Chapter 7 discusses the two current, major curricula for entry into practice, that is, the associate degree in nursing (ADN) and the baccalaureate/BSN. Both of these programs have been in existence since the mid-20th century, replacing the hospital-based diploma programs that continue to exist, but are decreasing in numbers. This chapter describes generic (entry-level) baccalaureate programs as well as fast-track baccalaureate programs for college graduates and RN-to-BSN programs. The old issue of entry into practice rears its ugly head as the ADN and baccalaureate are examined; however, with the need to produce more nurses as rapidly as possible to meet health care demands and the need for higher education in nursing, the author of Chapter 7 describes curricula that embrace both programs and foster career ladder opportunities.

Chapter 8 Curriculum Planning for Specialty Master's Nursing Degrees and Entry-Level Graduate Degrees

Chapter 8 reviews the history of master's-level graduate education from the beginning, when additional education for administrators and educators was recognized, to the need for further education for clinical specialties and eventually, for primary care roles as nurse practitioners. The various current master's programs are described including the RN to MSN, entry-level MSN (for nonnursing college graduates; American Association of Colleges of Nursing [AACN], 2017a), the clinical nurse leader, advanced practice programs, and functional roles such as nursing administrators, educators, and managers. Issues related to master's programs are raised such as the remaining question about entry into practice, at what level advanced practice belongs, and the standardization and regulations for advanced practice through licensing, accreditation, certification, and education.

Chapter 9 Planning for Doctoral Education

The traditional place for advanced practice roles such as the nurse practitioner, nurse anesthetist, nurse midwife, and clinical nurse specialist has been at the master's level. However, the DNP degree is replacing the master's in response to the AACN recommendation that the DNP be the terminal practice degree by 2015 (AACN, 2004). This position and the IOM's (2010) recommendation for doubling the number of nurses with doctorates by 2020 led to an explosive growth of DNP programs across the nation, starting first with postmaster's degrees and moving to the BSN to DNP program. The launch of the DNP (AACN, 2017b) was met with much controversy from inside and outside of the profession related to the role of nurses with doctorates. An issue raised by nursing was the many different nursing doctoral degree programs and titles that confused the public and the profession itself.

Graduate programs are particularly hard hit by the looming shortage of doctorally prepared teachers as faculty members age and retire and the numbers of new graduates from doctoral programs do not meet the demand. Nursing education programs vary in their hiring practices. There remains a preference in hiring PhD-prepared faculty for baccalaureate and higher degree programs (Oermann, Lynn, & Agger, 2015). An issue related to doctorally prepared faculty is the debate that continues about the (DNP) versus the research-focused degrees (DNS/PhD) and their places in nursing education. Tenure-track positions are often reserved for those with a research-focused doctorate, who can generate funding from their research agenda. However, a counterargument is that the DNP prepares nurses for applied research, translational science, and evidence-based practice and they could compete in tenure-track roles. It is also argued that DNP gradu-ates are the experts in the practice role and can be role models for the students. There are persuasive arguments on both sides but the majority of those expressing opinions agree that for either degree, there are implications for collaboration of practice and research. Also agreed upon is that, for those nurses planning to teach in schools of nurs-ing, it is essential to have additional knowledge and skills (courses) in education, for example, curriculum development, instructional strategies, educational technology/simulation, and student and program evaluation.

CHAPTER 10: A PROPOSED UNIFIED NURSING CURRICULUM

Chapter 10 raises the continuing issues related to the numerous points of entry into practice in nursing as it responds to the demand from the health care system and the recommendations of experts in the field. For nurses who are educated at higher levels, a few nursing programs offer multilevel nursing education whereby students can enter at the lower division of higher education, step out to become licensed, and at a later date return for upper division and graduate levels of nursing education. However, these days, these types of programs are few and far between, but at the same time, most baccalau-reate programs have accelerated pathways for diploma and associate degree nurses to continue their education to receive a bachelor's and/or for them to transition directly into an MSN.

A proposed unified nursing curriculum is presented that offers a nonstop program from baccalaureate to doctorate parallel to a "step-out" program that allows students to step out of the program, become licensed, practice, and return without penalty to con-tinue their education as their personal and professional goals change. The chapter ends with a list of characteristics for nursing education in the future that promotes the prep-aration of nursing leaders, policy initiators, faculty, researchers, and advanced practice clinicians and practitioners. Educated nurses of the future will be prepared to work col-laboratively with other professions in delivering safe, high-quality, and evidence-based services to the consumer.

CHAPTER 11: DISTANCE EDUCATION, ONLINE LEARNING, INFORMATICS, AND TECHNOLOGY

When planning for distance education programs, a needs assessment is indicated and Chapter 11 offers an overview of the factors to consider along with its costs and plan-ning for a budget. Current formats for delivering the curriculum through satellite campuses and web-based online learning are described and their advantages and disadvantages are discussed. The tremendous growth and impact of informatics on nursing education are reviewed including simulated clinical experiences, high- and low-fidelity mannequins and anatomical models, standardized patients, and the utilization of information systems and electronic records. The chapter reminds the reader that the distance education programs should match the curriculum's mission and goals to assure their quality and integrity.

Research findings related to the efficacy of distance education programs are reviewed as well as a discussion of the trends and issues that should be identified and raised. Some current issues raised include the challenges for providing cost-effective programs, the increasing market of learning management systems, and the maintenance of quality through evaluation processes including meeting professional and accreditation stan-dards. Additional issues include intellectual property rights, student to faculty ratios, and maintaining privacy for both students and faculty.

CHAPTER 12: PROGRAM EVALUATION AND ACCREDITATION

Chapter 12 reviews common definitions, concepts, and theories in evaluation that apply to nursing curricula and program evaluation. Nursing education evaluation is evolving from an emphasis in the past on the use of models of evaluation in education to the adaptation of business and health care models to measure productivity, outcomes, cost-effectiveness, and quality. Chapter 12 discusses accreditation agencies, their purpose, and their role in total quality management. While accreditation is voluntary, it carries certain advantages for the institution and its students and graduates. For example, an accredited institution demonstrates to the public that it meets quality standards or criteria set by education and the profession, and therefore increases its marketability. For students and graduates, an accredited program signifies that they are eligible for certain financial aid programs and, in most cases, admission to an institution of higher education for the next degree level(s).

Owing to many accreditation standards, educational programs usually have master plans of evaluation in place to facilitate the process of collecting and analyzing data. One flaw in many of the master plans is the lack of specific plans to follow-up on the analysis and its recommendations. Implementing strategies to act on the recommendations closes the loop between data collection and actions for change in the curriculum, thus maintaining an up-to-date and vibrant program. Educators have a responsibility to participate in program approval and review processes in academe by membership on institutional committees as well as for the nursing program. These kinds of activities contribute to faculty's professional development and the ability to keep abreast of changes occurring in education and the profession that call for modifications of program outcomes, and accreditation and regulatory standards and criteria.

CHAPTER 13: PLANNING FOR ACCREDITATION

Chapter 13 presents a case study illustrating a nursing faculty's preparation for an accreditation site visit. In the United States, there are three accreditation bodies for nursing programs. The Accreditation Commission for Nursing Education (ACEN) provides accreditation for certificate, diploma, or professional degree programs. The Commission on Collegiate Nursing Education (CCNE) provides accreditation for BSN, MSN, post-master's certificates, and DNP programs. The National League for Nursing (NLN) Commission for Nursing Education Accreditation (CNEA) accredits nursing programs from the PN/VN level to the clinical doctorate. In addition, there are two accrediting agencies for nurse midwives and nurse anesthetists. PhD programs are not accredited by a nursing accreditation program but are usually housed in institutions of higher education that have regional accreditation. Chapter 13 provides an overview of accreditation processes for nursing education programs and a case study is presented that describes the processes a nursing faculty undergoes for preparing for an accreditation visit, including preparation of the self-study.

CHAPTER 14: RESEARCH AND EVIDENCE-BASED PRACTICE IN NURSING EDUCATION

Chapter 14 discusses the need for research in nursing education for evidence-based practice. It reviews Boyer's (1990) and AACN's (2014) statements on the scholarship of teaching that serve as guiding principles for faculty to conduct research and produce scholarship that deepens our understanding of education and learning processes. The temptation for faculty is to rely on tried and true strategies for developing curricula and instructional strategies. However, with the rapid changes in the health care delivery system and the impact of technology, educators must provide curricula that are responsive to changes and prepare nurses for the future. Nurses must be able to think critically and creatively, use and generate technology for safe and quality patient care, collaborate with other health professionals and the clients they serve, provide leadership for health care policies, and participate in or conduct research that, in the end, produces high-quality health care. Each chapter of this text reviews the classic and recent literature related to curriculum development and evaluation in nursing. Chapter 14 summarizes studies in the literature that offer ideas for further study and uses the NLN's *Research Priorities for Nursing Education* (2016) to suggest topics for further study and research. It is hoped that many studies are replicated for their generalizability and usefulness to nursing educators and that new research findings lead toward evidence-based practice in education and practice.

WHENCE WE CAME AND WHERE TO GO

Chapter 1 reviews the history of nursing education from the mid- to late 1800s to the 21st century. It is interesting to see the visions of nurse leader educators over the centuries that called for a unified approach to curriculum development in nursing and placement of nursing as a discipline and science into academic institutions of higher learning. It is equally interesting to see the influence that international wars and the major changes in the health care system and society had on nursing education. Nursing education programs found that with governmental help, they could accelerate nursing programs into institutions of higher learning and produce graduates for high-demand eras. Advanced practice roles at the master's level came about as high technology and managed care systems began to change the health care delivery system and research-focused doctoral programs came about as nursing sought its professional identity and began to build its scientific body of knowledge. The explosive growth of the DNP in the last decade as the terminal degree in nursing for advanced practice is remarkable. As the graduates of these programs increase and impact the health care system at the same time that the political atmosphere is calling for legislative changes that affect the health care delivery system, the role of nursing becomes even more crucial. Some of the major challenges facing nursing education for the future are discussed in the following sections.

THE FUTURE EDUCATIONAL PREPARATION FOR NURSING

The IOM's (2010) recommendations regarding nursing's future had an impact on nursing education. That, coupled with the AACN (2004) statement on the DNP as the entry for advanced practice nurses, might be called the "tipping points" for change in nursing education in the 21st century. Gladwell (2002) introduced the concept of tipping points as "little things that happen that result in making a big difference." Although the IOM recommendations and AACN's position are not "little things," they influenced change. While the minimum level of education to practice as an RN is an associate's degree, the IOM, the American Nurses Association (ANA), and the Tri-Council for Nursing are in strong support of the BSN being the minimum requirement for entry to practice. The literature identifies better patient outcomes when the nurse is a BSN or higher. Haskins and Pierson (2016) conducted a systematic review examining 30-day mortality rates and patient outcomes when care is provided by BSN-prepared nurses. Results of the meta-analysis identified that patients had a 5% lower odds of 30-day mortality when cared for by a BSN or higher educated nurse. Additionally, there was a noted 6% lessening of failure to rescue. Both of these findings were statistically significant.

Associate degree and baccalaureate nursing programs' collaboration for curricula that provide seamless entry into the bachelor's degree for associate degree students/graduates are increasing exponentially, as are BSN to doctorates. There are articulation agreements with community colleges offering bachelor's degrees (depending on state regulations) and those that are looking beyond. Giddens, Keller, and Liesveld (2015) discuss the development of a new educational model to increase the number of BSNs into the workforce. The New Mexico Nursing Education Consortium created a model that allows for parallel degree tracks. Students who are eligible and attending a community college can apply to one of two parallel degree tracks. Those who apply to the BSN track are admitted to both the community college and a "designated partner university." Courses are taken between both schools; students register for courses at both institutions. The BSN degree is awarded by the partner university, as New Mexico does not allow for community colleges to grant bachelor degrees. Due to the number of community colleges in the state, universities may serve as partners to multiple community colleges. These partnerships allow for sharing of resources such as faculty and space. Additionally, the curriculum is shared for both the ADN and BSN degree tracks. The curriculum was developed for the BSN program and modified to meet the goals and standards for associate degree education. This allows the BSN to meet CCNE accreditation standards and the ADN track to meet ACEN standards. This innovative model increases access for nursing students in New Mexico to earn a BSN, while still preserving the option of ADN education.

The growth of DNP programs and the increase in enrollments in research-focused doctorates indicate an expansion in the workforce of nurses prepared at the doctorate level who will be the scientists, faculty, advanced practice heath care providers, and nursing leaders (Murphy, Staffileno, & Carlson, 2015). It is a forecast of the role that nursing will play in leading health care policy changes for the benefit of the population and providing evidence-based practice built upon collaborative translational science and research.

A key component of professional education is the faculty who is responsible for developing and implementing curricula that prepare nurses for the future. It is agreed that over the recent past, the focus of instruction changed from teacher-centric to participative, learner-centric modalities. As mentioned previously, nursing is in the process of producing additional doctorally prepared nurses who will serve as faculty members for the newer models of education. Some will be advanced practice nursing leaders who focus on translational science, while others will be researchers exploring and identifying new knowledge for the science of nursing. They will encounter the same challenges facing current educators to fulfill the role of academic faculty, that is, teaching, service, and scholarship/research. The enigma to be solved is how faculty roles are defined to, first, provide high-quality instruction that prepares professionals who meet current and future health care needs and, then, to meet the other faculty expectations, that is, remain current in practice, provide service, and maintain research and scholarship.

NURSING INFORMATICS AND TECHNOLOGY

Throughout the chapters of this text, nursing informatics, clinical simulations, and technology applications are discussed as they apply to curriculum development and evaluation. Previous reviews in this chapter alluded to the need for alignment of these advances to the curriculum plan (organizational framework and student-learning outcomes). Personal digital assistants (PDAs), which seemed a modern technological advancement only yesterday, rapidly became outdated as smartphones and tablets allow for rapid access to databases for health care information. Technology-enhanced classrooms (smart classrooms) provide opportunities for teaching and learning through the integration of technology, such as computers, specialized software, audience response technology, networking, and audio/visual capabilities. It is hard to imagine the future and additional expansions of technology and their application to nursing and education. Thus, it becomes the responsibility of nursing educators to become or remain sophisticated in the use of informatics, clinical simulations, and other applications. While there are numerous studies on the application of these strategies in nursing education, there remains the need for replication of studies and comparisons of programs across the country to validate their effectiveness and to provide information on best practices. For example, the following studies are illustrations of best practices. Njie-Carr et al. (2017) reviewed the literature on the "flipped classroom technique" and found that it produced effective learning. Gamification (Looyestyn et al., 2017), audience response systems (ARS), applications (Montenery et al., 2013), and simulated clinical experiences (Rodriguez, Nelson, Gilmartin, Goldsamt, & Richardson, 2017) provide strategies to enhance student learning.

CAREER PATHWAYS AND PROMOTING PROFESSIONAL DEVELOPMENT FOR THE FUTURE

Career Ladder Pathways in Nursing

Nursing, as a profession, prides itself on providing career ladder opportunities through experience in the workforce and progression of degree opportunities from the licensed practical nurse/licensed vocational nurse (LPN/LVN) to the doctorate. Entry into practice as RNs remains multilayered with graduates of diploma, ADN, BSN, and entry-level master's degrees eligible for licensure. These multiple pathways continue to confuse the public and those seeking education to become RNs. Baccalaureate schools of nursing have a long history of offering user-friendly programs for RNs, doing away with past practices of requiring the RNs to repeat lower division nursing courses and integrating them into classes with generic BSN students. The RN-to-BSN or RN-to-MSN programs are for the most part accelerated, usually with 1 year of full-time study to earn the baccalaureate and for the RN-to-MSN programs, 2 to 2.5 years of full-time study. Courses are geared toward adult learning strategies with classes scheduled 1 day a week, while others offer the program totally online, or a combination of both. The majority of programs have part-time options as well.

For some time, ADN and diploma graduates did not have an incentive to return to school for their baccalaureate or higher degrees owing to, among other factors, the absence of differentiation of practice in the worksite. However, current data reveal employers prefer those graduates with a BSN over their ADN counterparts. Auerbach, Beurhaus, and Staiger (2015) found a shift in employment settings. There was a drop in the percentage (65%–60%) of ADN-prepared RNs employed in hospitals; the percentage of BSN-prepared RNs grew during the same period from 67% to 72%. Similarly, in 2016 AACN conducted a survey to examine new graduates' employment rates among BSN graduates. Findings indicated that employers within the communities preferred hiring BSNs and 70% of BSN students had been offered positions prior to graduation.

Schools of nursing bear the responsibility for evaluating the credentials of applicants with prior education or degrees not in nursing. There is a need for flexibility in granting credit for courses equivalent to those pre- and corequisites in nursing and nursing courses (for RNs with degrees not in nursing) to enter into the curriculum and to complete the next academic level. Examples are RNs with baccalaureates or master's in other disciplines and nonnurses with baccalaureates or higher degrees who matriculate directly into master's programs rather than repeating the baccalaureate. Of course, RNs need upper-division–level nursing courses or their equivalent and nonnurses need nursing courses equivalent to the baccalaureate but offered at the graduate level prior to entering master's or doctorate-level nursing courses.

The advantages to the entry-level doctorate program are numerous. It would facilitate high school graduates' entry into a nursing program with graduation 8 years away, thus producing expert clinicians, researchers, and educators who are relatively young in age. The 8-year total curriculum plan provides the time for in-depth education, clinical practice, and the production of quality graduates prepared for practice, teaching, and research roles. If the profession embraces this transformation of nursing education, then it must come to grips with the reality that there are roles for personnel such as the LPNs/LVNs. It is logical that these programs fall into the community college genre, thus raising the specter of the "civil war" in nursing yet again. These authors leave that debate to the nursing educators reading this text and the nursing profession over the next few decades.

Although this text focuses on curriculum development and evaluation in nursing in the United States as we contemplate the future with its promise and challenges, there is a need to envision a broader, global perspective about nursing and the education required for its professionals. Cyberspace communications give us the ability to share knowledge and expertise with colleagues in health care and discover commonalities and differences that enrich the profession and lead to improved delivery of health care. International colleagues share the same concerns of U.S. nursing educators for preparing quality health professionals to meet the needs of the world's populations from the poorest nations to the richest.

SUMMARY

This chapter summarized each of the previous chapters in the text and raised issues from each topic. While the world order, the national society, and the health care system change rapidly, it is difficult to predict the future. There are prevailing trends that should have an impact on the development and evaluation of nursing curricula over the next decade. If nursing chooses not to respond to these changes, the profession will continue to be splintered with less opportunity for it to help to shape public policy toward optimal health care for the populace. Nursing educators have a responsibility to work with their colleagues in practice and research to develop curricula that prepare nurses for the future, who are competent and caring, excellent clinicians and practitioners, leaders and change agents, and scholars and researchers. A nursing education system for the future will have the following characteristics:

1. Clearly defined levels of education and differentiated practice in the health care system based on education and experience
2. Entry into practice for staff nurse positions following a 3-month residency in a selected arena of practice
3. Quality institutions of higher education that specialize in the preparation of staff nurses for entry into evidence-based practice in a timely fashion
4. Quality institutions that focus on the faculty role of excellence in teaching, community service, research, and the translation and application of knowledge from nursing science and related disciplines
5. Quality institutions of higher education that specialize in the preparation of nurses to provide evidence-based advanced practice nursing and interprofessional services for individuals, families, communities, and aggregates
6. Students, graduates, and faculty who are active participants and generators of new knowledge in nursing and related disciplines' research
7. Quality institutions of higher education that specialize in the preparation of nurse leaders who will influence health care policy and change the health care system for the benefit of the populations they serve

8. Academic and health science centers that specialize in nursing research and advancement of nursing science through translational science and evidence-based practice; testing of theories; the development of new theories, concepts, and models; and educational innovations on the national and international levels

DISCUSSION QUESTIONS

- Given the rapid changes in the health care and educational systems and the ongoing shortage of nurses, what changes in nursing education do you envision within the next 5 to 10 years?
- What strategies for changing nursing education worked in the past and how can they apply to needed changes in nursing education today? What are the lessons from the past that prohibited nursing from moving its educational agenda forward? How can today's nurse educators use these lessons to bring about change?

LEARNING ACTIVITIES

Student-Learning Activities

Synthesize the information in this text into a "Dream School of Nursing." Develop a curriculum that prepares nurses for practice 10 years hence, keeping in mind that practice and the setting in which it is delivered will be different. Let your imagination run wild!

Faculty Development Activities

Hold a faculty meeting focused on brainstorming and let creative thoughts flow freely. List the characteristics of the ideal nurse prepared to practice 5 to 10 years hence. Examine these characteristics and decide how a curriculum can be developed that provides the kind of education necessary to prepare this kind of nurse. Focus on creativity and newer theories of learning. Compare these ideas to your existing curriculum. How can it be transformed into the one you envision and still meet accreditation and professional standards and criteria?

References

American Association of Colleges of Nursing. (2004). *AACN position statement on the practice doctorate in nursing.* Retrieved from http://www.aacnnursing.org/Portals/42/News/Position-Statements/DNP.pdf

American Association of Colleges of Nursing. (2014). Defining scholarship for the discipline of nursing. Retrieved from http://www.aacnnursing.org/News-Information/Position-Statements-White-Papers/Defining-Scholarship

American Association of Colleges of Nursing. (2017a). Degree completion program for registered nurses: RN to master's degree and RN to baccalaureate programs. Retrieved from http://www.aacnnursing.org/News-Information/Fact-Sheets/Degree-Completion-Programs

American Association of Colleges of Nursing. (2017b). DNP fact sheet. Retrieved from http://www.aacnnursing.org/Portals/42/News/Factsheets/DNP-Factsheet-2017.pdf

Auerbach, D. I., Buerhaus, P. I., & Staiger, D. O. (2015). Do associate degree registered nurses fare differently in the nurse labor market compared to baccalaureate-prepared RNs? *Nursing Economics, 33*(1), 8–12, 35.

Boyer, E. L. (1990). *Scholarship reconsidered: Priorities of the professoriate.* Princeton, NJ: The Carnegie Foundation for the Advancement of Learning. Retrieved from http://depts.washington.edu/gs630/Spring/Boyer.pdf

Giddens, J., Keller, T., & Liesveld, J. (2015). Answering the call for a bachelors-prepared nursing workforce: An innovative model for academic progression. *Journal of Professional Nursing, 31,* 445–451

Gladwell, M. (2002). *The tipping point. How little things can make a big difference.* New York, NY: Little, Brown.

Haskins, S., & Pierson, K. (2016). The impact of the bachelor of science in nursing (BSN) degree on patient outcomes: A systematic review. *Journal of Nursing Practice Applications & Reviews of Research, 6*(1), 40–49.

Institute of Medicine. (2010). *The future of nursing: Leading change, advancing health.* Washington, DC: National Academies Press.

Looyestyn, J., Kernot, J., Boshoff, K., Ryan, J., Edney, S., & Maher, C. (2017). Does gamification increase engagement with online programs? A systematic review. *Public Library of Science One, 12*(13), 1–19.

Montenery, S., Walker, M., Sorensen, E., Thompson, R., Kirklin, D., White, R., & Ross, C. (2013). Millennial generation student nurses' perceptions of the impact of multiple technologies on learning. *Nursing Education Perspectives, 34*(6), 405–409.

Murphy, M. P., Staffileno, B. A., & Carlson, E. (2015). Collaboration among DNP- and PhD-prepared nurses: Opportunity to drive positive change. *Journal of Professional Nursing, 31,* 388–394.

National League for Nursing. (2016). *NLN research priorities in nursing education 2016–2019.* Retrieved from http://www.nln.org/docs/default-source/professional-development-programs/nln-research-priorities-in-nursing-education-single-pages.pdf?sfvrsn=2

Njie-Carr, V. P. S., Ludeman, E., Lee, M. C., Dordunoo, D., Trocky, M. M., & Jenkines, L. S. (2017). An integrative review of flipped classroom teaching models in nursing education. *Journal of Professional Nursing, 33*(2), 133–144.

Oermann, M. H., Lynn, M. R., & Agger, C. A. (2016). Hiring intentions of directors of nursing programs related to DNP- and PhD-prepared faculty and roles of faculty. *Journal of Professional Nursing, 32*(3), 173–179.

Rodriguez, K. G., Nelson, N., Gilmartin, M., Goldsamt, L., & Richardson, H. (2017). Simulation is more than working with a mannequin: Students' perceptions of their learning experience in a clinical simulation environment. *Journal of Nursing Education and Practice, 7*(7), 30–36.

APPENDIX

Case Study

Sarah B. Keating

A fictitious case study is presented in this Appendix to illustrate a needs assessment and the development of a proposed curriculum based on the assessment. It includes the collection of data related to external and internal frame factors, their analyses, a curriculum decision based on the findings, and a proposed program of study.

CHAPTER OBJECTIVES

Upon completion of the Case study, the reader will be able to:

- Analyze a needs assessment of two fictitious schools of nursing considering expansion of their degree programs through a collaborative arrangement
- Identify gaps in the data collected for the needs assessment and other possibilities for development from the data analysis
- Practice curriculum development based on the case study's needs assessment by refining the proposed program or developing a new one

EXTERNAL FRAME FACTORS

Description of the Community

An existing baccalaureate and higher degree nursing program whose home campus is located in a suburban town of 20,000 adjacent to a large U.S. state capital with a population of more than 1,000,000 is about to undertake a needs assessment to determine if the program should expand. The U.S. home institution is a private, sectarian, multipurpose higher education institution. It has a long history of liberal arts education and recently developed a partnership with a higher education university in Kenya, Africa, that is supported by the same religiously based organization. Presently, the Kenyan university offers a bachelor of arts in general studies (BA) and is the home institution to a bachelor of science in nursing (BScN) program with master's degrees in business and education that are available online. The purpose of the partnership between the two universities is to increase and diversify the student population, to develop exchange programs, and to promote international higher education. The U.S. institution's home campus has several professional schools including business, education, engineering, nursing, and the performing arts with baccalaureates and master's degrees in those majors and there are three doctorate programs, in education (PhD), business administration (DBA), and nursing practice (DNP). The undergraduate population numbers 8,000 and there are 3,000 graduate students. There is a total of 850 on-campus faculty members with 350 of them part time. In the past 5 years, the institution and specifically, its professional schools, increased the number of online course offerings.

Nursing faculty and administrators are aware of the continuing and projected nursing workforce shortage in the nation and in the region, the changes in the health care system and their effect on the nursing workforce, and the trend for increasing the basic entry level of nursing education to the baccalaureate. They have anecdotal information that employers of nurses prefer baccalaureate or higher degree nurses owing to the complexity of the acute care setting, the shortages of nurses prepared to practice in primary care and community settings, and the Institute of Medicine's (IOM, 2010) recommendation on *The Future of Nursing* that recommends the baccalaureate as the threshold for professional nursing.

Responding to this need, 3 years ago the nursing program developed a track in the baccalaureate program for RNs to complete their BSN degrees totally online in addition to its on-campus undergraduate bachelor's program (BSN). At the same time, it expanded its master's family nurse practitioner (FNP) and adult/geriatric acute care nurse practitioner (AANP) advanced practice options into a DNP program. The majority of the master's and DNP theory courses are offered online and the DNP is open to master's-prepared advanced practice nurses as a DNP completion track. The master's program offers post-baccalaureate community health nursing (CHN), and administration (ADM) tracks, as well as an entry-level clinical nurse leader (CNL) program for nonnursing college graduates. The ADM and CHN master's and the completion DNP are totally online. The graduate program recently experienced an increase in applications from nurses in practice in the United States and from the graduates of the BScN program of the parent institution's partner in Kenya.

The nursing program is clinically affiliated with a religious-based health care organization of the same denomination as its parent organization. The health care organization is a managed care system and has nationwide and regional facilities and some international services in East Africa and Kenya. It is supportive of the nursing program and offers clinical sites for student practice. It has scholarship or loan forgiveness programs for its staff and for students who come to its facilities after graduation. Recently, there has been interest in the graduate program from other nations' health care systems and nursing programs that are affiliated with the supportive religious organization. With this information in hand, the dean of nursing asks the faculty to conduct a needs assessment for expanding the nursing program by increasing enrollments for entry-level nurses and/or expanding the graduate program to provide additional advanced practice nurses both nationally and internationally. The dean appoints the two associate deans of nursing to serve as leaders of a needs assessment task force.

Using the guidelines for assessing external and internal frame factors (see Chapter 3, Tables 3.1 and 3.2), the task force initiates a needs assessment. The U.S. campus includes the town, nearby city, six major suburban areas, and an adjacent three-county rural area. The major industries and employers near the home campus include the state government, two alternative energy manufacturers, several food-processing plants, a large inland port, a railroad center, a rocket engineering and manufacturing plant, the primary and secondary educational systems, and several large health care systems that serve the city, suburbs, and rural neighbors. In addition to the home campus nursing program, a state-supported baccalaureate and higher degree program with a nursing program is located in the city. There are three state-supported community college nursing programs and there is one large university-based medical center with a PhD nursing program. Other than the home campus DNP program, there are no other DNP programs in the nearby region.

Results from statewide achievement tests reveal that the city's Kindergarten through 12th grade system ranked in the 60th percentile. Most of its students prefer to remain in the local area and the majority of those who continue schooling after high school (40%) go to the local community colleges. Fifty-five percent of the suburban students continued their education in either community colleges or higher educational institutions; however, only 15% of students in rural areas continued their education after high school.

The public transportation system within the region includes buses and a light rail system. Three major highways intersect with the city, providing easy access for automobile travel. There is a middle-sized airport with commuter planes and major airlines and AMTRAK services are available. Greyhound Bus has a terminal in the city with buses providing interstate transportation. There is one major daily paper, several suburban papers, at least 25 radio stations, five major television stations, TV cable service, and telecommunication services for computer access. There are four major health care systems. There are public health clinic services for those who do not have health coverage and who are eligible for state-supported health care programs. The city has an elected city council with a mayor, while the smaller incorporated cities are managed through part-time mayors and city councils with full-time city managers. The counties have elected boards of supervisors and each has a sheriff department supplemented by state highway patrol services.

The campus in Kenya is located outside of the largest major metropolis and capital of the nation in a rural countryside. The campus is somewhat isolated by its location and the surrounding countryside by its boundary of fences and walls with security systems in place. The campus is located about 10 miles outside of the capital city and there is a weekly, daily bus service that leaves at 7 a.m. in the city and departs campus at 5 p.m. Students needing transportation on other days and times must provide their own transportation. The adjacent cosmopolitan city has an international airport, public transportation consisting of minibuses, buses, and trains. It is a media hub for Kenya, East Africa, and international broadcasting groups.

The Kenyan government operates the constitution of 2010 with the president as chief executive, a deputy president, an attorney general, and about 14 cabinet secretaries. Kenya has a legislature, senate, and judiciary arm. The country is divided into 47 counties that are decentralized and have separate governments. The official language in Kenya is English (from its time as a British colony) and the national unifying language is Kiswahili (Swahili). The population of Kenya is about 49 million with 40% of the population under 24 years and 55% in the 25 to 54 years of age group. The life expectancy is 59.5 years. Eighty-three percent of the population is Christian, 11% Muslim, 1.7% Traditionalists, and the remainder other (Central Intelligence Agency [CIA], 2017).

Agriculture is Kenya's main economic resource and it is an economic and transportation hub for East Africa. Tourism is another attraction; however, terrorism incidents over the past few years led to a decrease in tourism. The lack of infrastructure within the country due to a weak government hampers its economic growth (CIA, 2017). Kenya's educational system consists of an 8-year public, government-supported, primary school system for children starting at 6 years of age followed by a secondary system that runs for 4 years. Its purpose is twofold: to provide education for children who will terminate their education at age 18; and to provide for those who intend to continue into higher education. The country has five public universities with an emphasis on technology and science. There are other private universities with a variety of degree offerings that are supervised by the commission on higher education (Embassy of the Republic of Kenya, 2017). Three of the universities in the city, including the institution's partner, offer nursing programs that award the BScN, and one offers a master's degree in nursing. (The majority of nurses in Kenya have a diploma in nursing.)

The government of Kenya has been attempting to institute universal health care; however, it lags behind the rest of the world in providing care for its citizens (Okech & Lelegwe, 2016). The major components of the health care system include the Ministry of

Health at the national level which is divided into the Ministry of Medical Services and the Ministry of Public Health and Sanitation. Health facilities are distributed publicly and through private and faith-based organizations regionally, with the most sophisticated services available in the major cities and at the national level. The tertiary National, Referral, and Teaching Hospitals (NRTH) such as Kenyatta National Hospital in Nairobi have premier levels of services. The next level of care is found in the secondary county hospitals, followed by primary hospitals. Beneath the primary level there are health centers, dispensaries, maternity centers, and nursing homes, and at the base, community health services at the village, household, and family levels. As is common in most countries, private care provides the highest quality of care, while public services are crowded and difficult to access, especially in rural areas (Okech & Lelegwe, 2016; Turin, 2010).

Preliminary Conclusions

The infrastructure of the home campus region and the population base for potential student and health care services support the existing campus program and could accommodate additional nursing students and graduates. The Kenyan campus infrastructure supports the nursing program and there is potential for growth.

Demographics of the Populations

The total population of the city adjacent to the U.S. home campus is a little over 1.2 million. The racial breakdown for the urban region by percentage is as follows: White: 45.3, Native American: 1.3, African American/Black: 8.6, Asian: 10.9, Hispanic: 12.6, two or more races: 6.3, and other race: 15.0. The age distribution is as follows: 19 years and younger: 30.2%, 20 to 34: 23.0%, 35 to 44: 15.0%, 45 to 59: 15.9%, 60 to 74: 10%, and 75 and older: 5.9%. Of the population, 77.3% hold a high school diploma and 23.7% have a baccalaureate or higher. The unemployment rate is 5.6%. The median household income is $41,200. In contrast, the populations of the three surrounding counties are quite different. The racial breakdown averages over 70% White, 7% African American, 2% Native American, 9% Asian, 12% Hispanic, and 1% other. The average median income is $51,000 and less than 5% households are below poverty level. The average age distribution in the counties reveals a somewhat older population than the city. About 23% of the counties' residents hold a high school diploma, 17% hold baccalaureates, and 31% had some college education but no degree.

The population of Kenya is 49 million and reflects an overall increase as births exceed deaths; if external migration continues, there will be a decrease of 11,000 per year (Country Meters, 2017). There are about eight African ethnic groups in Kenya with their specific languages spoken in rural areas and in places where they live. In addition to the African tribes, there are Asian, Arab, and European groups. The population of the multicultural, cosmopolitan city near the campus is over 3.5 million. Half of its population lives in slums; however, the other half live in high-income estates or good housing with new apartment buildings rising in response to the economic growth and resultant expanding middle income group.

Unemployment rates in Kenya are high (40%), particularly among the young, and are leading to the high rates of emigration to seek better employment opportunities. Major employment sectors in Kenya include agriculture with Kenya exporting tea, coffee, fruits, and vegetables; the service industry to support tourism; telecommunications; and mining for soda ash, salt, gold, and some precious stones. Poverty in both rural and urban areas remains high, for example, two-thirds of Nairobi's population live in the slums. As mentioned previously, children must enroll in the publicly supported school system from age 6 until the end of the secondary school system, around age 18. However, parents must pay for books, supplies, uniforms, and transportation putting a burden on the poor, and thus the dropout rates from primary to secondary schools are high. Owing to the mandated primary education, the literacy rate is 87% and there has been an improvement in the rates of education for females.

Preliminary Conclusions

Overall, the population surrounding the home campus in the United States is growing and is economically stable. Its diverse ethnic population meets the program's goal to increase cultural diversity in its student population. There is a large percentage of individuals who are educated beyond high school and who are potential students, faculty, and staff for the program. The situation in Kenya is vastly different. Emigration rates for the young are high and completion rates for secondary education that provides potential students are low. Higher education opportunities are very limited owing to the lack of available programs and financial support.

Political Climates and Bodies Politic

The town in which the U.S. home campus is located has a mayor and a town council, while the capital city has a mayor and city council. The Democrats are the political party in control for both the town and city. The adjacent counties have mayors and council governments for the smaller cities and boards of supervisors for the county government that are predominantly Republican. A review of the political climate reveals that while there are no major health issues currently, key members of the governing bodies and political action groups are aware of the nursing program and its role in the preparation of health professionals for the region. The director of extended education felt that most of the cities' and counties' populations were aware of the parent institution from the college's media campaign. Extended education runs spot announcements on the radio and advertisements in the local newspaper, usually a month before the semesters start. The director described his role on the committee on higher education for the city council, which gives him the opportunity to meet other key educators in the community. It was his overall impression that the reputation of the institution and its quality were gaining in the community.

Although the parent institution's board of regents has only one representative in the public government, the president of the college meets periodically with ad hoc committees of the city councils and boards of supervisors to discuss higher education issues that affect their populaces. He told the survey team that the institution enjoys a high regard in the town and city (students provide income for local businesses) and as a private, high-quality educational institution faculty from the university are often called in as consultants on issues in the region.

The dean of the nursing in Kenya shared that he and the dean of pharmacology hold positions in the faculty governance (the senate) and that they also serve on the advisory board for the academic vice president. Nationally, nursing is well respected and is beginning to increase its educational preparation at the BScN and master's levels, although the predominant nursing workforce is diploma prepared. Kenyan law allows independent practice for RNs who must be reviewed and licensed by the National Council. The president of the college is well aware of the need for nurses and in his role as member of the advisory board to the Commission on Higher Education is educating the commission about the need to raise expectations for the level of preparation for nurses. He serves on the Advisory Board of the Kenyan National Commission for Higher Education that accredits all private higher education institutions in the country. (Public institutions are not required to be accredited by the commission.) Through his membership, he is aware of changes and issues in the government and the political milieu that could affect the institution. At the same time, he is able to have some influence in decisions that affect higher education.

Preliminary Conclusions

The faculty team concluded that key members of the body politic and the public surrounding the U.S. home campus recognize the quality of the institution and are familiar with its programs. The presidents of both institutions and the director of extended education in the United States have key roles in promoting the universities in the community. In Kenya, the nursing program is respected on the university campus and the dean holds influential positions on campus. Nursing as a profession is respected nationally in Kenya, for example, nurses can practice independently.

The Health Care Systems and Health Needs of the Populaces

There are four major health care systems serving the U.S. home city and surrounding home campus region. Data from the websites of the American Hospital Association, the National Association for Home Care, the Morbidity and Mortality Weekly Reports (www .cdc.gov/mmwr/international/relres.html), the state health department's health statistics, and GIS Inventory maps (www.gisinventory.net/index.php?page_id=624) are collected to compare the region's health indicators to national and statewide data. One of the systems is a large nonprofit health care organization that has a nationwide network. There are two nonprofit regional health care systems providing enrollees with a wide array of services. One is sponsored by the same religious-based organization as that of the nursing program's parent institution. The other is a federation of former independent nonprofit community hospitals that merged to share resources for cost savings. There is one public hospital in addition to the state-supported university medical center.

The Veterans Administration (VA) has a large medical center with acute care for all specialties (except maternity and pediatrics, which it subcontracts to other regional hospitals), outpatient services, a nursing home unit, and a rehabilitation center. It prefers RNs with baccalaureates for staffing and employs master's- and DNP-prepared CNLs, clinical specialists, acute care and primary care nurse practitioners, managers, and administrators. It provides clinical practice sites for both undergraduate and graduate students in the region and encourages its staff to continue its education with released time and educational stipends as incentives. It is especially supportive of the master's CNL program and uses many of the school's graduates including administrators and DNP graduates in advanced practice roles. There are three for-profit agencies and there is one nonprofit visiting nurse association for home health care and hospice care. Most school districts have one school nurse; there is a nurse practitioner with four RNs assigned to the city jail; and three of the major industries have occupational health nurses.

The major health care problems of the populace match those of the morbidity and mortality statistics of the state and the nation. The population is aging and thus, the need for health services for seniors and chronic diseases is expected to rise. The systems appear to meet the acute care needs of the populace. Additional nurse practitioners are needed in the near future to staff primary care services owing to the increased numbers of insured clients.

The majority of staff nurses are associate degree graduates. All of the large health care systems employ clinical specialists or acute care nurse practitioners and those with primary care services employ nurse practitioners. The university-based medical center has an all RN staff and employs more clinical specialists and acute care nurse practitioners than the other systems. The public health clinics use public health nurses prepared at the baccalaureate and master's levels for follow-up visits and for health promotion and disease prevention programs. Nurse practitioners staff the few primary care clinics. The visiting nurse organization uses both public health nurses and RNs for home visiting and hospice services. The administrators reported that they welcome nursing students and have existing clinical placement agreements with the regional nursing schools. The affiliating system was especially open to having additional students in their agencies and indicated that the program's students would receive priority placements.

Kenya's health care system is organized from the top down and health care services are distributed regionally. The city adjacent to the university has a large teaching hospital where private and public health care at the tertiary care level is provided and which provides clinical experiences for the nursing students. Counties provide the next level of care; however, the quality of care drops significantly. In smaller regional health centers, complex health problems are referred to the larger institution with the health centers focusing on primary care, counseling, and maternity and child health services. Only 20% of Kenyans have health insurance and over half of the population lives in poverty. Major health problems include malaria, communicable diseases, HIV (although rates have slowed somewhat), malnutrition, high maternal and infant mortality rates, poor sanitation, and lack of affordable medications. Kenya has a shortage of health professionals and they are poorly distributed throughout the country (Child Fund International, 2017).

Preliminary Conclusions

There is a wide variety of health care agencies with a plethora of potential clinical experiences available for students enrolled in the U.S. home campus nursing program. Nursing administrators welcomed the idea of expanded programs to increase the numbers of baccalaureate and higher degree nurses in the region. Health care problems and needs of the populace are not unique and match the existing content of the curriculum. Kenya has major health and socioeconomic problems to address and, except for large metropolitan areas, tertiary health care services are limited and of lesser quality. With so many Kenyans living in poverty, minimal health insurance coverage of the population, major health problems requiring primary care, maternal child health, and community/public health services, and the concomitant shortage of nurses, there is a critical need to expand nursing education opportunities.

Characteristics of the Academic Settings

A survey of the U.S. schools' websites provides the types of nursing programs and tracks offered, enrollments, graduation rates, licensure examination (National Council Licensure Examination [NCLEX]) pass rates, and where the majority of graduates works. In the area, three community colleges offer associate degrees in nursing (ADNs) and the state-supported school offers an entry-level bachelor of science in nursing (BSN) program as well as an RN-to-BSN program. It has two master's specialty tracks: one in education and an FNP program. The three community colleges are about equal in size and their total enrollments approximate 150 with 50 graduates each year. Their qualified applicant pool numbers 350 each, although they believe they may be drawing from the same applicant pool. The vast majority of their graduates remains in the local area to practice in acute care, nursing homes, or home health agencies. The state-supported school has a total enrollment of 300 students in the basic BSN program, 60 RNs in the RN-to-BSN program, and 90 in the graduate programs. The master of science in nursing (MSN) nurse practitioner program is the most popular with the educational tracks enrolling approximately 10 students each year. The basic BSN program graduates approximately 65 each year. About 80% of its graduates remain in the area to practice. The qualified applicant pool for the basic BSN program is 350 and again, the administrator believes some of the applicants may be in the same pool as the ADN programs.

The U.S. university academic health sciences center currently has medical, dental, pharmacy, and nursing programs. It is a research extensive institution and therefore offers a research-focused degree (PhD) in nursing. Graduates of the nursing program hold positions as researchers in medical centers and as faculty in schools of nursing. It has about 36 students enrolled in the program in various stages of doctoral study, graduates about 10 students each year, and admits approximately 8 to 10 students per year.

In the city near the Kenyan campus, there are seven private universities and one state-supported university that has a BScN and MSN program. Two of the private universities have BScN programs that are in competition for applicants to the partner university. The campus is about 10 miles outside one of the major cities in Kenya. It has a traditional campus with academic, ADM, library, sports and recreational complexes, and student housing. It holds accreditation by the Kenyan Commission on Higher Education and regional accreditation from one of the accreditation commissions in the United States. It is an international campus and students from other countries enroll in its programs with many coming from those nations affiliated with the sponsoring religious organization. Recently, the Kenyan government fostered a partnership with private universities to support Kenyan students' tuition at private institutions. There are four major areas of study in the institution including the Colleges of Social Studies and Humanities, Science and Technology, Health Sciences, and Engineering and Agriculture. Within the College of Health Sciences are the Schools of Pharmacology and Nursing. Nursing awards a BScN in basic nursing practice and is accredited by the National Council of Kenya (NCK; for nursing). There are 100 students in the undergraduate program with 25 graduating each year. It experiences about 100 applications each year.

Preliminary Conclusions

In the United States, the region has six nursing programs, three ADN, two baccalaureate and master's degree programs (includes the home campus), one DNP program offered on the home campus, and one PhD in nursing program. There appears to be an adequate qualified applicant pool for the regional programs. In Kenya, there are three higher degree in nursing programs that are in competition with the partner school; however, there is an adequate applicant pool each year.

The Need for the Program

In the region of the U.S. home campus, the nursing workforce has 1,450 RNs of whom 1,250 are employed. The four major health care systems report a vacancy rate of 10% and the schools, public health clinics, and home care agency report a total of 50 vacant positions. The number of vacancies does not account for the numbers of nurses in the workforce who plan to retire within the next 5 years. In addition to entry-level positions, 100% of the administrators of the nursing services programs told the team that they anticipated increasing their staff owing to the growing demand and complexity of health care. The administrators indicated a preference for baccalaureate-prepared nurses and when informed about the entry-level master's, RN-to-BSN online program, and the DNP program, their interest increased, especially if the programs are accelerated.

In Kenya in 2012, there were 19,592 nurses employed in 4,287 health care facilities. It was difficult to estimate the numbers of nurses needed in Kenya as private institutions do not report to the Ministry of Health (National Council, 2012). The ratio of nurses in Kenya in 2017 was around 80 per 100,000 population, compared to approximately 782/100,000 in the United States (American Association of Community Colleges, 2017).

Preliminary Conclusions

There is a documented need for entry-level nurses in the United States and an increased need for baccalaureate-prepared graduates and advanced practice nurses. There is a shortage of nurses at all levels to meet the health care needs of the population in Kenya. The needs thus far match the types of options of the home campus nursing program and there is a need for all levels of nurses in Kenya. Since the university in Kenya has only the entry-level BScN, there are possibilities for expansion in their program for RNs to BSN and possibly a master's program through collaboration with the home campus online.

The Nursing Profession

In the United States, nursing is responding to the IOM (2010) recommendations calling for advanced nursing education and to the effects of the Affordable Health Care Act (U.S. Department of Health and Human Services, 2017) that resulted in more of the population having health insurance. According to the American Association of Colleges of Nursing (AACN, 2017), the numbers of students enrolled in BSN, particularly in degree completion programs, master's, and the doctorate in nursing practice increased significantly.

In the United States, about 60% of the employed nurses work in acute care, the remainder are in community-based agencies. About 60% of the working nurses have an ADN or diploma, 31% have a BSN, 8% have a master's, and less than 1% have a doctorate. It was difficult to match the educational preparation of the nurses to the type of position they held although anecdotal information demonstrated that the majority of master's-prepared nurses were top administrators (vice presidents), clinical specialists, CNLs, or nurse practitioners. The BSN nurses were employed in public health, schools, home care, or as case managers or administrators.

The latest information on the nursing workforce in Kenya came from the Kenya Nursing Workforce Report (National Council, 2012). At that time, hospitals employed 67.9% of the nursing workforce, dispensaries 17.7%, and 3.1% were in government management offices. Of the nursing workforce, 13% had postbasic specialty training and 79.5% received basic midwifery training. Out-migration was a problem with over 1,200 nurses applying to migrate between 2008 and 2012 although the rate has been decreasing. Enrollments in schools of nursing increased and in 2012, there were 4,294 enrolled with 278 in certificate programs, 3,568 in diploma programs, and 400 in BScN programs. In 2012, there were 83 training institutions with about 80% of their graduates passing the registration examination. Of newly registered nurses, 74.2% were diploma prepared, 19.6% were certificate (enrollees in diploma or BScN programs), and 6.2% were BScN.

Preliminary Conclusions

In the United States, there is a shortage of nurses in the region, state, and nation. The majority of the workforce practices in acute care and is prepared at the ADN level, although enrollments in baccalaureate and higher degree programs are increasing. The current workforce in the United States does not meet the preferred need for baccalaureate and advanced practice–prepared nurses. The existing regional schools of nursing cannot meet the current demand for nurses and employers of nurses forecast an increasing need in the future. In Kenya, there is a critical shortage of nurses and particularly those prepared at the baccalaureate and higher degree levels. Seventy percent of the workforce is employed in acute care with only 17.7% employed in dispensaries in spite of the need for nurses in primary care, maternal and child health, and public health nursing roles to match the health needs of the populace.

Regulations and Accreditation Requirements

The U.S. program is due for a Commission on Collegiate Nursing Education (CCNE) reaccreditation visit in 2 years. CCNE requires that educational programs planning new programs must submit a substantive change report to the commission no earlier than 90 days prior to implementation or no later than 90 days after its implementation. The U.S. nursing program has approval of the state board of nursing. The board must approve any expansions of the program that affect any of the licensure or state certification requirements and must be presented to the board at least 6 months in advance. Board guidelines include a list of qualified faculty, adequate student services including library facilities, approved clinical facilities, and adequate classroom and learning laboratories.

The nursing program on the Kenyan campus is accredited by the NCK. Schools in Kenya must submit an application form and a copy of the curriculum. Faculty teaching in degree programs must have at least a master's degree and 2 years of clinical training, while those teaching in diploma programs must have at least a baccalaureate, 2 years of clinical practice, and preparation in education and curriculum development. Schools are inspected to ensure that standards are maintained such as tutor capacity, physical facilities, transportation, bed capacity, and bed occupancy.

Both parent institutions in the United States and Kenya have regional accreditation. New degree programs must be preapproved by the agency at least 6 months prior to the enrollment of the first class. The criteria for approval are much the same as the state board of nursing. In addition to the requirements of the board, the regional agency looks for evidence of infrastructure feasibility and educational effectiveness. The usual turn-around time for a response to a proposal is 2 months.

Preliminary Conclusions

Both the parent institutions and the nursing programs are accredited regionally and nationally. The home campus nursing program is accredited by the State Board of Nursing. If the faculty and administrators of the home campus revise or develop new tracks in the program or develop a partnership with Kenya, the proposal for the changes must be completed and submitted to the State Board of Nursing and the regional accrediting agency at least 6 months prior to start-up of the program. A description of the program should be submitted to CCNE and the NCK in Kenya 90 days prior to its initiation.

Financial Support

The assessment team prepares a report and business case on the financial resources of the parent institution and the nursing program. The parent institution has an endowment fund of over $120 million. It has an active alumni association and raises at least $2 million each year for scholarships. Its capital operating costs match that of the tuition and fees income each year. It has several million-dollar grants from private and federal sources for research in science and for program development in education. The nursing program has one federal grant ($600,000) for the DNP program, $10,000 from the federal advanced education nursing traineeships, one health care system grant for $10,000 for preparing RNs to BSNs, and several scholarship funds totaling $5 million in endowments. The financial-aid programs include a statewide tuition assistance program for needy students, the federally sponsored work-study programs and traineeships, PELL grants, nursing loan programs, and a forgivable loan program from a health care agency for students who agree to work for that agency for 2 years upon graduation. In addition, there are numerous private scholarships that are available to nursing students from external sources. The university in Kenya has an endowment fund through the religious-based organization of $10 million (U.S. equivalent dollars). Industry in Kenya in the metropolitan areas provides tuition support for students majoring in agriculture, engineering, and business. The health care organization where students have clinical experiences offers three full scholarships for students in nursing.

The U.S. comptroller ensures the team that the institution will provide a business plan for the nursing program to calculate start-up costs and the economic feasibility of an expanded program and that he will share it with his counterpart in Kenya. If the program appears to be economically sound, the institutions will provide the start-up costs. The four major health care systems indicate to the assessment team that they will continue to provide clinical sites, and scholarships or loans for nursing students are possible.

The affiliate system has some labs that students could use for clinical skills practice and they are quite interested in scholarship programs or forgivable loans for students who commit to a 2-year contract upon graduation.

The dean of nursing in Kenya indicates that he will investigate additional resources for nursing students such as the Ministry of Health and the sectarian health care system that provides clinical experiences for students. He reminds the team that the Kenyan government recently put a tuition assistance program in place for students in private institutions of higher education.

Preliminary Conclusions

The parent institutions in the U.S. and Kenya and the nursing programs are financially stable. There is the promise of start-up funds and professional consultation from the home campus for a business plan if the decision to expand the program is realized. In addition to the traditional economic resources, there are potential sources of income and support from the health care systems in both places and the government in Kenya recently put a tuition assistance program in place for students enrolled in private institution.

INTERNAL FRAME FACTORS

Description and Organizational Structure of the Parent Academic Institutions

The most recent accreditation reports for the CCNE and the board of nursing, the regional accreditation report, and the report for the National Council of Kenya (NCK) provide a description including the organizational structure for both universities and schools. The home school of nursing shares offices, classrooms, and several laboratories with the science department. In addition, it has one clinical skills lab, one low- and one high-fidelity simulation lab that are under its control. Nursing represents about 4.5% (350 BSN and 100 master's, and 60 DNP) of the student body and was the first professional school in the university. The institution averages an enrollment of 8,000 undergraduate students each year with the graduate school enrollment at 3,000. It has six schools: Arts and Sciences (40% of the enrollment), Business Administration and Economics (20%), Computer Science (10%), Education (10%), Extended Education (4%), and Nursing. All but the Arts and Sciences school have graduate programs and Education is a graduate-only school. The highest degree that the institution awards is the doctoral degree (PhD, DBA, and DNP) and it awards the bachelor of arts, bachelor of science, master of arts, and master of science degrees.

Although the original purpose of the university had strong liberal arts and religious foci, the institution became multipurpose with the addition of the professional schools. The School of Extended Education offers distance education programs in business administration, computer sciences, and education from the home campus and works collaboratively with nursing on the RN-to-BSN program. Each school has a dean and the school of nursing dean has been in his position for 12 years and therefore has a strong voice in the council of deans. There is an academic provost to whom the deans report. The president is its chief executive officer. There is a comptroller, a dean of student affairs and enrollment services, directors of human resources, the library, and information services and instructional support.

The academic senate is composed of two representatives from each school's faculty, three members-at-large, undergraduate and graduate student representatives, a presidential appointee, and the academic provost. There are three major committees of the senate: curriculum, graduate, and faculty affairs. There is one nursing faculty member on the graduate committee, one nurse is chair of the faculty affairs committee, with another, a member-at-large of the senate. The school of nursing faculty and the senate curriculum committee must approve new academic programs and curriculum revisions. If the proposals emanate from graduate programs, the graduate committee recommends approval after review and sends them to the senate with recommendations.

The school of nursing faculty numbers 40 full-time tenured/tenure-track faculty and 15 part-time clinical faculty, not including the dean, and five administrative support staff (approximately 1 to 11, faculty to student ratio). There are two administrators for instructional support and information systems. A part-time clinical instructor serves as the clinical placement coordinator. There are two associate deans, one each for the graduate program and the undergraduate program. The three track coordinators for the BSN, Master's, and DNP program have 20% released time for these functions. The part-time faculty's teaching role occurs primarily in supervising students during their clinical experiences. The faculty members teach in both undergraduate and graduate programs, although some are predominantly assigned to one or the other depending on their clinical expertise and academic preparation. Seventy-five percent of the full-time tenure track faculty members have doctorates and there are currently three enrolled in doctoral programs. The school of nursing faculty meets once a month during the academic year and there are four major committees: curriculum, graduate, peer evaluation, and student affairs. All program and curriculum revisions must be approved through the appropriate nursing committee structure, approved by the faculty-as-a-whole, with final administrative review and approval by the dean. Approved proposals are forwarded to the appropriate senate committee that makes recommendations to the senate that votes for approval or disapproval. Upon approval of the senate, the provost completes a final review and makes recommendations to the president.

The dean of nursing in Kenya provided an organizational chart for his university and the school of nursing. Like the home campus, the university as a private, sectarian institution has a strong reputation in the region and with its accreditation by the Commission on Higher Education in Kenya as well as the U.S. regional accreditation carries high regard in academic circles. The university numbers a total of 6,000 students (5,500 undergraduate and 500 graduate) with nursing accounting for 2% (100 students) of the total and pharmacology 3% for a total of 5% for the College of Health and Human Services, social studies and humanities, 25%; science and technology, 20%; and agriculture and engineering, 50%. There are 260 full-time faculty members and 40 part time. In nursing, there are 10 full-time and 5 part-time faculty members with an approximate 1 to 8 faculty to student ratio. The part-time faculty members supervise students in the clinical settings. There are 1½ administrative assistants and one clinical faculty coordinator who staffs the learning lab. All of the full-time faculty members have master's degrees and the part-time faculty members have BScNs that meet the requirements of the National Council. The faculty meets as a whole once a month and task forces are assigned ad hoc according to program needs. For curricular changes, an ad hoc committee reviews proposals, refines them and then presents them to the faculty for approval. If approved, a proposal moves to the curriculum committee of the university senate that, upon approval, moves it forward for full senate approval. The vice president for academic affairs makes a recommendation to the president who must approve or disapprove the program. A nursing faculty member serves on the senate and the dean of nursing is a member of the president's advisory council.

Preliminary Conclusions

Both universities have strong reputations for high-quality liberal arts and professional educational programs and the nursing programs and their faculty members have significant roles within the institutions. There are clear hierarchal lines of communication for administrative decisions and for gaining curriculum and program approval. While the nursing schools account for only a small proportion of the total academic offerings, they are highly regarded by others. The schools have representatives on the governing senates and the deans of nursing have influential roles in the administrative systems.

Mission and Purpose, Philosophy, and Goals of the Parent Institution

Owing to the institution's religious base, both nursing programs' missions are congruent with those of their parent institutions' missions and goals that focus on the preparation of compassionate and responsible citizens for society and professionals who provide services to the community.

Preliminary Conclusions

The nursing programs' missions and purposes, philosophies, and goals are in congruence with those of the parent institutions.

Internal Economic Situation and Its Influence on the Curriculum

When conducting the assessment of the external frame factors, faculty found that both schools of nursing are financially stable. The U.S. comptroller will develop a business case for a proposed program, and there are potential external funding resources for new programs should they start. The sponsoring religious organization and its health care system both in the United States and in Kenya indicated an interest in donating some start-up funds and possible scholarships. However, this requires released time for faculty to write the grants. It is calculated that two faculty members from the U.S. campus and one from Kenya each need 10% released time for the next semester to write these grants. The comptroller refers both deans to their respective provost/vice president who agree to provide a total of $10,000 in the United States and $5,000 equivalent dollars in Kenya for faculty to write grant proposals.

A concern of the deans and faculty is the need to provide released time for curriculum development when and if expansion is approved. This would involve at least three faculty members and would take about 5% of their workload in assigned time activities to develop or revise the existing curriculum. The comptroller suggests that the deans place this on their agendas when the next year's budgets are proposed.

Preliminary Conclusions

The schools of nursing are economically stable. Their administrations indicate support for developing a business case for an expanded and/or revised program. The provost and the vice president will provide funds for the next semester for faculty to write grants for program development. The deans will include the cost for faculty-released time for curriculum development into next year's budget.

Resources Within the Institution and Nursing Programs

Since proposed changes or new programs must match the resources of the existing programs and yet meet the needs of students who may be at a distance from the schools, the assessment team surveys resources needed for possible distance outreach. The home campus classrooms, learning and computer laboratories and classrooms, although not under the U.S. school's control, are adequate in size and number for the current on-campus student enrollment. There is a need to upgrade the clinical practice laboratory and add at least one additional simulation lab with high-fidelity mannequins. The library has one of the largest holdings in the region for nursing journals and texts as well as for other disciplines. The director of the library and the administrators for information systems and instructional support services meet with the team and indicate that nursing will continue to have access to these technologies.

The Kenya school of nursing shares general classrooms with the total university and has no problems with scheduling lecture classes. There is one science lab that is shared with the school of pharmacy and nursing has its own skills lab with four hospital beds, mannequins, and equipment; a low-fidelity lab to practice additional skills; and a computer lab with 10 computers donated from the health care system. The university library is well stocked with texts and journals from the arts and sciences and recently, through a grant from industry, increased its online access to over 100 databases including PubMed, Cumulative Index to Nursing and Allied Health Literature (CINAHL), and EBSCO Information Services. For the present undergraduate students, the campus offers adequate learning labs, classrooms, and library facilities although a new high-fidelity simulation lab would help meet clinical skills demands as health care becomes more complex. As mentioned before, the schools of business and education have online programs for students, thus the infrastructure for web-based learning has been initiated. The Kenyan faculty representative indicated an interest in web-based learning and is currently enrolled in a U.S. online doctoral program. She is interested in exploring possibilities for nursing to collaborate with the schools of business and education in distance education. The dean and the faculty member met with the deans of business and education and information systems and instructional support administrators to share information about the possibility of expanding their program in collaboration with the U.S. campus. The deans are interested in the proposal and agree to meet again when plans are in place to initiate a program.

In the United States, the team meets with the director of enrollment services and discusses recruitment, student records, counseling services, financial aid programs, and work-study options for nursing students. The proposed program calls for at least one additional staff member in enrollment services for all of the services mentioned previously. The faculty member in Kenya discusses possible expansion of the nursing program with student services. Since it is more than likely, the expansion will be web based; additional recruitment, financial aid, and online access to databases are indicated.

Preliminary Conclusions

Current facilities and services for the schools of nursing are adequate for the on-campus programs in the United States and in Kenya, including the current online programs in the United States. However, the following is a list of needs if the program expands, or an outreach web-based program is decided upon.

Home Campus	Kenya Campus
Upgrade clinical skills lab	High-fidelity simulation lab
High-fidelity simulation lab	Additional staff for student services
Additional staff for web-based learning, and other student services	Faculty development for web-based program
Additional faculty depending on enrollments	Additional faculty depending on enrollments
	Expansion of web-based systems

Potential Faculty and Student Characteristics

The team agrees that a full-time coordinator for a new program or additional faculty for expanded program(s) is necessary during the planning stages as well as for managing the program when it commences. If tracks are expanded, and depending on enrollments, additional faculty members will be added with increased released time for the coordinators of the expanded programs. Educational levels, clinical expertise, scholarship and research, and teaching experience qualifications of new faculty must be matched to the needs of new programs, university expectations, and accreditation standards. If the Kenyan program adds graduate tracks, it will need master's and preferably doctorate-prepared faculty. At the present time, the dean in Kenya has his doctorate and one faculty member is earning her doctorate in nursing practice online from an American university. The size of the faculty will be determined by the choice of program, specialty, prelicensure program or not, and the delivery mode of the program. Currently, the faculty to student ratio of 1 to 11 on the home campus and 1 to 8 in Kenya is acceptable.

Like the faculty, the characteristics and size of the student body depend on the decision to expand or to offer new programs and the types of programs. A calculation is necessary for the critical mass of number of students needed to meet the cost of mounting the program. With these factors in mind, the team looks at enrollment patterns over the past 5 years. The undergraduate program enrollments have been stable; however, the applicant pool decreased on the home campus by 5%. The entry-level MSN program applicant pool increased by 15%. The DNP program is very popular and the admission rate was about 20% (30 admissions to 150 applicants) with a waiting list for up to 1 year. Graduates of the home campus BSN program have priority for admission to the DNP program with up to 15 admitted each year. In Kenya, the applicant pool for the BScN increased slightly over the past 2 years. There have been increased inquiries about a graduate program. Establishing a partnership with the Kenya School of Nursing would require additional staff on both campuses to coordinate recruitment and admission activities.

Preliminary Conclusions

While the current overall nursing faculty to student ratio is good for both schools, any new or expanded programs will require additional faculty and staff depending on enrollments and the nature of the programs. Support staff for the programs, admissions, and enrollment services will be necessary. Applications to the existing programs on both campuses remain steady and in fact, are increasing for the graduate-level programs on the home campus. The applicant pool remains steady in Kenya and there have been increased inquiries for a graduate program.

See Appendix Table 1 for a summary of the findings for external and internal frame factors of the needs assessment.

SUMMARY OF THE NEEDS ASSESSMENT

A needs assessment of external and internal frame factors revealed a positive environment for an expanded program when compared to the desired outcomes of the guidelines for assessing external and internal frame factors found in Chapter 3, Tables 3.1 and 3.2. Both physical environments of the universities in the United States and Kenya are supportive of the schools of nursing and the surrounding communities have resources available to the academic communities. The universities hold U.S. regional accreditation and the Kenyan university is accredited by the Commission on Higher Education in Kenya. Both schools of nursing are accredited nationally: in the United States, by CCNE and in Kenya, NCK. The schools of nursing are highly regarded on the home campuses, their missions and goals match those of the institutions, and the administrators and faculty of the programs hold influential positions on campus and in the community. Because of the efforts on the part of the institutions' leaders and faculty in the community, the broader body politic supports the universities and the schools of nursing.

Competition from neighboring schools of nursing seems negligible owing to the large applicant pool, and the need for nurses and the PhD program in the United States has the potential for providing faculty from its graduates. Potential applicants to all U.S. programs reflect a diverse population and the applicant pool in Kenya is steady but the

APPENDIX TABLE 1   Analysis of the Case Study's Needs Assessment: External and Internal Frame Factors and Decision Making

External Frame Factors	Findings			Conclusions
	Positive	Negative	Neutral	
Community Description	Size, location, and infrastructure of the home region support potential expansion. In Kenya, the infrastructure of the BScN program is supportive and there is potential for growth.			*Positive* In the United States, the community location and support systems, including the online program, can accommodate an expansion of the program. The Kenyan program has infrastructure support.
Demographics	There is an adequate diverse regional applicant pool in the United States and the economy is stable. There is a pool of potential faculty and staff in the United States. The applicant pool for the Kenyan BScN is good.	In Kenya, graduation rates from secondary schools are low and there is a high emigration rate of the educated youth.		*Positive* Applicant pools for the home campus and Kenya are good. In the United States, there is a diverse population in the region. In the United States, there is a pool of potential faculty. *Negative* The potential applicant pool for an expanded BScN program in Kenya is uncertain.
Political Climate and the Body Politic	The parent institution and Kenyan campus are recognized in their respective communities. Representatives in leadership positions from both campuses have influential contacts in the community.			*Positive* Both nursing programs and their parent institutions are respected in their communities. Relationships with leaders in both locales are influential and good.

Health Care System and Health Needs of the Population	There is a wide variety of health care agencies for learning experiences. Nursing administrators favor and support BSN or higher degree programs. Health care needs match curriculum content. There is a critical need to expand nursing education in Kenya.	Multiple health and social problems face the population of Kenya.	*Positive* The health care system is supportive and offers many learning opportunities for students. Health care needs match the existing curriculum. There is a critical need for nurses to meet the health care needs of the Kenyan population. *Negative* There is a critical need to address the health care and social needs of the population of Kenya.
Academic Settings	Adequate diverse applicant pool for all six U.S. area schools. The Kenyan campus offers only BScN and has an adequate applicant pool.		*Positive* In the United States, there is an adequate, diverse applicant pool. In Kenya, there is an adequate applicant pool to the BScN.
Need for the Program	In the United States, there is a need for additional entry-level nurses in light of current and future shortages. There is a demand for BSN+ prepared nurses. Existing program offerings match the demand. In Kenya, there is a need for all levels of nursing, specifically, degree prepared.		*Positive* An expanded program could meet the regional and Kenyan demand for additional nurses at the professional entry-level and advanced practice levels.

(continued)

APPENDIX TABLE 1   Analysis of the Case Study's Needs Assessment: External and Internal Frame Factors and Decision Making (*continued*)

External Frame Factors	Findings			Conclusions
	Positive	Negative	Neutral	
Nursing Profession			There is a shortage of nurses prepared at the baccalaureate and higher degree levels in the United States. There is a critical shortage of nurses in Kenya. The majority of nurses in Kenya are prepared at the diploma level.	*Neutral* As stated in the need for the program, nursing workforce shortages at higher degree levels continue in the United States. There is a critical shortage of nurses in Kenya. The majority of nurses are prepared at the diploma level in Kenya.
Regulations and Accreditation	Both parent institutions and the nursing programs are accredited.		A proposal for a new degree program must be submitted to the regional accrediting body and the State Board of Nursing.	*Positive* Both parent institutions and the nursing programs are accredited. *Neutral* Proposals must be submitted to the accrediting and regulating bodies in advance of initiation if the assessment of external and internal frame factors is favorable toward an expanded program.
Financial Support	Financial reports indicate economic health and stability in both places. The parent institution will provide start-up funds. At least two health care systems offered financial assistance.		There are other potential financial resources to be investigated.	*Positive* The financial picture is good. *Neutral* There are future potential resources that need to be explored further.

Internal Frame Factors	Findings			Conclusions
	Positive	Negative	Neutral	
Description and Organizational Structure of the Parent Institution	Both schools are held in high regard by their parent institutions. Organizational and hierarchal communication lines are clear for curriculum approval. There are nursing representatives on the senates. The deans have influence in the universities.			*Positive* The organizational structures and administrators are supportive. The deans have influence in the universities. Nursing representatives are on the senates.
Mission and Purpose, Philosophy, and Goals of the Parent Institution	Both nursing programs' missions, purposes, philosophies, and goals match those of their home institutions.			*Positive* The nursing programs' missions, purposes, philosophies, and goals match those of their home institutions.
Internal Economic Situation and Its Influence on the Curriculum	Both schools are economically stable. There is administrative support and funds for grant proposals. A business plan will be developed.			*Positive* A business plan will be developed. The schools are financially stable. There are funds for grant writing.
Resources Within the Institution and Nursing Program	Current facilities are adequate on both campuses. Library resources are adequate. A web-based system exists in the United States.	On-campus facilities may need updating if entry-level programs are added. Additional staff and faculty may be required.	There is potential for a web-based system in Kenya.	*Positive* Current facilities are adequate on both campuses. Library resources are adequate. A web-based system exists in the United States.

(continued)

APPENDIX TABLE 1   Analysis of the Case Study's Needs Assessment: External and Internal Frame Factors and Decision Making (*continued*)

Internal Frame Factors	Findings			Conclusions
	Positive	Negative	Neutral	
				Negative On-campus facilities may need updating if entry-level programs are added. Additional staff and faculty may be required. *Neutral* There is potential for a web-based system in Kenya.
Potential Faculty and Student Characteristics	Faculty to student ratios are good. Faculty are qualified. Applications to the programs are increasing except for the entry-level BSN on the home campus.		Additional faculty and staff will be necessary with program expansion.	*Positive* Faculty is qualified. Present faculty ratios are good. Overall, application rates are good. *Neutral* Additional faculty and staff will be necessary if the program expands.
Overall Conclusions				28 Positive 4 Negative 7 Neutral

population base for entry-level baccalaureate programs is small. The health care systems indicate a need for nurses prepared at the baccalaureate and higher degree levels and continue to support both schools of nursing. Health care needs are very high in Kenya and there is a shortage of nurses. In addition, with the great majority of nurses prepared at the diploma level, there is a need for degree programs for the existing workforce. The potential for a collaborative online program exists as Kenya has experience with master's education in business and education and the United States. RN-to-BSN, master's, and doctorate programs are all online.

The financial health of both institutions is good and there are possible additional resources available for program expansion. There are multiple grants and scholarships available to nursing programs and students in the United States and there is tuition support from the national government in Kenya as well as possible scholarships from the health care systems. Both schools of nursing currently have adequate classrooms, clinical labs, and technology support; however, if the Kenyan program were to offer web-based courses, it would need to link to the existing web system for business and education. Library and instructional support systems are adequate at this time, although additional staff and faculty may be needed if enrollments increase and there is an increased need for technical support.

The organizational structures of the two universities are such that faculty members develop the curriculum and the governing bodies of the universities (the senates) review and approve the proposals prior to administrative approval by either the provost (U.S.) or academic vice president (Kenya) and finally, the presidents with assent from the respective boards of trustees. The parent institution indicated support by offering to develop a business case and start-up funds should the faculty recommend an expanded program and it will work with the Kenyan campus. The provost and the academic vice president promised funds for faculty to write grants for program development.

Final Decision Statement

Based on the needs assessment of the external and internal frame factors that surround the schools of nursing on the U.S. campus and in Kenya, the needs assessment team recommends the development of a partnership between the two schools to maintain the viable offerings in the U.S. curriculum and to increase the numbers of baccalaureate and higher degree level nurses in Kenya through web-based education.

The assessment team offered several recommendations to the deans for their consideration and action based on the analysis and summary. Possible strategies for developing specific plans to implement the recommendations were included:

1. Open the online RN-to-BSN program to diploma graduates in Kenya.
   a. The School of Nursing in Kenya should take the lead in recruitment and enrollment services for Kenyan nurses to enroll in the online U.S. program.
   b. The U.S. campus provides its expertise and experience in online education so that the campus in Kenya assumes responsibility for its own program at least 3 years following its implementation.
2. Expand the RN-to-BSN program into an accelerated RN-to-MSN online program for both schools.
   a. Review both schools' baccalaureate programs to ensure that core concepts and content meet accreditation and professional standards.
   b. Review the current master's program and its options for an accelerated master's for RNs.

3. Open the online DNP advanced practice tracks to Kenyan BScN graduates.
   a. If there is interest in the program from Kenya, add up to five slots in the program with at least three targeted for qualified BScN graduates.
   b. Explore the possibility of an additional advanced practice track in maternal/child health to meet the critical health care needs of Kenya and its potential in the United States.

CASE STUDY: CURRICULUM FOR ACCELERATED RN-TO-MSN PROGRAM

The following is a description of a curriculum that opens the U.S. RN-to-BSN program to diploma-prepared RNs from Kenya and revises the RN-to-BSN program to accelerate both U.S. and Kenyan students into the master's ADM or CHN tracks. The administrative track prepares leaders for management roles in the health care system that applies to both nations. The CHN track prepares professional nurses to provide high-level, coordinated community/public health nursing care. It includes public health sciences that are especially useful to nurses in Kenya where rural areas, poverty factors, and inadequate infrastructures cause major health problems. It was decided that the RN-to-BSN and the accelerated RN-to-MSN programs have priority and will serve as a pathway, at a later time, to the DNP program. Opening the RN-to-BSN track to Kenyan nurses will require consultation, planning, and coordination with the dean and faculty in Kenya and the financial officers on both campuses. For this case study's purposes, the following is a sample curriculum plan for the RN to MSN, online, CHN track.

After a review of the existing missions, visions, and overall goals of the two parent universities and the schools of nursing, both faculties find them similar and broad enough to encompass the existing end-of-program objectives for the RN-to-BSN and master's CHN programs. The overall master's end-of-program outcome serves as the guide for the student-learning outcomes (SLOs) throughout the RN-to-MSN program and states, "the master's prepared nurse provides advanced practice nursing and interprofessional leadership within the evolving and complex health care system to prevent disease, promote health, and elevate care for groups, communities, and populations in various settings."

In order to move into graduate-level courses, RNs complete the equivalent of upper-division–level BSN courses having completed lower division courses in their entry-level nursing programs (ADN or diploma). Individual assessment of the RNs' associate degrees or diplomas must take place to ensure that the lower-division courses or their equivalents have been completed. The U.S. home campus has articulation agreements with the regional associate degree programs so that ADN graduates directly transfer in credits. For the remaining RNs, if prerequisite discrepancies are found, individual academic plans are made to either enroll in equivalent courses or receive credit for them through challenge or portfolio through their home campus in the United States or Kenya. It should not take any longer than 1 or 2 semesters for them to complete the prerequisites.

It is planned that the accelerated RN-to-MSN program will take 3 years, full time to complete (a part-time option will be available). The first year (Level 1) is 1 calendar year (three semesters) and students complete the equivalent of upper-division nursing courses in the BSN program. Therefore, the level objectives for Level 1 of the program are the same as the SLOs for the basic BSN. The outcomes are those that already exist on the U.S. campus and were compared to the Kenyan BScN nursing program and found to be similar enough to be approved by the Kenyan nursing faculty, the academic senates, and the administrations of the parent institutions. They are consistent with the AACN Baccalaureate Essentials for Professional Nursing Practice (2008).

The RN-to-MSN Level 1 student will:

1. Apply a liberal education and the sciences to the practice of professional nursing.
2. Demonstrate leadership in providing high-quality care and patient safety in the health care system.
3. Provide professional nursing care that is based on the translation of evidence.
4. Manage information and technology in the provision of quality patient care.
5. Participate in health promotion and disease prevention practice to improve population health.
6. Influence health care policy, financing, and regulations as they affect professional nursing practice.
7. Improve health care outcomes through interprofessional communication and collaboration.
8. Demonstrate professional values that include altruism, autonomy, human dignity, integrity, and social justice.
9. Respect the variations of professional practice that apply to the care of individuals, families, groups, communities, and populations across the life span.

To meet the SLOs, the RNs take many of the same courses that junior and senior students in the BSN program take; however, like the RN-to-BSN students, the courses are offered online. The courses are pathophysiology, genetics, health assessment, interprofessional health care practice: communication and collaboration, introduction to nursing research, nursing leadership, CHN theory and practice, and analysis of the health care system. The practicum takes place in the nurses' home communities under the supervision of the faculty and mentorship of an approved, qualified CHN mentor in the community. A professional nursing course is the first course that RNs take to bridge concepts from lower-division to upper-division courses. Three advanced science courses are included in preparation for the master's tracks, which for the community/public health nursing track, are Public Health Sciences, Biostatistics, and Epidemiology.

After completing Level 1 courses, the RNs spend two semesters in the first level of the MSN program (Level 2, of the RN-to-MSN program). They select the advanced practice option in which they wish to major, that is, ADM or CHN. Upon completion of Level 2, the student moves to Level 3.

Note the adaptation of the objectives in italics for the CHN track. Similar adaptation occurs for the ADM track.

The RN-to-MSN Level 2 student will:

1. Integrate knowledge from the sciences and humanities into advanced nursing practice in the care of groups, communities, and populations.
   - *Integrate knowledge from the sciences, humanities, and public health sciences into advanced nursing practice in the care of groups, communities, and populations.*
2. Provide nursing leadership in health care organizations and systems.
   - *Same*
3. Participate in patient safety and quality improvement strategies in the care of groups, communities, and populations.
   - *Same*
4. Translate scholarship and research into advanced practice nursing.
   - *Translate scholarship and research into advanced practice nursing in the community setting.*
5. Apply informatics and health care technologies to advanced practice nursing.
   - *Same*

6. Advocate for change in health care systems and policy that benefits the health of groups, communities, and populations.
   • *Same*
7. Participate in interprofessional collaboration to improve group, community, and population health outcomes.
   • *Same*
8. Provide advanced practice nursing strategies for clinical prevention and health promotion for groups, communities, and populations.
   • *Same*

The RN-to-MSN Level 3[a] student will:

1. Apply knowledge from the sciences and humanities to advanced nursing practice in the care of groups, communities, and populations.
   • *Integrate knowledge from the sciences, humanities, and public health sciences into advanced nursing practice in the care of groups, communities, and populations.*
2. Provide leadership in health care organizations and systems.
   • *Same*
3. Initiate patient safety and quality improvement strategies in the care of groups, communities, and populations.
   • *Same*
4. Integrate scholarship and research into advanced practice nursing.
   • *Integrate scholarship and research into advanced practice nursing in community settings.*
5. Apply informatics and health care technologies to advanced practice nursing.
   • *Same*
6. Institute change in health care systems and policy that benefits the health of groups, communities, and populations.
   • *Same*
7. Provide leadership for interprofessional collaboration to improve group, community, and population health outcomes.
   • *Same*
8. Improve the health of groups, communities, and populations through advanced practice nursing strategies for clinical prevention and health promotion.
   • *Same*

[a]These outcomes are the same as the end of program outcomes/objectives of the MSN program.

MSN students have core courses in nursing theory, research, health care systems policy, and advanced pathophysiology, pharmacology, and health assessment. Their specialty courses consist of three core science courses and three didactic courses with clinical preceptorships for each. Students complete 600 hours of supervised clinical practice by the end of the program. In addition, students complete a project as a capstone experience. A sample program of study for the MSN, CHN track program follows the summary.

SUMMARY

The faculty agrees that the level objectives for the RN-to-MSN programs come from the SLOs (end-of-program objectives) and are learner focused; contain the content of what is to be learned; and specify when they are to be completed and to what extent. The level objectives imply mastery of the content; they must be met by the end of course-work for each level, and are arranged in sequential order. All of the objectives are measurable and serve as guides for developing course objectives, and for collecting data for formative (course, faculty, and level reviews) and summative evaluation (program review and accreditation).

SAMPLE PROGRAM OF STUDY MSN, CHN TRACK

Level 1: Nursing Courses (equivalent to BSN program outcomes) and Core Public Health Courses

Semester 1	Semester 2	Semester 3
Pathophysiology (3)	Interprofessional Health Practice (3)	Nursing Leadership (3)
Professional Nursing (2)	Practicum (2)	Practicum (2)
Health Assessment (2)	Analysis of the Health Care System (3)	Community Health Nursing (2)
Practicum (1)	Introduction to Nursing Research (3)	Practicum (4)
Genetics (3)	Biostatistics (3)	Epidemiology (3)
Public Health Sciences (3)		
Total credits 14	*14*	*14*

Level 2: MSN Advanced Community Health Nursing Courses

Semester 1	Semester 2
Nursing Theory (3)	Translational Research (3)
Advanced Pathophysiology (3)	Advanced Pharmacology (3)
Advanced Health Assessment (1)	Leadership and Political Action (2)
ªPracticum (2)	ªPracticum (1)
Total credits 9	*9*

Level 3: Advanced Community Health Nursing Courses

Semester 1	Semester 2
Community Health Nursing (3)	Community Health Nursing (3)
ªPracticum (3)	ªPracticum (3)
Interprofessional Leadership in the Community (2)	Capstone (3)
ªPracticum (1)	
Total credits 9	*9*

ª600 hours of supervised clinical practice @ 4 hours/credit.

DISCUSSION QUESTIONS

1. As you read the case study, what gaps in the information did you identify and what additional data would you like to have? Were there redundancies or too much information in the data that you viewed as unnecessary to the needs assessment?
2. What in your opinion are the pros and cons of collaboration with another school of nursing in a region, nationally, internationally?

SUGGESTED LEARNING ACTIVITIES

Student Project

Identify another possible collaborative program that the two schools of nursing in the case study could develop. Summarize the data that justifies development of the program and identify any gaps in the data that you believe need further assessment. Develop a program of study for your selection.

Faculty Project

Analyze the needs assessment from the case study and determine how easy or difficult it would be for you to collect similar data for your nursing program. Do you believe nursing programs should routinely conduct needs assessments for evaluation purposes and to identify the need for changes in the future? Why or why not?

References

American Association of Colleges of Nursing. (2017). Standard data reports. Retrieved from http://www.aacnnursing.org/News-Information/Surveys-Data/Standard-Data-Reports

American Association of Colleges of Nursing. (2008). *The essentials of baccalaureate education for professional nursing practice*. Washington, DC: Author.

American Association of Community Colleges. (2017). *Nursing demographics*. Retrieved from http://www.aacc.nche.edu/Resources/aaccprograms/health/Documents/nursing_demographics.pdf

Central Intelligence Agency. (2017). The world fact book. Retrieved from https://www.cia.gov/library/publications/the-world-factbook/geos/ke.html

Child Fund International. (2017). Struggles facing the Kenyan health care system. Retrieved from https://www.childfund.org/Content/NewsDetail/2147490088

Country Meters. (2017). Kenya population. Retrieved from http://countrymeters.info/en/Kenya

Embassy of the Republic of Kenya. (2017). Education in Kenya. Retrieved from https://kenyaembassy.com/aboutkenyaeducation.html

Institute of Medicine. (2010). *The future of nursing: Leading change, advancing health*. Washington, DC: National Academies Press.

National Council. (2012). *Kenya nursing workforce report: The status of nursing in Kenya. 2012*. Retrieved from http://www.nursing.emory.edu/_includes/docs/sections/lccin/Kenya_Nursing_Workforce_Report.pdf

Okech, T. C., & Lelegwe, S. L. (2015). Analysis of universal health coverage and equity on health care in Kenya. *Global Journal of Health Science, 8*(7), 218–227.

Turin, D. R. (2010). Health care utilization in the Kenyan health system: Challenges and opportunities. *Inquiries Journal, 2*(9), 168.

U.S. Department of Health and Human Services. (2017). Key features about the Affordable Care Act by year. Retrieved from https://www.hhs.gov/healthcare/facts-and-features/key-features-of-aca-by-year/index.html#

Glossary

Accelerated programs: programs consisting of intensive full-time study with no breaks, giving students the opportunity to finish the program in a shorter time than traditional programs. They include accelerated RN to BSN, RN to MSN programs, and entry-level BSN and MSN programs for graduates with bachelor's (or higher) degrees not in nursing.

Accreditation: a process that education programs undergo to receive recognition for meeting basic standards or criteria set by national, regional, or state organizations. Although it is voluntary, most programs undergo accreditation to demonstrate their quality to the consumers (students, parents, alumni, and employers) and to meet certain requirements for financial aid and academic requirements.

Adult learning theory, andragogy: a model of instruction geared toward adult learning that takes into account the adult's autonomy, life experiences, personal goals, and need for relevancy and respect.

Articulation agreements: renewable agreements negotiated to ensure equivalency between college and university courses, support educational mobility, and facilitate the seamless transfer of academic credit between ADN and BSN programs (AACN, 2014).

Asynchronous: learning activities that occur at various times.

Behaviorism, behaviorist learning theory: a group of learning theories, often referred to as stimulus-response, that view learning as the result of certain conditions that stimulate the responses (behaviors) that follow.

Benchmark: a reference point in similar organizations/institutions that is used to compare quality and to identify gaps that drive improvement measures.

Body politic: the people/power(s) behind the official government within a community. It is composed of the people and major political forces that exert influence within the community.

Brain-based learning: learning that is enhanced by creating conditions where the brain learns best such as relaxed alertness, immersion in complex multiple experiences, and actively engaging in experiences that help develop meaning.

Clinical nurse leader: master's prepared generalist who evaluates, assesses, and coordinates care for clients or groups of clients across all settings within a microsystem (AACN, n.d-a).

Cognitive learning theory: focuses on learning as an internal process including thinking, understanding, information organizing, and consciousness (Aliakbari, Parvin, Heidari, & Haghani, 2015).

Concept analysis/mapping: a detailed analysis of a concept and its relationships within the curriculum depicted into a map with arrows signifying relationships.

Concept-based curriculum: a theoretical or organizational curriculum model that guides the development of the program and makes it unique; it unifies the curriculum and creates a coherent approach across courses and levels (Ervin, Bickes, & Schim, 2006).

Constructivism, constructivist learning theory: a learning perspective that argues that individuals construct much of what they learn and understand, which produces knowledge based on their beliefs and experiences.

Content mapping: similar to concept mapping, it tracks specific content's placement throughout the curriculum.

Continuous quality improvement (CQI): a system designed to provide for ongoing evaluation, analysis of findings, and implementation of plans for improvement within an organization.

Critical thinking: "all or part of the process of questioning, analysis, synthesis, interpretation, inference, inductive and deductive reasoning, intuition, application, and creativity. Critical thinking underlies independent and interdependent decision making" (American Association of Colleges of Nursing [AACN], 2008, p. 37).

Curricular framework: an organizational or conceptual framework that guides the development and evaluation of the curriculum plan according to the program mission/vision, overall goal, philosophy, and student learning outcomes, and responds to professional educational standards.

Curriculum: the formal plan of study that provides the philosophical underpinnings, goals, and guidelines for delivery of a specific educational program.

Deep learning: allows students to dig deeper into complex and challenging learning situations. It is intentional and creates new meaning for the learner (Candela, 2016).

Demographics: data that describe the characteristics of a population, for example, age, gender, socioeconomic status, ethnicity, education levels, and so on.

Distance education: any learning experience that takes place a distance away from the parent institution's home campus.

Doctor of nursing practice (DNP): a doctorate degree that "prepares nurse leaders at the highest level of nursing practice to improve patient outcomes and translate research into practice" (AACN, n.d-b).

Educational taxonomies: provide the terminology on which to focus for the main domains of learning: cognitive, psychomotor, behavioral, and affective.

End-of-program objectives (see also Student learning outcomes): reflect the framework of the curriculum and define the specific expectations or competencies of graduates upon completion of the nursing program.

Entry-level master's/generic master's/accelerated master's for nonnurses/second-degree master's programs: programs that prepare nonnursing college graduates for eligibility to take NCLEX. Programs vary from generalist degrees to specialty or functional roles.

Entry-level/generic programs: programs that prepare students for eligibility to take the licensure examination (NCLEX) for RNs. The programs include diploma, associate degree, baccalaureate, master's, and doctoral levels. Students entering master's entry-level programs have a baccalaureate in another field as a minimum. Students in entry-level programs do not have previous education in nursing.

Evidence-based practice: discipline-specific (nursing) practice that is research based and reflects the entirety of nursing practice and research.

Flipped classroom: a reversed instruction model in which students complete preclass assignments and use in-class time for active learning activities (Williams, 2012).

Formal curriculum: the planned program of studies for an academic degree or discipline.

Formative evaluation: evaluation "intended by the evaluator as a basis for improvement" (Scriven, 1996, p. 4). The assessment that takes place during the implementation of the program or curriculum. It can also be viewed as process evaluation. In education, this type of evaluation is often linked to course or level objectives.

Frame factors: the external and internal factors that influence, impinge upon, and/or enhance educational programs and curricula. As a conceptual model, they serve to collect, organize, and analyze information that is useful for the development and evaluation of curricula. There are two major categories of frame factors, external and internal factors:

> **External frame factors**—factors outside of the home institution in which the nursing program is housed.

> **Internal frame factors**—factors within the institution and in the nursing program that influence the curriculum.

Goal: overall statement(s) of what the program prepares the graduates for. Statements are usually long term and stated in global terms.

Goal-based evaluation: evaluation based on the stated goals of the entity undergoing evaluation. It is frequently used in education and tied to the stated goals, purpose, and end-of-program objectives (student learning outcomes) of the program or curriculum.

Goal-free evaluation: a method to assess and judge some thing or entity. The evaluator has no prior knowledge of the entity (program or curriculum) that he or she is evaluating. The person must be an expert in the field of evaluation and the type of entity that is evaluated. The value of this type of evaluation is that it is relatively bias free.

Graduate education: education that takes place after completion of the baccalaureate, that is, master's and doctorate levels.

Humanism, humanistic learning theory: an approach to teaching and learning that assumes people are inherently good and possess unlimited potential for growth; therefore, it emphasizes personal freedom, choice, self-determination, and self-actualization.

Hybrid distance education: utilizes a blend of synchronous and asynchronous formats for learning.

Immersion (as in web-based with immersion): the student comes to the home campus for one or more days during a semester or academic year to test and participate in hands-on practice, utilizing standardized patients, simulation manikins, and task trainers. Students are able to interact face to face with faculty and peers of their cohort during this time.

Informal curriculum: sometimes termed as the hidden curriculum, cocurriculum, or extracurricular activities; planned and unplanned influences on students' learning.

Institutional accreditation: a comprehensive review of the functioning and effectiveness of the entire college, university, or technical institution. The state mandate or institutional mission provides the lens used to guide the review.

Learning: "change in behavior (knowledge, attitudes, and/or skills) that can be observed or measured and that occurs . . . as a result of exposure to environmental stimuli" (Bastable & Alt, 2014, p. 14).

Massive open online courses (MOCCs): open enrollment for access to online higher education courses with some offering to academic credit if certain course requirements are met.

Mission statement: the institution's beliefs about its responsibility for the delivery of programs through teaching, service, and scholarship.

M1 and M2 master's programs: the size of master's programs according to the Carnegie classification of educational institutions.

Multiple intelligences: presents seven constructs of intellects: bodily kinesthetic, visual-spatial, verbal-linguistic, logical-mathematical, musical-rhythmic, interpersonal, and intrapersonal (Gardner, 1983).

Needs assessment: the process for collecting and analyzing information that can influence the decision to initiate a new program or revise an existing one.

Nonsectarian: not associated with a religious organization.

Objectives: the steps necessary for reaching the overall goal of the program that include a description of the learner, a behavior that is measurable, a timeframe, at what level of competency, and the topic or behavior expected.

> **Course objectives:** have the same properties as end-of-program and midlevel objectives but apply to specific courses and relate to and lead toward midlevel and end-of-program objectives.

> **End-of-program objectives:** highest level of learner behaviors that demonstrate the characteristics, knowledge, and skills expected of the graduate and relate to the overall goal. They focus on the learner and must include a behavior that is measurable, a timeframe, at what level of competency, and the topic or behavior expected. These can also be defined as student learning outcomes.

> *Example:* X School of Nursing prepares competent, compassionate nurse clinicians and leaders who serve the health care needs of the people of the state and the health care systems.

> **Level (intermediate) objectives:** Have the same properties as end-of-program objectives but occur midway through an educational program and are usually higher than the first-level objectives.

> **Student (individual) learning outcomes:** All of these objectives are student or individual learning outcomes and should be learner-centered and describe what behavior (outcome) is expected.

> *Example:* At the end of the Health Assessment course, the student will present a complete health assessment of a client that includes an accurate health history, a write-up of all components of the physical examination, a list of problems and actual or potential nursing diagnoses, and a plan for follow-up of the problems and diagnoses.

Pedagogy: teaching methods; although it originally applied to methods used to educate children, it can be used to apply to all age groups.

PhD program or, in the case of nursing, the PhD or DNS: degrees that emphasize nursing theory and research and educate nurses prepared to conduct research and foster the development of new knowledge in health care and nursing.

Private educational institution: an institution supported through private funding.

Problem-based learning (PBL): a mechanism for teaching students that focuses on clinical problems and professional issues that the nurse may face in practice.

Program approval: a process whereby regulating bodies review programs to ensure consumer safety. Nursing education programs are subject to state regulations that are usually administered by the state board of nursing.

Programmatic or specialized accreditation: focuses on the functioning and effectiveness of a particular program or unit within the larger institution (e.g., medicine, nursing).

Public institution: an institution whose main financial support comes through governmental funds.

Quality: measured as "purposeful, transformative, exceptional, and accountable" (Schindler, Puls-Elvidge, Welzant, & Crawford, 2015, p. 8).

Quality assurance: the process of collecting data on how well the institution or program meets its defined standards, criteria, goals, and mission.

Regional accreditation agency: one of seven private, voluntary accreditation agencies within six defined regions of the United States, formed for the purpose of peer evaluation and setting of standards for higher education.

Regulatory: a form of approval, recognition, or accreditation required by a federal, state, or provincial government agency.

R1, R2, and R3 doctoral programs: the level of research conducted in doctoral programs according to the Carnegie classification of educational institutions.

Satellite campuses: programs that offer the curriculum as a whole or in part on off-campus sites from the parent institution. While they may incorporate technology and the Internet, learning still takes place in classrooms with in-person participation of the instructor and students.

Scholarship of teaching: application of teaching activities to scholarship that includes four components: discovery, integration, application, and teaching (Boyer, 1990).

Sectarian: associated with or supported by a religious organization.

Simulation: allows students to participate in activities that mimic real-life scenarios or situations.

Standardized patients: individuals who have been trained to portray a patient with a specific medical condition; often hired to teach and evaluate students' performances in a simulated clinical setting.

State-regulatory agencies: agencies that recognize or approve colleges, universities, or programs for operation within the state as governed by state statutes.

Student learning outcomes (see also End-of-program objectives): reflect the framework of the curriculum and define the specific expectations or competencies of graduates upon completion of the nursing program.

Summative evaluation: a holistic approach to the assessment of a program that uses results from formative evaluation (Scriven, 1996). Summative evaluation takes place at the end of the program and measures the final outcome.

Synchronous: learning activities that take place simultaneously.

Team-based learning: a structured, active learning strategy involving a sequence of three key phases: preclass preparation; readiness assurance process; and application.

Total quality management: continuous assessment of an educational program, correcting errors as they occur, thus improving the quality of the program.

Translational science: research findings that are translated and applied into practice.

Undergraduate education: postsecondary education from the associate degree (traditionally 2 years) to the baccalaureate (traditionally 4 years) levels.

Virtual learning environment (VLE): educational programs offered online in cyberspace.

Vision statement: a statement that is outlook oriented and reflects the institution's plans and dreams about its direction for the future.

Web-based learning: education offered online and the student interacts with faculty and other students via computer.

References

Aliakbari, F., Parvin, N., Heidari, M., & Haghani, F. (2015). Learning theories application in nursing education. *Journal of Education and Health Promotion, 4*(2). doi:10.4103/2277-9531.151867

American Association of Colleges of Nursing. (n.d.-a). Clinical nurse leader toolkit. Retrieved from http://www.aacnnursing.org/Education-Resources/Tool-Kits/Clinical-Nurse-Leader-Tool-Kit

American Association of Colleges of Nursing. (n.d.-b). Developing a DNP program tool kit. Retrieved from http://www.aacnnursing.org/Education-Resources/Tool-Kits/DNP-Tool-Kit

American Association of Colleges of Nursing. (2008). *The essentials of baccalaureate education for professional nursing practice.* Washington, DC: Author.

American Association of Colleges of Nursing. (2014). Articulation agreements among nursing education programs. Retrieved from http://www.aacnnursing.org/News-Information/Fact-Sheets/Articulation-Agreements

Bastable, S., & Alt, M. (2014). Overview of education in health care. In S. Bastable (Ed.), *Nurse educator: Principles of teaching and learning for nursing practice* (4th ed., pp. 3–30). Burlington, MA: Jones & Bartlett.

Boyer, E. L. (1990). *Scholarship reconsidered: Priorities of the professorate.* Princeton, NJ: The Carnegie Foundation for the Advancement of Learning. Retrieved from http://depts.washington.edu/gs630/Spring/Boyer.pdf

Candela, L. (2016). Theoretical foundations of teaching and learning. In D. Billings & J. Halstead (Eds.), *Teaching in nursing: A guide for faculty* (5th ed., pp. 211–229). St. Louis, MO: Elsevier Saunders.

Ervin, N. S., Bickes, J. T., & Schim, S.M. (2006). Environments of care: A curriculum model for preparing a new generation of nurses. *Journal of Nursing Education, 45*(2), 75–80.

Gardner, H. (1983). *Frames of mind.* New York, NY: Basic Books.

Schindler, L., Puls-Elvidge, S., Welzant, H., & Crawford, L. (2015). Definitions of quality in higher education: A synthesis of the literature. *Higher learning research communication, 5*(3), 3–13.

Scriven, M. (1996). Types of evaluation and types of evaluators. *Evaluation Practice, 17*(2), 151–161.

Williams, C. (2012). Flipped class method gaining ground. *District Administration, 48*(1), 64.

Index